W9-COB-287

Michigan State University
Department of Epidemiology

Clinics in Developmental Medicine No. 151
CEREBRAL PALSIES:
EPIDEMIOLOGY AND CAUSAL PATHWAYS

© 2000 Mac Keith Press
High Holborn House, 52–54 High Holborn, London WC1V 6RL

Senior Editor: Martin C.O. Bax
Editor: Hilary M. Hart
Managing Editor: Michael Pountney
Sub Editor: Pat Chappelle

Set in Times and Avant Garde on QuarkXPress

The views and opinions expressed herein are those of the authors and do not necessarily
represent those of the publisher

Accuracy of referencing is the responsibility of the authors

First published in this edition 2000

British Library Cataloguing-in-Publication data:
A catalogue record for this book is available from the British Library

ISSN: 0069 4835
ISBN: 1 898683 20 4

Printed by The Lavenham Press Ltd, Water Street, Lavenham, Suffolk
Mac Keith Press is supported by Scope

Clinics in Developmental Medicine No. 151

Cerebral Palsies: Epidemiology and Causal Pathways

FIONA STANLEY
TVW Telethon Institute for Child Health Research
and The University of Western Australia
Perth, Australia

EVE BLAIR
TVW Telethon Institute for Child Health Research
Perth, Australia

EVA ALBERMAN
Department of Environmental and Preventative Medicine
St Bartholemew's and the London Medical School
London, England

2000
Mac Keith Press

Distributed by 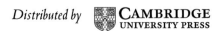 **CAMBRIDGE**
UNIVERSITY PRESS

AUTHOR'S APPOINTMENTS

Fiona J. Stanley

Director, TVW Telethon Institute for Child Health Research; *and* The Variety Club Professor of Paediatrics, The University of Western Australia, Perth, Australia

Eve Blair

Senior Research Officer, TVW Telethon Institute for Child Health Research; *and* Research Officer to the Western Australian Cerebral Palsy Register, Perth, Australia

Eva Alberman

Professor Emeritus, Department of Environmental and Preventive Medicine, Wolfson Institute of Preventive Medicine, St Bartholemew's and The Royal London School of Medicine and Dentistry, London, England

CONTENTS

GLOSSARY

Several terms are used imprecisely in the language of perinatal medicine. This leads to poor communication, making comparisons between studies and individuals difficult, and encourages illogical thinking. This glossary defines the terms, particularly the epidemiological terms, and the acronyms used in this book. The rationale for our choice of meaning is also given in some instances in the hope of encouraging standardized use.

Aetiology of disease. The route by which a diseased state is arrived at. *See also* Cause.

Age of complete ascertainment. The age at which a Register counts persons described as having cerebral palsy in order to calculate occurrence rates.

Antecedent of disease. Used epidemiologically to refer to factors which confer an increased probability of subsequent disease if they are present. Use of the term does not imply why or how the factor confers a greater probability of disease. Specifically, while a cause of a disease must be an antecedent, an antecedent may not always be a cause (Blair 1996).

Apparently life-threatening event (ALTE). Previously referred to as near-miss sudden infant death syndrome (SIDS).

Association. Denotes that the probability of the occurrence of one factor varies with the occurrence of a second factor. If the probability increases with the existence of the second factor the association is positive, if the probability decreases the association is negative.

Attributable to. Was caused by. *See also* Cause; Population attributable risk.

Bias. Deviation of results or inferences from the truth, or any factor or process that causes such a deviation. There are many sources of bias, and epidemiologically the term does not necessarily imply that the deviation was the result of prejudice or subjective factors.

Birth asphyxia.
    Birth refers to the intrapartum period, usually taken as the onset of labour to either the complete expulsion of the infant, or to the departure from the delivery suite.
    Asphyxia is the process whereby hypoxia causes some chronic ill effect. It is a vague term in which neither the duration nor the severity of the ill effect is specified; however, the ill effect is understood to be more than compensatory responses to the hypoxia which reverse with restoration of normal oxygenation.
    Acidosis is indicative of hypoxia and is therefore evidence for, but not sufficient evidence of, asphyxia. It is seldom possible to be certain from clinical signs whether birth

asphyxia has occurred. Intrapartum signs of fetal distress followed by abnormal neonatal neurological signs and signs of hypoxic damage to other organs, particularly the heart and kidneys, are compatible with birth asphyxia, but are not specific to it. Any such signs may be the result of damage occurring before labour, unless it can be demonstrated that the fetus was undamaged immediately before labour (Blair 1993). *See also* Fetal distress; Signs of birth asphyxia.

Bivariate exposure analysis. Statistical analysis where the effects of two exposures on the outcome are estimated simultaneously. Two exposures create three independent variables: each exposure occurring in the absence of the other, and the two exposures occurring together.

Blinding. Keeping pertinent knowledge from participants in an intervention trial in order to avoid systematic bias resulting from human manipulation. Blinding is possible at three points. Blinding outcome assessors involves concealing from the assessor pertinent aspects of the clinical history of the patient until the assessment of the outcome is completed and the results documented. Blinding subjects involves concealing from the subject the identity of the intervention that they are receiving, *e.g.* whether they are receiving the putatively active drug or a placebo: it is often more difficult to conceal the identity of therapeutic interventions than of pharmacological interventions. Blinding care providers involves concealing from the care provider the identity of the intervention administered to each subject.

Case. A subject with the outcome of interest.

Causal pathway. The sequence of causes leading to the outcome of interest.

Cause of disease. A cause is any factor that contributes to the occurrence of a disease, without necessarily being sufficient cause in itself.

CMV. Cytomegalovirus. A herpes infection of the TORCH group (q.v.). It is common, there is no available vaccine, and infection during pregnancy, particularly primary infection, has been associated with cerebral palsy (see Chapter 6).

CNS. Central nervous system.

Cohort study. An observational epidemiological study in which a defined cohort of persons is followed over a period of time without intervention from the investigator. Such studies may be conducted *prospectively*, defined and followed into the future, so that exposure measurement cannot be systematically biased by a knowledge of the outcome, as is possible in *retrospective* cohort studies in which the period of observation is already completed at the initiation of the study.

Confidence interval. The range of values in which there is a specified probability, often

95%, that the true value will lie. Thus for a 95% confidence interval there is a 5% chance that the true value lies outside this range, while for a 90% confidence interval 10% will lie out of the given range. For a given probability, the confidence interval decreases (and the precision of the estimate increases) as the number of subjects increases.

Confounder. This is an epidemiological term to denote a factor that is associated with both an exposure and the outcome of interest. Stratification of the analysis by the confounder will result in the true odds ratio associated with the exposure of interest being obtained within each stratum and this will differ from the odds ratio obtained without stratification. However, a factor on the causal path between an exposure and the outcome of interest is *not* a confounder and must not be adjusted for, although it will be associated with both (Weinberg 1993). An understanding of causal mechanisms is therefore necessary before assigning confounder status.

Control. (1) *As a noun:* In case–control or intervention studies, controls are persons with whom the cases (case–control) or experimental treatment group (intervention) are compared. Hence a controlled study is one in which the group of interest is compared with another group. (2) *As a verb:* In statistical analysis, to control means to take into account or to adjust for additional factors which may affect the relationship between two factors.

Crossover trial. A method of evaluating treatments in which subjects are submitted to both the experimental and control interventions: *i.e.* they cross from one treatment arm to the other. The subject's outcome under one set of conditions is compared with the outcome of the same subject under the other set of conditions. While this reduces the problem of variability between experimental and control subjects, since the two interventions cannot be applied simultaneously, the subject may change between when the observations are made under intervention and under control conditions. It is not suitable for interventions with long-term or permanent effects.

Defensive medical practice. Medical practice in which the choice of treatment is guided by the wish to avoid future blame should an adverse outcome occur.

Descriptive study. Describes existing distributions of variables without regard to cause or other hypotheses; antonym = analytic study.

Distribution. The frequencies of the categories or (quantitative) values of a measurement made on a group, *i.e.* the proportions of the group belonging to each category or having each value (or range of values) possible for the measurement.

ECG. Electrocardiogram.

ECMO. Extracorporeal membrane oxygenation, performed for cardiorespiratory failure.

Ecological study. A descriptive study in which the units of analysis are populations rather than individuals.

Effectiveness. The extent to which an intervention brings about its intended effect when deployed in the field.

Efficacy. The extent to which an intervention can bring about its intended effect under ideal conditions.

Epiphenomenon. When considering the relationship between an exposure and an outcome, an epiphenomenon is another outcome of the exposure of interest that is not on the causal path between that exposure and the outcome of interest. Thus if an exposure results in two outcomes, A and B, where A and B are not causally related, outcome A is the epiphenomenon when considering outcome B and vice versa.

Equipoise. A state of balance. In the context of alternative therapeutic interventions for a given clinical condition, equipoise is a state of complete uncertainty as to which intervention is superior and is a necessary prerequisite for the ethical conduct of a randomized controlled trial.

Evidence-based practice. Practice based on scientifically sound evidence, as opposed to tradition or authority. Sometimes assumed to infer practice based on the results of systematic reviews (q.v.), though other forms of scientifically sound evidence are possible.

Exposure. An exposure is any factor which *may* have some relevance to disease aetiology. The term includes genetics, demographic characteristics, toxic or lifestyle exposures and therapeutic interventions. Thus, epidemiologically, social class, race and gender are considered exposures, as well as exposures to environmental hazards or pharmaceutical interventions. Exposures constitute one of the three components of any epidemiological study, along with subjects and outcomes.

EPTB. Extremely preterm birth. This should be defined on each occasion as it is variably defined in the literature. The World Health Organization suggests a classification cut-off point at <28 completed weeks of gestation (see Chiswick 1986; cf. VPTB). The biological rationale could be that around 28 weeks of gestation neuronal myelination commences, as does the ability to mount a glial response (scarring) to neuronal damage. However, both these are continuous processes, without a clear-cut age of initiation or recognition.

Fetal distress. Abnormal fetal behaviour, typically:
(a) Alterations in the fetal heart rate [tachycardia (>160 bpm); bradycardia (<120 bpm)—considered severe if the rate drops below 60 bpm]; delay in the recovery of fetal heart rate following uterine contractions; lack of response to uterine contractions; or reduced beat to beat variability of the heart rate.

(b) Passage of meconium: this is a poor predictor of suboptimal outcomes, particularly in term infants.

Fetal distress is compatible with the occurrence of birth asphyxia (q.v.) and is frequently taken as an indication that it has occurred; however, fetal distress may have many causes and is not specific to birth asphyxia. Fetal distress occurring during the intrapartum period is also called *intrapartum stress* or, sometimes misleadingly, *signs of birth asphyxia*.

Generalizability. The range of situations to which the conclusions of research may properly be applied. It is not appropriate to apply conclusions to situations which have not been examined. Therefore, in order to explore the generalizability of conclusions a wide range of situations needs to be examined. Typically this involves including research subjects with a wide variety of characteristics and observing the effects of those characteristics on outcomes.

Gold standard. A true or reliable measurement or observation. Irrefutable evidence. Also used as the antonym of surrogate. For example, the gold standard evidence for an intra-ventricular haemorrhage is seeing blood in the ventricles at autopsy, in contradistinction to surrogate evidence obtained from cerebral imaging or blood in the cerebrospinal fluid at lumbar puncture, from which an intraventricular haemorrhage may be inferred, although, since it is only an inference, this conclusion may be erroneous.

Iatrogenic. Refers to an unfavourable factor resulting from a clinician's professional activity which may be either an unintended effect or the foreseeable side-effect of an activity anticipated to result in net benefit.

Incidence. The rate at which a condition arises in a population during a specified time period. It is measured as the number of new cases occurring in the specified time period divided by the number of persons at risk. There are two ways of measuring incidence. The *incidence rate* has units of time^{-1} and is calculated using for the denominator, the sum of the duration of time for which each individual was at risk of the disease. The *cumulative incidence* is a proportion and is calculated using for the denominator the mean number of persons at risk during the specified time period, often estimated as the mid-period number of persons at risk. Incidence (as opposed to prevalence, q.v.) is measured by those interested in aetiology and prevention. For cerebral palsy the reported incidence is usually a cumulative incidence. For an irreversible condition, such as cerebral palsy, the difference between the incidence and prevalence is dependent on the difference in mortality rates between those with the condition and the population from which they arise.

Intellectual disability. Defined as an intelligence quotient (IQ) level <70, which generally reflects a global mental deficit. Categorized as *mild* (IQ 50–69), *moderate* (IQ 35–49), *severe* (IQ 20–34) and *profound* (IQ <20).

Interobserver agreement/reliability. The extent to which observations (of the same thing) made by more than one observer agree. Often measured as Cohen's kappa which gives the proportion of observations in agreement in excess of that expected to occur by chance alone.

Intra-observer agreement/reliability. The extent to which repeated observations of a single observer agree, measured as for interobserver agreement.

Intrapartum. The period during labour and delivery, ideally taken as the onset of labour to the complete expulsion of the child.

Intrapartum stress. Fetal distress occurring in the intrapartum period.

IVH. Intraventricular haemorrhage. Bleeding into the cerebral ventricles.

IUGR. Intrauterine growth restricted/restriction. IUGR implies that some *pathological* factor has prevented the achievement of optimal intrauterine growth. It is not equivalent to SGA (small for gestational age, q.v.) where there may be no pathology. IUGR is not easily clinically defined. Possible indicators of IUGR (in contradistinction to SGA) include low ponderal index, falling weight percentiles on serial ultrasound study, or reduced or absent end diastolic flow on Doppler ultrasound blood flow studies. The quantitative criteria from which it is inferred should be defined.

Learning disability. A CNS deficit which impedes the process of learning, *e.g.* attention deficit disorder.

Level one facility. In this book this refers to an obstetric facility that is not on the same site as any specialized neonatal care facilities. *See also* Tertiary facility.

Marker. An indicator of a factor of interest which is not directly that factor of interest. It is a surrogate factor, an associated measure or indirect evidence pertaining to a factor or an event and can be contrasted with a *gold standard* (q.v.).

Meta-analyses: symbols used in figures. Each horizontal line represents the results of one study (the shorter the line, the more certain the results). The diamond represents the pooled estimate of all studies, with its width being proportional to the confidence limits. The sizes of the blocks representing the odds ratio for each study are proportional to the weight (q.v.) that the study contributes to the pooled estimate.

Minimization. Refers to methods of allocating subjects to treatment arms that do not rely solely on chance but seek to minimize the differences in distributions of known or suspected determinants of the outcome between the treatment arms. It is preferable to randomization where there is an insufficient probability that randomization will create treatment groups with similar distributions of preexisting determinants of the outcome.

Models of causation. Models or patterns of factors that lead to disease, examples of which are: (a) the single sufficient cause, (b) multiple independent causes, and (c) the causal pathway.

MRI. Magnetic resonance imaging. A versatile technique for imaging brain structures which may be performed at any age. It requires expensive equipment including a large and powerful magnet into which the subject must be introduced and there remain motionless for the duration of the scan. Successful MRI imaging therefore requires subject compliance, or sedation or general anaesthesia.

MRS. Magnetic resonance spectroscopy. A spectroscopic technique allowing remote identification of chemical composition, including oxygenation status.

Multicentre study. A study in which subjects are recruited from several geographically distinct locations. The rationale for this logistically complicated exercise is to increase sample size: it may be the only way to amass sufficient numbers of cases of rare diseases. Care needs to be taken if there is the possibility of systematic differences in the disease of interest between the locations.

Multifactorial. Involvement of several factors, not all necessarily involved in each individual.

Multiple pregnancy. A pregnancy carrying more than one embryo/fetus.

Multivariate analysis. Statistical analysis where the effects of several factors associated with the outcome are estimated simultaneously. This allows adjustment for confounding factors and known determinants of the outcome when estimating the effect of one or more exposures of interest. It is a competitive situation; thus if a variable that is perfectly correlated with the outcome is included in the analytical model (as, for example, an early sign of the disease), the association with other variables will be reduced to insignificance.

NCPP. National Collaborative Perinatal Project. A cohort study of approximately 54,000 births in 12 US hospitals between 1959 and 1966 in which the children were followed longitudinally to the age of 7 years. The unique combination of sample size and length of follow-up has allowed several unique observations pertinent to the epidemiology of the cerebral palsies. However, because it preceded the introduction of neonatal intensive care it is uninformative about the epidemiology of the cerebral palsies in very preterm infants.

Neonatal encephalopathy. A clinically defined syndrome of disturbed neurological function in the earliest days of life, manifested in the term infant by difficulty with initiating and maintaining respiration, depression of tone and reflexes, abnormal level of consciousness and/or seizures. This condition should not be termed hypoxic–ischaemic encephalopathy unless it is certain that hypoxia–ischaemia was the cause. *See also* Birth asphyxia.

NIRS. Near infra-red spectroscopy. A spectroscopic technique that can distinguish oxygenated from deoxygenated haemoglobin.

Observational study. A study in which there is no intervention from the investigator. It includes descriptive and analytical (case–control or cohort) studies. Antonym = interventional or experimental study.

Odds. The ratio of the probability of an occurrence to the probability of non-occurrence. For example, if of 100 very preterm infants, 10 have cerebral palsy, the odds of cerebral palsy are 10:90 (11%), in contrast to the probability of cerebral palsy of 10/100 (10%).

Odds ratio. The ratio of two odds. This measure of association between exposure and outcome is estimated in case–control studies rather than the relative risk, because the denominator data (the number of people at risk of being counted in the numerator) is not measured. Where incidence is low the odds ratio approximates to the relative risk.

PAR. Population attributable risk (also known as *attributable proportion, attributable risk, attributable fraction, aetiologic fraction*). This statistic estimates the amount of a disease attributable to a certain factor and implies that this amount of the disease would be avoided if that factor were removed. It is estimated from the strength of association with the factor and the prevalence of the factor in the population. However, the estimated value needs to be interpreted with care, particularly if the proportions attributed to each of several factors are estimated and added. The concept can be meaningfully applied only if the factor is indeed causal; moreover, the estimated value presupposes single sufficient causes. When several PARs are estimated simultaneously, their sum generally overestimates the proportion attributable to the sum of those exposures, as is readily evident when the estimated sum exceeds 100%. This demonstrates the interdependence of potentially causal factors and provides further support for the concept of causal pathways to disease. A more reliable method of estimating the proportion of a disease attributable to a group of exposures is to estimate the strength of association with a single variable (a variable representing all exposures in the group of interest). If the exposures in the group form steps of a causal path it is not meaningful to divide this attributable proportion between exposures within the group.

Parity. The number of previous pregnancies carried by a woman up to the gestational age at which a birth is statutorily defined.

Peto odds ratio. A way of combining odds ratios widely used in statistical analysis.

Pilot study. Exploratory research to define the subjects, exposures and outcomes.

Plurality. The number of fetuses carried in a multiple pregnancy. Also termed *multiplicity* or *order* of the pregnancy

Pre-eclampsia (synonyms: *pre-eclamptic toxaemia, toxaemia of pregnancy*). The clinical criteria for pre-eclampsia are not standardized. They include a pregnancy-induced elevation of maternal blood pressure as well as some degree of proteinuria (synonym, albuminuria). Pre-eclampsia should be differentiated from *pre-existing maternal hypertension*, on which it may be superimposed, and also from *isolated pregnancy-induced hypertension* that is not associated with proteinuria. However, pre-eclampsia forms a subset of all pregnancy-induced hypertension, and the few cases of *eclampsia*, in which pre-eclampsia has progressed to maternal convulsions, are usually included in the pre-eclamptic group unless specifically differentiated.

Pregnancy-induced hypertension. Pregnancy-induced elevation of maternal blood pressure with or without other symptoms of pre-eclampsia.

Prevalence. In a given population, the prevalence of a condition is the proportion of the population experiencing the condition at a specified point in time. Knowledge of prevalence is most useful in planning service provision.

Preterm birth. Without further qualification this refers to births before 37 completed weeks of gestation.

Proportion of expected birthweight. The ratio of the observed birthweight to the 50th percentile birthweight for a population of babies delivered at the same gestational age and defined nonpathological determinants of birthweight, such as infant gender, maternal race and height.

PVH. Periventricular haemorrhage. Bleeding into the white matter surrounding the cerebral ventricles.

QT (Ward–Romano) syndrome. An autosomal dominant inherited disorder marked by specific ECG abnormalities which may lead to recurrent syncope and/or sudden death.

Randomization. The act of allocating subjects to therapeutic interventions at random. Once the subject is entered into a therapeutic trial (*i.e.* has met the criteria for trial entry and agreed to participate) there is no further selection to determine which intervention they should receive. Randomized controlled trials are used when it is not known which of two or more clinical strategies gives greatest benefit (equipoise). In order to make a fair comparison, each strategy should be applied to groups identical with respect to factors determining outcome. Since not all of these factors are known, the only means of equalizing the distribution of unknown factors is to rely on chance, which will have an increasing probability of creating equal groups with increasing numbers of subjects randomized. Random allocation achieves two ends: it avoids systematic bias in the allocation of subjects to treatments and, given enough subjects, avoids random bias in allocation. The number of subjects considered sufficient is not estimatable (the greater the number the less random bias there is likely to be) but increases with increasing variability between subjects with respect to factors determining outcome. There are many clinical situations involving uncommon and heterogeneous diseases where an insufficient number of subjects is available for there to be any reasonable probability of creating two equal groups by random allocation. In such cases, methods must be employed that minimize differences in distributions of known confounders in the two groups, while maintaining avoidance of systematic bias in allocation—*see* Minimization.

Randomized controlled trial. A clinical trial in which two or more interventions (which may include *no treatment*) are compared and eligible subjects are allocated to the intervention groups at random.

Relative risk. The ratio of a risk in one population to the same risk in another population—often a population exposed to a factor of interest relative to a population not exposed to that factor. It is used as the measure of association between exposure and outcome in cohort studies.

Risk. The probability of occurrence of an outcome, usually a suboptimal one.

Risk factor. A factor associated with the outcome of interest. It does not necessarily imply that the association is causal.

Sample size estimates. The number of subjects that need to be included in a study in order to answer a particular question can be estimated in advance, if the following are available:

(a) A specified research question [typically the effect of an intervention (cohort study) or of an exposure (case–control study) on the frequency of a specified outcome], a specified research design and specified criteria for subject selection.

(b) Known frequency of outcome in the absence of intervention (cohort study) or of exposure in controls (case–control study) among subjects meeting the criteria for subject selection.

(c) An estimate of the magnitude of the effect of the intervention or exposure on outcome.

(d) A defined level of confidence required of the estimate.

The precision of the sample size estimate depends on the accuracy of (c), the accuracy with which the result can be guessed in advance.

It is not possible to determine a sample size for exploratory studies that are not designed to answer one particular question, *i.e.* for feasibility or pilot studies. As a guide to a reasonable sample size for exploratory studies, the sample size required to answer the most completely defined research question may be used.

Screening test. An initial examination of persons apparently without a particular condition performed in order to identify those who are more likely to have the develop the condition. To be effective there should be a diagnostic test available for those who screen positive. Screening tests are useful where sensitivity is high, where they are more acceptable (cheaper, less time consuming or invasive) than the diagnostic test, and where there is an effective early treatment or intervention for the condition in question.

Sensitivity. The sensitivity of a test is the proportion of cases of a particular disease which the test identifies as cases; also known as *true positive rate* (cf. Specificity). Calculated as:

$$\frac{\text{Number of cases of disease testing positive for the disease}}{\text{Number of cases of disease tested}}$$

Sibship. A group comprising all births to an individual woman. This includes stillbirths, intrapartum and postnatal deaths, as well as surviving children.

SIDS. Sudden infant death syndrome. Unexplained death of an infant who was previously considered well. *See also* Apparently life-threatening event.

Signs of birth asphyxia. Intrapartum and neonatal signs compatible with, but not specific to, birth asphyxia (q.v.). These include signs of intrapartum stress (q.v.), intrapartum and immediate postnatal metabolic acidosis, neonatal encephalopathy, and neonatal renal, cardiac and respiratory dysfunction.

Small for gestational age (SGA). Implies that the fetus or newborn infant is smaller than other fetuses or babies of the same gestational age. There is no necessary implication of pathology or of growth restriction, although SGA is strongly associated with IUGR (q.v.) and for this reason is often used as a surrogate measure for it. The criterion defining small is variable and must be defined for each quantitative discussion along with the reference population considered and any factors other than gestational age that have been adjusted for. Thus, one of the most common definitions of SGA is below the 10th birthweight percentile of the total population of geographical region X adjusted for gestation week and gender.

Specificity. The specificity of a test is the proportion of subjects without a particular disease which the test correctly identifies as not having the disease; also known as *true negative rate* (cf. Sensitivity). Calculated as:

$$\frac{\text{Number of subjects without disease testing negative for the disease}}{\text{Number of subjects without disease tested}}$$

SPECT. Single photon emission computed tomography.

Standard deviation (SD). A measure of dispersion or variation of a distribution of values. The mean of the distribution gives the value around which the distribution is centred, and the SD is a measure of how widely values are dispersed around this centre. It is calculated as the positive square root of the variance, where the variance is given as the sum of the squares of the difference between each value and the mean.

Standard error (SE). The standard deviation of an estimate, used as a measure of precision of the estimate.

Systematic review. A review of the evidence available for a given subject, in which the evidence is systematically sought by methods that are precisely documented, such that if it were replicated by another reviewer the same results and conclusions would be obtained. A review unaffected by the personality of the reviewer.

Sometimes used to infer a review conducted under the auspices of the Cochrane Collaboration, which has documented precise guidelines as to the conduct of reviews in their Handbook (Mulrow and Oxman 1997) and which monitors the reviewing process from conception to dissemination through a network of review groups each with multiple editors.

Tertiary facility. In this book, an obstetric care unit that includes a neonatal intensive care unit with the facility to intubate and ventilate newborn infants.

Topography. Bodily distribution of motor impairments.

TORCH. Acronym representing the four vertically transmitted viral infections: toxo-plasmosis, rubella, cytomegalovirus and herpes.

VPTB. Very preterm birth. This should be defined on each occasion as it is variably defined in the literature. The World Health Organization suggests a classification cut-off point at <32 completed weeks of gestation (see Chiswick 1986; cf. EPTB). This criterion has a biological rationale pertinent to cerebral palsy aetiology in that the risk of germinal matrix haemorrhage is high before 32 weeks and declines thereafter as the germinal matrix disappears. However, cerebral maturation is continuous, and it is preferable to conduct analyses using gestation as a continuous variable. Where statistical considerations result in categorizations of gestational age, the effect of changing boundary values should be examined, *e.g.* do conclusions vary if the definition of the very preterm category varies between, for example, 30 and 34 completed weeks of gestation?

Weight. As an attribute of a study contributing to a meta-analysis of several studies, the weight indicates the contribution of that study to the pooled estimate. It is dependent on the proportion of the total number of study subjects it contributes and, on occasion, on its relative scientific quality.

"I thought the following four [rules] would be enough, provided that I made a firm and constant resolution not to fail even once in the observance of them.

"The first was never to accept anything as true if I had not evident knowledge of its being so; that is, carefully to avoid precipitancy and prejudice, and to embrace in my judgment only what presented itself to my mind so clearly and distinctly that I had no occasion to doubt it. The second, to divide each problem I examined into as many parts as was feasible, and as was requisite for its better solution. The third, to direct my thoughts in an orderly way; beginning with the simplest objects, those most apt to be known, and ascending little by little, in steps as it were, to the knowledge of the most complex; and establishing an order in thought even when the objects had no natural priority one to another. And the last, to make throughout such complete enumerations and such general surveys that I might be sure of leaving nothing out.

"These long chains of perfectly simple and easy reasonings by means of which geometers are accustomed to carry out their most difficult demonstrations had led me to fancy that everything that can fall under human knowledge forms a similar sequence; and that so long as we avoid accepting as true what is not so, and always preserve the right order of deduction of one thing from another, there can be nothing too remote to be reached in the end, and too well hidden to be discovered."

(René Descartes, 1637)

ACKNOWLEDGEMENTS

We are grateful to many people for their support, guidance, encouragement and contributions to the writing of this book.

After our decision to rewrite *The Epidemiology of the Cerebral Palsies*, originally published in 1984, encouragement for the enterprise came from our many international colleagues working in epidemiological research in the cerebral palsies. These include Ann Johnson and her team in Oxford; Karin Nelson at NIH; Judith Grether in California (who also read Chapter 6); Alan Leviton (who read Chapter 7) and Jennifer Pinto-Martin, Olaf Dammann and Karl Kuban from Boston's neuroepidemiology network; Bengt and Gudrun Hagberg from Sweden who continue in retirement to provide data and good ideas; Peter Pharoah, Richard Cooke and the Mersey team; Ian McGillivray who provided data from his study in Avon, England, as did Linda de Vries from her study in Holland. Mervyn and Ezra Susser from New York provided useful insights and wisdom about causal thinking. Nigel Paneth from Michigan, Bill Silverman from California, Jack Sinclair from Canada, Caroline Crowther and David Henderson-Smart, both from Australia, read chapters and commented on ideas. From Australia, Nadia Badawi, Jenny Kurinczuk and John Keogh provided data and feedback on concepts, Beverly Petterson commented on Chapter 10 and Sarah Love on Chapter 13. The Western Australian Cerebral Palsy register data was provided by Linda Watson, whose tireless work for cerebral palsy research should be acknowledged here. She helped with Chapter 4, with many of the tables and figures, and collected and organized the data concerning the registers in the Appendix. We are grateful to all the individuals listed in the Appendix under Cerebral Palsy Registers Worldwide who kindly provided information about their registers. Barbara Moore handled the mammoth task of obtaining the references; Colleen Moylan and Natalia Bilyk helped with the manuscript and the figures and tables. We thank them all for their knowledge, their experience and their time.

Members of the TVW Telethon Institute for Child Health Research put up with the absences of their Director (FJS) on Mondays (and other times) and carried out additional work to enable her to spend time on the book.

The Institute of Public Health in Cambridge hosted FJS on study leave in 1997 when work on the book commenced. We would also like to thank Wesfarmers for their continued support for the Institute and this project.

Finally we are all working mothers or grandmothers and feel grateful to our families for their love and support through the writing and rewriting of this book. Our commitment arises from a deep concern for the hardships faced by people affected with cerebral palsy and their families and our hope that they may benefit from good quality research.

FIONA STANLEY
EVE BLAIR
EVA ALBERMAN
September 1999

1
INTRODUCTION

"Epidemiology is fundamentally a search for patterns." (Smithells 1970)

This book is a sequel to *The Epidemiology of the Cerebral Palsies*, published by Mac Keith Press some 15 years ago (Stanley and Alberman 1984). The earlier book aimed to review the epidemiological literature concerning this diverse group of motor disabilities and to encourage good epidemiological methods in their investigation. It focused on prevalence and aetiology, concentrating particularly on those groups with causes which were not obviously postneonatal, although one chapter was dedicated to that group. The book involved several authors for its 12 chapters and was greatly facilitated by a meeting in Bristol in 1981 on childhood disabilities.

The current volume is a response to the many developments in the field of cerebral palsy research since the early 1980s that are outlined below. It was also stimulated by a meeting, organized by Adrien Mossinger in collaboration with Judith Lumley, Nigel Paneth and Henning Schneider, in Berne in March 1996 (Ackermann-Liebrich *et al.* 1996), and considerably helped by the friendly communications between perinatal and paediatric epidemiological researchers over the last 20 years. During these decades, excellent meetings organized by the International Cerebral Palsy Association, the Little Foundation, Scope (formerly The Spastics Society) and Mac Keith Meetings have enabled researchers to keep in touch.

Why a new book?
THE EPIDEMIOLOGY OF THE CEREBRAL PALSIES IS CHANGING (see Chapters 4 and 6–11)
Both the epidemiology of the cerebral palsies, and our perceptions of it, are changing. Traditional beliefs that cerebral palsy was largely a disease of the intrapartum period has been challenged, fuelled by the enormous increase in obstetric litigation, encouraging the search for alternative causes in term infants. Concurrently there have been changes in the patterns of occurrence, particularly amongst the new cohorts of very preterm survivors. These have resulted from changes in obstetric and neonatal care that have decreased the risk of perinatal mortality particularly at earlier gestations and in very low birthweight (VLBW) infants (see Chapter 4), from changes in maternal characteristics, and from the more widespread use of successful treatments for infertility. Infertility treatments have resulted in increases in multiple births, particularly those of higher orders, which carry an increased risk of early delivery and of cerebral palsy (see Chapter 10).

Reports of temporal trends in the proportion of all births which are delivered preterm are not consistent. Little change has been seen in Western Australia (Fig. 1.1). Decreases have been reported in France (Breart *et al.* 1995) and Finland (Rantakallio *et al.* 1991), and increases in an inner city tertiary medical centre in the USA (Amini *et al.* 1994). However,

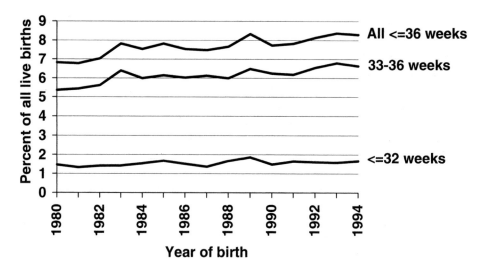

Fig. 1.1. Preterm births by gestational age in Western Australia, 1980–1994. (F. Stanley and L. Watson, unpublished data.)

generally the data suggest little improvement in these proportions in most countries, both developed and developing (Guyer *et al.* 1997, Di Renzo *et al.* 1998).

Influences increasing rates of preterm delivery, such as the increased multiple birth rate and greater use of iatrogenic early delivery for maternal or fetal disease, are being balanced by influences reducing it, such as improved maternal health and more optimal parity distributions.

Since the rate of cerebral palsy tends to increase as the gestational age at delivery decreases (see Chapter 4), the greater proportion of surviving preterm infants increases their proportion of cerebral palsy. However, the extent to which changes in survival following preterm birth has influenced cerebral palsy rates within gestational age strata is the subject of much discussion. On the one hand, some causes of preterm birth may themselves be causes of cerebral palsy (Leviton 1987). On the other hand, very preterm newborn infants are vulnerable to cerebral damage resulting from vascular and respiratory instability in the neonatal period: if this were the predominant route to cerebral palsy in very preterm infants, gestation-specific rates would be very dependent on the quality of neonatal care (see Chapters 4 and 6).

New Ways of Categorizing and Using Cerebral Palsy Data (see Chapters 2 and 3)
New and different ways of classifying outcomes as well as exposures are being explored. Our data sets should be developed to maximize flexibility of classification to answer the variety of epidemiological questions.

We have debated at length how we should define and aggregate the cerebral palsies for epidemiological studies. We now offer Chapter 2, which suggests that maximum epidemiological advantage will be obtained by all-inclusive registering of cases of motor (and other) disability, allowing selection of cases pertinent to particular questions. Chapter 3 suggests that intelligent ways to categorize childhood disability will vary with the objectives of the research as well as with what data are available. It is now universally acknowledged that the cerebral palsies are heterogeneous as regards to cause, clinical features, severity and associated disabilities and that motor disability may be just one adverse consequence of an underlying cause, *e.g.* congenital rubella syndrome.

Cerebral palsy is defined by clinical description only. It is not informative of aetiology, pathology or prognosis. To measure valid time trends it is important to have a stable definition over time. Thus all conditions that have traditionally been included in cerebral palsy data collections should continue to be included so that trends over time can continue to be monitored. The growing number of specific causes of cerebral palsy that are now recognizable, such as chromosomal and metabolic defects, raises questions about the usefulness of the term 'cerebral palsy' from an aetiological perspective. We even debated whether this book should retain the term 'cerebral palsy' in the title, but finally decided that it succinctly and uniquely conveys a lot of information. One purpose of this book is to encourage a more uniform understanding of the information that it conveys.

MORE DATA ARE AVAILABLE ON THE CEREBRAL PALSIES
More registers are being established (see Appendix), more studies are being conducted on the cerebral palsies, their precursors and other childhood disabilities, and these are suggesting new or refined causal hypotheses, several of which were reported at the Berne meeting (Ackermann-Liebrich *et al.* 1996). The older beliefs concerning the causes of cerebral palsy are being challenged using sound research methods that seek to avoid bias and control for confounding variables.

New and improving imaging techniques for the human brain are being developed. More widespread use of neonatal ultrasound imaging in preterm infants with follow-up to ages at which cerebral palsy can reliably be ascertained, together with epidemiological analysis, have suggested that certain images suggestive of white matter damage are strong predictors of later cerebral palsy. If these are the first accurately measurable signs of the neuropathological lesion, they may be used as proxy measures of cerebral palsy in studies of the neonatal period. Computerized axial tomography (CAT), magnetic resonance imaging (MRI) and single photon emission computed tomography (SPECT) may greatly aid the understanding of the cerebral pathology underlying cerebral palsy. It is not yet clear to what extent it is possible to use scans done at a time when cerebral palsy has been identified, to ascertain the timing and pathology of earlier cerebral malfunction. Insults of known timing with cerebral palsy outcomes, which can be used as gold standards to compare with the results of imaging, are very seldom available. Better clinical data are needed to test the sensitivity, specificity, and positive and negative predictive values of these techniques. Inter- and intra-observer reliability also needs to be measured. This book will refer to imaging studies only briefly because their use in cerebral palsy epidemiology is in its infancy, but they may have an important role in the clarification of cerebral palsy aetiology in the future.

DATA ARE SYSTEMATICALLY REVIEWED AND MORE EASILY ACCESSIBLE

Interpretation of scientifically sound studies is facilitated by the development of the science of systematic reviews, following the vision of Archie Cochrane who in 1979 wrote: "It is surely a great criticism of our profession [medicine] that we have not organised a critical summary, by specialty or subspecialty, adapted periodically, of all relevant randomised controlled trials." Over the years following Cochrane's statement, randomized controlled trials concerning care during pregnancy and childbirth have been systematically reviewed, spearheaded by Iain Chalmers in Oxford (Chalmers 1989). This proved to be the first step in what is now a major international collaborative effort encompassing many aspects of medical care (Henderson-Smart and Crowther 1997) known as the Cochrane Collaboration. All evidence (published and unpublished) of the effects of health care is systematically sought and reviewed and selected and/or weighted on the basis of scientific validity before collation to avoid the bias perhaps unavoidable in unsystematic reviews. New evidence is incorporated as it becomes available and obsolescence is now avoided by electronic dissemination. Results are presented in a standardized pictorial format (as well as text), enabling accurate interpretation at a glance, with a view to encouraging up-to-date evidence-based clinical and health care practices. "If this is not done, important effects of health care (good and bad) will not be identified promptly, and people using the health services will be ill-served as a result. In addition, without systematic, up-to-date reviews of previous research, plans for new research will not be well informed. As a result, researchers and funding bodies will miss promising leads, and embark on studies asking questions that have already been answered" (Cochrane Collaboration 1997).

Enthusiasts of particular new management strategies have tended to review the evidence pertaining to that strategy non-systematically. These reviews are prone to biased data selection and interpretation and tend to encourage inappropriate use of the new strategies. An example was the introduction of electronic fetal heart rate monitoring in labour on the grounds that it would prevent cerebral palsy (see Chapter 12).

Throughout this book we endeavour to adhere to the principles of systematic review and refer to the systematic reviews that have been accomplished. While there are some randomized controlled trials of perinatal therapies that have included follow-up to an age at which cerebral palsy can be reliably recognized (Grant *et al.* 1989, Allan *et al.* 1997), there are disappointingly few (Johnson 1997, Tarnow-Mordi and Brocklehurst 1997). If these trials are to provide useful information to clinicians about the overall effect of their interventions, we must continue to lobby for them to be funded to follow subjects for longer periods. Meanwhile, indications of the impact of the new perinatal interventions on population cerebral palsy rates can be provided by population-based cerebral palsy registers; these issues are discussed in Chapters 4 and 12.

THE MEDICAL MANAGEMENT OF PREGNANCY, CHILDBIRTH AND NEONATES HAS CHANGED SINCE 1984 (see Chapter 12)

Many medical management strategies have been introduced or used more liberally, including antenatal steroids for fetal lung maturation, tocolytics, continuous electronic fetal monitoring, caesarean section, neonatal intubation and ventilation, lung surfactants, prophylactic indomethacin and extracorporeal membrane oxygenation (ECMO). Many are of consequence primarily for very preterm births and may be the principle reasons for the continuing decline in very preterm perinatal mortality, discussed in Chapter 4, although continuous electronic monitoring in labour and caesarean section are used across the whole gestational age spectrum. Some of these strategies have been rigorously evaluated by randomized controlled trials. Systematic reviews of their impact on immediate outcomes are available on the Cochrane Database. As mentioned already, these studies can be informative only if followed up to the age of cerebral palsy recognition, although some proxy measures, such as ultrasound evidence of cerebral white matter damage, are reasonable predictors of cerebral palsy (see Chapter 7). Cohort and randomized controlled studies evaluating the impact of these management strategies on cerebral palsy occurrence, either individually or together as part of the package of neonatal intensive care, are rare. Thus, often the extent to which they may be influencing rates of cerebral palsy is measurable only by using registers and other epidemiological studies that use less rigorous methods with greater opportunities for misinterpretation (see Chapter 12).

Using data from cerebral palsy registers, it can be seen that there has been no significant decline in the total population rates of cerebral palsy over the period during which these management strategies have been introduced.

LITIGATION FOLLOWING CEREBRAL PALSY OUTCOMES HAS INCREASED

The popular belief that cerebral palsy was caused mostly in the intrapartum period and was therefore avoidable by modern obstetrics fuelled the increase in litigation against obstetricians (Freeman and Freeman 1992) both in numbers of cases and in the amounts awarded. Obstetrics and gynaecology now accounts for the highest proportion of indemnity payments of any medical specialty, almost one third of which are for brain damaged babies (Tito 1996). The dramatic increase in insurance premiums and the psychological impact of litigation on those involved in obstetric care has had an adverse impact on obstetric services. It has caused obstetricians to either leave the profession or practice defensively, and costs have increased to cover both their insurance premiums and the additional services entailed in defensive practice. This has occurred as a result of an overestimate of the likelihood of obstetric malpractice causing—or failing to prevent—intrapartum cerebral damage. Furthermore, the litigation itself focuses attention on the intrapartum period, away from factors and events occurring earlier in development, where it is now believed that perhaps 80 per cent of cerebral palsy pathology is initiated (see Chapter 8).

As a result, many lay and some medical people still believe that cerebral palsy is predominantly a currently avoidable perinatal problem. The results of accurate data analysed by rigorous epidemiological methods must be disseminated to inform the public, particularly prospective parents, that perinatal care cannot ensure the delivery of the perfect baby. Table 1.1 lists data from Western Australia showing expected rates for adverse pregnancy outcomes.

The changing gestational age profile of cerebral palsy suggests that very preterm cerebral palsy rates may depend on neonatal care and infertility management as well as obstetric care. This has created intense interest in population rates such as those available from registers and has demonstrated their usefulness to perinatal care providers and health service

TABLE 1.1
Anticipated pregnancy outcomes*

Of all conceptions
>15% (45,000) will miscarry

Of all births
5% (14,500) will have a birth defect
6% (17,340) will be preterm, more than three weeks before the due date
0.2% (580) will have cerebral palsy by age 5
0.4% (1156) will have intellectual disability by age 6

*Rates from Western Australia data bases applied to the Australian population, that is with good levels of obstetric and neonatal care. Numbers in parentheses refer to the number estimated to occur in Australia every year. (Adapted from Stanley *et al.* 1994.)

planners. However, rates are only the starting point in the search for causes and hence for evidence-based preventive strategies.

THE PARADIGMS OF CAUSATION ARE CHANGING: CAUSAL PATHWAYS TO THE CEREBRAL PALSIES (Chapters 5–11)

In the past, aetiological research sought sufficient causes by attempting to identify single factors with a strong and unconfounded association with cerebral palsy outcomes. The archetypal example might be a dramatic intrapartum catastrophe resulting in an apparent stillbirth, rescued by vigorous resuscitation and maintained by intensive care. However, sufficient causes have been recognized for only a small proportion of those cases not post-neonatally acquired, prompting more creative approaches to causation.

A significant proportion of cases exhibit a plethora of single or multiple antecedents that are unimpressive compared with the severity of asphyxia known from animal experimentation to be necessary to cause permanent damage to a normal brain, a severity that more often results in death (Myers 1972, Williams *et al.* 1993). In many cases no antecedents at all are recognized. These observations, together with the Rhesus iso-immunization example (see Chapter 5), led to the suggestion that cerebral palsy may seldom result from single sufficient causes but more often be the end result of causal pathways comprising a number of less dramatic factors (Nelson 1986, Blair and Stanley 1993). If each step of the pathway is dependent on previous steps, or influenced by them, a range of preventive strategies becomes possible, enabling the most acceptable to be chosen.

A causal pathway is a sequence of interdependent events culminating in disease. The interdependence may take two forms:

(1) Earlier factors may increase the probability of later factors: for example, very preterm birth predisposes to cerebral haemorrhage by exposing the fragile very preterm infant to an extrauterine environment. Very preterm birth is not in itself a sufficient cause of cerebral palsy: most children born very preterm do not have cerebral palsy. However, without such an early birth the infant would have been much less likely to be exposed to a number of factors, such as fluctuations in blood pressure and oxygenation, that may be more immediate causes of cerebral haemorrhage and ultimately permanent cerebral pathology.

(2) Alternatively, the pathological effect of later factors can be dependent on the presence of earlier factors while not being a direct result of them. For example, Morton *et al.* (1991) reported a series of cases of cerebral palsy among the Amish of North America. These were neurologically damaged during an infection in infancy, but the pathological effect of the infection was dependent on their genetically inherited metabolic defect.

Causal pathways are discussed in detail in Chapters 5–11. We believe that this way of thinking about aetiology is crucial, both to elucidate cause and allow a scientific approach to prevention, and to avoid focusing on single factors as has happened with birth asphyxia. This will avoid negative effects on both care and research.

MANAGEMENT AND THE PRINCIPLES OF EVALUATION
Chapter 13 is devoted to the epidemiological issues surrounding evidence-based practice in the management of the cerebral palsies. The awareness of the need for evidence-based management is growing, and controlled trials are now being reported. The problems of small sample size and the considerable heterogeneity in clinical expression complicates our attempts at scientific assessment, while the incurable but non-fatal nature of the disease complicates the choice of outcomes by which to gauge effectiveness. However, it is now urgent to address the challenges in attaining valid evidence of effectiveness peculiar to this field, because the recent availability of potentially quite hazardous management strategies makes management by tradition and authority dangerous. In addition, there are increasing demands for financial accountability and cost effectiveness in health service provision generally.

A major aim of this book is to encourage clinicians of all persuasions (medical, nursing and allied health professionals) to use these principles both for research and in decisions about care.

The cerebral palsies—epidemiology and causal pathways

This book is unashamedly epidemiological. It is written by epidemiologists who have life-long interests in neurological and developmental disabilities but who are not qualified to write books on neurology, radiology, genetics, pathology, fetal physiology or embryology. However, as a major aim of epidemiology is to identify causes which must be biologically plausible, collaboration with those disciplines is essential. We have not reviewed the large numbers of papers in each of these areas that relate to the cerebral palsies but have tried to convey how each of these disciplines is contributing, or may contribute in the future, to our understanding of cerebral palsy aetiology by suggesting new aetiological hypotheses. We encourage researchers in these disciplines to work with those who have data sets pertaining to cerebral palsy, as for example has been done between epidemiologists and neuropathologists in Oxford (Gaffney *et al.* 1994). This will enable their powerful new techniques to be used to further elucidate cause, and thus work towards prevention of this sometimes devastating condition.

2
WHAT ARE THE CEREBRAL PALSIES?

"What's in a name?" (Shakespeare, *Romeo and Juliet*)

Traditional definitions

In May 1958 in a letter to the *Lancet*, members of the Little Club proposed the following definition for cerebral palsy: "a persisting qualitative motor disorder appearing before the age of three years, due to non-progressive damage of the encephalon occurring before the growth of the central nervous system is complete." (Mac Keith and Polani 1958). The authors of this letter acknowledged the term 'cerebral palsy' was not exact, for the condition is clinically, pathologically and aetiologically heterogeneous. They recommended that in scientific usage, as more was learnt about each, the names of individual disease entities within the group should be used. However, they affirmed that the term was useful for research purposes and for common administrative usage, although a strict definition was necessary and should be adhered to. The statement remains as true today as when it was written, and a more recent definition added only minor qualifications: "an umbrella term covering a group of non-progressive, but often changing, motor impairment syndromes secondary to lesions or anomalies of the brain arising in the early stages of its development" (Mutch *et al.* 1992).

The long history of the descriptions and classifications of these conditions, contributed to by authors such as Little, Osler and Freud, was described by Ingram (1984) in our earlier book. All are consistent in describing the cerebral palsies as heterogeneous as regards cause, severity, outcome and clinical features.

An unusual feature of the term 'cerebral palsy' is that it refers only to clinical descriptions for which there is no definitive test. This implies that if the clinical symptoms disappear (Nelson and Ellenberg 1982, Taudorf *et al.* 1986) or if the brain lesion should turn out to be progressive, it is the diagnosis that is revised and not the natural history of cerebral palsy. It also follows that no subject meeting the clinical criteria should be excluded on the grounds of aetiology or pathology.

The definitions given at the beginning of the chapter, as well as later versions, have the advantage of simplicity but lack the precision required for reproducibility by different physicians. This problem was recognized by the members of the Little Club, who stated, "It should be possible for two observers to agree on the signs they find, however much they disagree on the probable anatomical changes producing the signs. But our two observers will discuss the problem more easily if they agree on the meaning of certain descriptive terms" (Mac Keith and Polani 1958). Such reproducibility becomes an important issue when registers are set up of patients of more than one or two different physicians. Although it has been shown that the reliability of the application of the term 'cerebral palsy' can be high if a small number of physicians have regular meetings to discuss individual cases (Blair and Stanley 1985), the comparability between its use in different places and over different times has been shown to be poor (Evans *et al.* 1986).

Areas of imprecision in traditional definitions
WHAT IS PROGRESSIVE?
By definition, the cerebral lesion neither resolves nor progresses. Since most cerebral lesions cannot be directly observed, inferences must be made from the clinical manifestation, which does change with age as well as with health, mood and fatigue. The challenge is to detect pathological progression or resolution against a background of change in clinical manifestation. There is no agreement on how long one must wait to exclude the possibility of progression, which could be very slow; or on the minimum age at which a motor impairment may be assumed to be both permanent and non-progressive.

Moreover, even the term 'progression' can be ambiguous. While there is general agreement that rapidly growing tumours and degenerative myelin disease are progressive and therefore excluded, the inclusion of subjects with other recognized diseases in which progression is a possible but not universal feature has been questioned. For instance, there are conditions where the clinical picture is produced by the cumulative detrimental effect of metabolic abnormalities, but this may be halted or avoided by appropriate therapy (Morton *et al.* 1991). Similarly the ischaemic cerebrovascular disease, moyamoya, predisposes to repeated cerebral insult (Soriani *et al.* 1993) and is a cause of acute hemiplegia—but no individual cerebral lesion is progressive. If an accumulation of static cerebral lesions due to moyamoya constitutes a progressive disease, does repeated child abuse resulting in an accumulation of cerebral lesions also constitute a progressive disease? In practice the answer will depend on the age at which the child is ascertained, and whether this is before or after the halting of the repeated insult.

SELECTION OF AGE LIMITS FOR REGISTERS
There is both a minimum age and a maximum age at which the label of cerebral palsy can be given, and both are arbitrary. The minimum is the age at which clinical signs can be assumed to be established, which will vary from one individual to the next. The maximum relates to the latest age a brain-damaging event can be considered to cause cerebral palsy as dictated by the definition—before the brain reaches maturity. Brain development is most rapid prenatally and in infancy but continues, albeit at a diminishing rate, throughout childhood. There is, therefore, no biological rationale for the choice of any particular age at which to define the brain as mature.

For the purpose of epidemiological registers, both the minimum age at which ascertainment of a birth-year cohort will be considered complete and accurate for inclusion in analyses, and the maximum age at which postneonatally acquired cerebral palsy cases will be included, must be decided. The minimum age of complete ascertainment will constitute the perceived balance between (a) the desire for timely statistics, (b) the exclusion of cases that resolve or are found to have a progressive syndrome, (c) the accuracy of the description of impairments, and (d) pragmatic considerations associated with case ascertainment.

9

This question of a minimum age at which cerebral palsy can be established with confidence is made more difficult as technological advances introduce further possibilities in the early detection of cerebral palsy. The feasibility of prenatal assessment of cerebral integrity is being explored by cerebral imaging (Govaert and de Vries 1997) and by ultrasound observations of spontaneous fetal movements (Rizzo *et al.* 1987). However, there is no evidence that either method will predict cerebral palsy with any validity. Recognition of cerebral palsy must therefore be delayed until motor development is established. This may be several months after birth in the most severe cases to several years in milder cases. Many current registers have chosen 5 years as their age of complete ascertainment, but this varies from 2 to 10 years (see Appendix).

The maximum age for inclusion of cases due to postneonatal causes is also 5 years in some registers, but this need not be the same as the age of complete ascertainment and will vary depending upon the aims of a particular register. If, for example, one purpose of a register is to establish the prevalence of motor disorders in children in a given age group, all cases occurring in children of those ages will be included. The postneonatally acquired group of cases differs from that of presumed congenital or perinatal origin in that, firstly, there is usually no doubt concerning aetiology, and secondly, there is evidence to suggest systematic differences in biological response to the cerebral pathology (Carr 1996). They are usually analysed separately or excluded from epidemiological studies, and it is important that it is made clear whether or not they are included.

A further issue for registers is whether to include a child with a firm diagnosis of cerebral palsy who dies before the age of complete ascertainment. Since death is most likely to occur in the most severely affected children, there is a good case for including them in a register. However, in such cases it cannot be assumed that they would not have been excluded by that age due to resolution of signs or recognition of a progressive syndrome. Some registers specify a minimum age of survival in order to be included as a case; this is 2 years in Mersey, England and in West Sweden and 3 years in the California data collection. Others accept all cases with a diagnosis of cerebral palsy regardless of age at death (see Appendix), thereby increasing the risk that some cases would not have met the criteria for inclusion had they survived, but reducing the loss of cases with more severe forms of cerebral palsy.

THE SEVERITY OF THE MOTOR IMPAIRMENT

It is generally accepted that the diagnosis of motor impairment requires the presence of neurologically detectable signs such as involuntary resistance to passive stretch or abnormal reflexes, and that clumsiness alone is not sufficient. The range of disability imparted by the impairment ranges from an imperceptible effect on movement (minimal) to complete absence of purposeful movement. A detectable effect on movement without significant loss of function is termed mild by at least one register (the Western Australian Register), and there is general agreement that the degree of severity required for inclusion lies within the minimal and mild categories. However, differentiation between these categories is subjective and these cases are likely to be under-ascertained because they are less likely to demand services. Some researchers therefore include only the more easily identifiable

TABLE 2.1
Diagnostic labels given to cases notified as cerebral palsy to the NE Thames Cerebral Palsy Register*

Main label	Number	%
No additional label	421	72.1
Chromosomal anomaly	6	1.0
Congenital cytomegalovirus infection	4	0.7
Genetic cause and/or known syndromes	18	3.1
Cerebral malformation	11	1.9
Cerebral atrophy/microcephaly	39	6.7
Hydrocephaly/ventricular dilatation	29	5.0
Periventricular leukomalacia/cysts or calcification	7	1.2
Porencephaly/other cerebral cysts	20	3.4
Other cerebral anomaly	3	0.5
Other label	26	4.5
Total	584	100.0

*Reproduced by permission from Williams and Alberman (1998).

groups who require aids such as walkers or orthoses (moderate impairment) or who cannot achieve function without aids such as wheelchairs or computers (severe impairment). This last group is very broad, and the addition of a profound category, to differentiate totally dependent persons from the largely independent wheelchair user would be useful for studies with objectives such as the measurement of mortality risk and the planning of service provision (M.J. Platt, personal communication 1998).

Inclusions and exclusions

There has been considerable discussion concerning the inclusion of cases that have been found to have specific and sufficient causes for the motor disorder. Different research groups and cerebral palsy registers have had differing policies in this respect, and most registers include cases with a variety of different additional diagnoses.

Table 2.1 is derived from data from an English register (Williams *et al.* 1996). The sample was population based and comprised 584 cases born between 1980 and 1986, excluding cases with no limb affected more than mildly and those where the onset had been after the second postnatal month. Data collection was by multiple-source ascertainment, from a large number of clinicians, of any case described as having cerebral palsy. The table shows the variety of differing diagnoses, or labels, which had been included (Williams and Alberman 1998).

A comparable, more intensively investigated, collaborative study from Sweden and Germany (Krägeloh-Mann *et al.* 1995) included a case with Proteus syndrome, another whose twin had had a fetal alcohol embryopathy, and one with congenital rubella embryopathy.

Such labels differ considerably in the degree to which they 'explain' the presence of the lesion leading to motor impairment. Thus, the presence of a chromosomal anomaly, single gene defect, other specific genetic condition or congenital infection may account for the occurrence of a cerebral malformation or maldevelopment. Alternatively, their presence

11

may simply increase the vulnerability of the fetus to nonspecific perinatal insults. Syndromes which interfere with blood clotting will clearly increase the risk of perinatal cerebral bleeding. The presence of cerebral cysts, whether stemming from the pre- or postnatal period, may indicate a history of a circulatory disaster, a risk to which multiple births are particularly prone. Motor impairments resulting from neural tube defects of the spinal cord are excluded by definition, but a diagnosis of spina bifida does not exclude the possibility of a coexisting impairment meeting the criteria for cerebral palsy. This can happen following operations for the defect if these are complicated by an infection. Similarly, cases with isolated hydrocephalus are sometimes excluded, although this is a cerebral defect sometimes associated with movement impairment and commonly results from the pathological sequence that follows cerebral haemorrhage in very preterm infants. These questions and other description of causal pathways are discussed in later chapters.

Most registers do not systematically report on the type of 'labels' discussed above, but these will certainly become more common over time as diagnostic resources develop, and will increasingly raise questions regarding the use of the term 'cerebral palsy' given the areas of imprecision that have been described (Badawi *et al.* 1998c).

How useful is the term 'cerebral palsy' today?
The usefulness of classifying a case under the descriptive umbrella term depends entirely upon the aims of making the classification. If the aim is to group cases of a similar clinical nature, perhaps for the purpose of planning for their care, or for trials of symptomatic treatment, aetiology may be irrelevant and the descriptive term remains of considerable value. If the objective is to study aetiology, it is clearly inappropriate to include those whose aetiology is already well understood. For studies of survival it is important to identify all cases but to study different aetiologies separately.

If the objective is to compare prevalence over time or in different places, or as a measure of pregnancy outcome, it is necessary to maintain a constant policy regarding exclusions across the samples to be compared. Such a policy must allow for the possibility that in many places and in earlier times, the newer diagnostic techniques may not have been available.

If the objective is to find an outcome to be used as a measure of obstetric and neonatal care, other questions arise. Pregnancy outcome has traditionally been measured in terms of mortality, but decreasing perinatal mortality has rendered this an insensitive indicator except at low gestations. Presumed congenital cerebral palsy has been suggested as an alternative index, but there is no logical reason to limit suboptimal outcome to non-progressive motor impairment of central origin. Results of brain imaging have confirmed that the cerebral anomalies responsible for motor defects may also be responsible for non-motor defects (Ipata *et al.* 1994, Eken *et al.* 1995), and genetic studies have revealed X-linked syndromes leading to motor impairment in affected boys, but intellectual disability and seizures in affected girls (Dobyns *et al.* 1996). Such findings reduce the justification for classifying motor disorders as a suboptimal pregnancy outcome separately from other consequences of congenital brain impairments such as seizures and cognitive, perceptual, sensory or behavioural impairments.

For the purpose of evaluating the quality of medical care, one needs information that will reflect the quality of care at the relevant time: *i.e.* preconceptional or prenatal, intra-partum or neonatal. For instance, cases of obvious prenatal origin should be excluded from studies evaluating delivery or neonatal care. Although this will reduce the numbers available for the study of subgroups, this would be compensated for by the inclusion of cases with other suboptimal neurological outcomes.

A separate question is whether the umbrella term has any usefulness in regard to measuring the general health of the population. Here the situation is different again, since this must encompass preconceptional and postnatal causes of ill-health, as well as those arising in pregnancy and the perinatal period. At any point in time causes of ill-health are the result of all that has gone before, including the quality of the environment, health behaviour and genetic constitution (see Chapters 5–12). Cerebral palsy is one of many conditions that may originate in part from any of these general causes. It could therefore usefully be added to the large number of adverse pregnancy outcomes which reflect the level of health of a population.

Why retain the term 'cerebral palsy'?
Because of the heterogeneity of the condition and our increasing understanding of some of its causes and related syndromes, we need to consider whether a case can be made for the retention of this umbrella term. Among the justifications for retaining it are that the conditions included make a significant contribution to long-standing and severe disability. Especially for young people this group of conditions is the most common, and it includes the most distressing of the most severely multiply disabling conditions. The term is now familiar to the public and policy makers, and it is important that its impact be retained.

In this era of information technology the term 'cerebral palsy' retains other advantages. It is short and unique. Search a databank using the keywords 'cerebral palsy' or even just 'palsy' and references will be found almost exclusively related to non-progressive motor impairment of central origin recognized in infancy or childhood. Keywords such as 'childhood impairment' or 'movement disorder' will identify a high proportion of references irrelevant to cerebral palsy as defined above. The term does convey considerable information, and while it is essential that it conveys the same information to everyone, its flexibility could be viewed as an added advantage. Examples of this flexibility, in terms of current common subgroupings of the cerebral palsies, their objectives, strengths and weaknesses, will be described in the following chapter.

3
THE CLASSIFICATION OF THE CEREBRAL PALSIES

On Monday, when the sun is hot
I wonder to myself a lot:
"Now is it true, or is it not,
"That what is which and which is what?"
(A.A. Milne 1926, *Winnie-the-Pooh*)

The previous chapter made it clear that the motor disorders included under the umbrella term of 'cerebral palsy' are heterogeneous. It also underlined the importance of defining objectives before attempting any classification for epidemiological purposes. For example, it was emphasized that if the objective is to compare historical and current time, stable definitions need to be maintained.

Subclassifications are also required to plan for service provision and evaluation, to carry out trials of symptomatic treatment, to use as measurable outcomes of quality of maternity care, and to execute aetiological and neuropathological studies with a view to prevention and/or prognosis.

Traditional classification by clinical description
It has been traditional, and is still usual, to classify different types of cerebral palsy by the clinical descriptions of the type, topography and severity of the motor impairment. These classifications were discussed in the previous book (Alberman 1984, Ingram 1984). Additional information on the presence of associated impairments and from data obtained by cerebral imaging may allow further subclassification. For studies which include cases being cared for by different clinicians, or for multicentre studies, the clinical manifestations must be described using standard and reproducible methods.

TYPES OF MOTOR IMPAIRMENT
Spasticity is the most common type of motor impairment with about 80 per cent of reported cases predominantly spastic. It is characterized by abnormal control of voluntary limb muscles and associated with an enduring positive Babinski reflex (indicating a lesion of the pyramidal tract), the presence of a clasp knife effect (sudden disappearance of abnormal resistance to passive stretch), and by exaggerated reflexes and/or clonus, sometimes in association with reduced truncal tone.

Dyskinesia is found more often in conjunction with spasticity than alone. It is characterized by the presence of involuntary movements which may be athetoid (writhing

14

movements) and/or dystonic (rigid posturing) and/or—now rarely—choreic (rapid, jerky movements).

Both *ataxia* and *hypotonia* are seen so frequently that they are seldom explicitly described unless they are the predominant motor impairment, a very rare situation (Dite *et al.* 1995, Blair and Stanley 1997). Isolated hypotonia frequently accompanies intellectual impairment and is not traditionally classified as cerebral palsy (Badawi *et al.* 1998c).

Different types of movement disorder may coexist. Although most workers will classify according to the predominant form, this may vary over time within any one individual.

TOPOGRAPHY

In all reported series of cases there are four commonly occurring distributions of spasticity. Several terms are used to describe these.

Quadriplegia denotes the involvement of all limbs with the arms being equally or more affected than the legs. Synonyms are *tetraplegia* and *double hemiplegia*, though the latter often implies lateral asymmetry.

Diplegia is used to describe more severe involvement of the legs than the arms. Some clinicians distinguish between *paraplegia* or *diplegia I* in which the arms are normal or minimally affected, and *diplegia II* in which the arms are perceptibly affected. In most series these subgroups are considered together as diplegia.

Left hemiplegia is the involvement of the left side of the body only, with the upper limb usually more affected than the lower limb. Its converse, *right hemiplegia*, is more common than left hemiplegia. Less symmetric distributions are also seen, giving rise to terms such as monoplegia or triplegia.

Table 3.1 demonstrates the variation between proportions classified to these groups in six well-established registers. A significant part of this variation is likely to represent variation in applying the descriptions rather than real differences in disease topography (see p. 17). The Western Australian Register classifies cases by the predominant cerebral palsy type (right or left hemiplegia, diplegia, quadriplegia, ataxia, athetosis, dystonia or hypotonia) with up to two additional codes to give a more complete picture of nonclassical spastic distributions and/or mixed forms of cerebral palsy. This enables the classification of topography by the *predominant pattern* for simple analyses or the *pure pattern* for differentiating non-classical distributions and mixed types, as shown in Table 3.1. The use of the limb-by-limb coding system in describing cerebral palsy, as discussed below, provides even more detailed information about the presence of all clinically observed signs and movement patterns.

SEVERITY OF THE MOTOR IMPAIRMENT OR RESULTING DISABILITY

In the previous book Jarvis and Hey (1984) discussed the impossibility of measuring the severity of the motor impairment objectively, because the disability it confers is so dependent on other factors, particularly cognitive ability. In practice, severity of impairment is usually inferred from functional ability. Jarvis and Hey called for a measure that ideally would be simple, inexpensive to administer, readily quantifiable, objective, easy to replicate and not requiring sustained motivation or marked intellectual ability. They noted that it would need to be standardized for age and that its distribution should be measured in healthy children.

TABLE 3.1
Distribution of types of cerebral palsy in six registers, excluding postneonatally acquired cases

CP type	W. Australia[1] 1975–90 (N = 756)		W. Sweden[2] 1983–90 (N = 383)	Mersey, UK[3] 1966–77 (N = 695)	Avon, UK[4] 1969–88 (N = 489)	E. Denmark[5] 1965–74 (N = 788)	N. Ireland[6] 1978–92 (N = 662)
	Predominant %	Pure %	Predominant %	Predominant %	Predominant %	Predominant %	Predominant %
Hemiplegia	36.2	33.1	33.7	27.0	36.2	26.8	37.0
Diplegia	31.6	18.0	44.9*	21.0	28.4	32.2	17.8
Quadriplegia	15.9	9.1	8.4	27.7	14.3	21.1	31.6
Non-classical spastic		16.0					
All spastic	83.7	76.2	87.0	75.7	78.9	80.1	86.4
Ataxia	7.0*	5.0	5.5	4.5		5.6	5.0
Dyskinesia	8.6	5.8	7.6	4.1		10.0	6.0
Hypotonia	0.6	0.5		2.0			0.2
Mixed							
—Mainly spastic		7.5		10.8**			
—Mainly non-spastic		4.9					
Other					21.1	4.3	
Unclassified				2.8			2.4

*Includes ataxic diplegia.
**Mixed CP associated with spasticity, not necessarily predominantly spastic.
[1]Unpublished data from Western Australian Cerebral Palsy Register.
[2]Hagberg et al. (1993, 1996).
[3]Pharoah et al. (1987).
[4]MacGillivray and Campbell (1995).
[5]Topp et al. (1997b).
[6]Parkes et al. (1998).

Since then this has been largely accomplished with the development of the Gross Motor Function Measure (GMFM) which has now been specifically applied to children with cerebral palsy (Palisano *et al.* 1997). While this is an excellent descriptive measure, its capacity as a sensitive evaluative instrument remains to be proved (see Chapter 13).

Decisions concerning whether and how to adjust severity scores for past and current treatment and associated impairments depend on the objectives of the study being undertaken. For planning services, a measure of the current functional capacity is required, however that capacity was obtained. For aetiological studies it may be important to note whether a particular function was achieved naturally or as a result of surgery, or whether cognitive disability hampers its achievement or assessment. Measurement of severity of impairment is also important when evaluating intervention strategies. While there are a few interventions that may have important effects on functions such as sitting and walking, most have a more limited effect, and positive gains in some functions may be accompanied by losses in others. Evaluative measures of severity of impairment must be sensitive to small changes in functional ability. Observers will often need to consider specific abilities separately, the relative desirability of each of which will be determined by the individual's circumstances and the presence of other impairments.

Inter- and intra-observer repeatability of clinical description
Within any subject the degree, and even the type of movement disorder may change over time. In the long term it will vary according first to the stage of motor development and later to ageing. In the short term it will vary with the level of health, fatigue, motivation, mood and environment. In addition to the differences in classification practices mentioned in relation to Table 3.1, considerable inter- and intra-observer variation between clinical descriptions of a given type, severity and even site of impairment is also found. This is particularly the case in the less common expressions of cerebral palsy. All these sources of variation create significant problems when these descriptions are used as the basis for comparison of cases in different places or over time, to monitor individual progress or to select subjects for multicentre studies.

Interobserver agreement may be improved by careful choice and standardization of the descriptive terms and observer education (Blair and Stanley 1985, Evans and Alberman 1985), but this is easier to accomplish in a single centre than nationally or internationally. Several cerebral palsy registers have used 'limb-by-limb' descriptions of type, distribution and severity of motor involvement. The important principle behind these descriptions is to allow separate coding for each limb and for the trunk and head as appropriate, and to represent the type of impairment and the degree of severity, as done in the Western Australian Register's data collection form shown in Figure 3.1. A second principle illustrated in this figure is to reduce interobserver variation resulting from differing interpretations of the specialist terms by using simple everyday language to describe signs. The form in Figure 3.1 is completed to represent a severely disabled child with a laterally asymmetric spastic quadriplegia, a hypotonic head and trunk and some associated athetosis: such cases do occur rarely and are difficult to describe using traditional descriptive terms. A very important feature of descriptive forms is the explicit and detailed instructions, which have been tested

WESTERN AUSTRALIAN CEREBRAL PALSY REGISTER
Description of motor and other disabilities

Name _____ Date of birth _____

Address _____

Centre _____ Record No. _____

Examiner _____ Date _____

MOTOR DISABILITY

```
┌─────────────────────────────────────────────────────────────────────────────┐
│  SEVERITY CODES                                                               │
│                                                                               │
│  Signs                     Function                                           │
│  Minimal    = 1 =   Motor signs present but no functional impairment.         │
│  Mild       = 2 =   Symptoms result in some functional impairment.            │
│  Moderate   = 3 =   Between mild and severe; eg, ambulant with walking frame. │
│  Severe     = 4 =   Little purposeful voluntary action, though function may   │
│                     be acquired, IQ permitting                                │
└─────────────────────────────────────────────────────────────────────────────┘
```

Use severity codes 1 - 4 in appropriate boxes to refer to function in (1) and to indicate severity of motor signs in (2) and (3).

		RUL	LUL	RLL	LLL	Head	Trunk
(1)	**Function:**	4	3	3	3	3	3

(2) **Signs Felt (tone):**

	RUL	LUL	RLL	LLL	Head	Trunk
Predominantly hypertonic	4	3	3	3		
With clasp-knife effect (yes/no)						
Predominantly hypotonic					3	3
Variable tone	4	3				

(3) **Signs Observed (abnormal movements):**

	At Rest	With excitement or intention
Short and jerky		
Slow and writhing		2
Tremor		2
Inco-ordination *(code only if this is the predominant motor dysfunction)*		
Movements resulting in abnormal postures and grimacing		

(4) Verbal description of motor disability including severity (as you would record in medical notes):

_____

_____

_____

_____

Fig. 3.1. The limb by limb approach to clinical description used by the Western Australian Cerebral Palsy Register. The form has been filled in to represent a severely disabled child with laterally asymmetric spastic quadriplegia, hypotonic head and trunk, and some associated athetosis.

and adapted to minimize inter- and intraobserver variation.

This limb-by-limb method of recording observations is more precise. It enables more accurate, detailed and flexible categorizations and allows the effects of changes in classification practices to be measured. For instance, the term hemiplegia may refer only to those in whom both limbs on one side are affected while the limbs on the other are apparently quite normal. Alternatively it may refer to those in whom three or all four limbs are affected, but the arm and leg on one side are more severely affected than those on the other. Such a distinction may have a substantial effect on classification categories, since those with four limbs affected may be included with quadriplegias or double hemiplegias or with hemiplegias. The use of severity codes for each limb also simplifies description of mixed signs such as spasticity occurring with athetoid movements.

Associated impairments

Recognized associated impairments include sensory defects, cognitive and learning disability, behavioural disorders, and the presence of seizures of different types. Several of these may coexist. These associated disabilities exacerbate the disability conferred by the motor impairment and may inhibit rehabilitation, particularly if they limit the utilization of therapy or aids. Their presence can be used to further subgroup cases. In a report combining the data on registered cases born between 1984 and 1989 from the Mersey, Oxford and Scottish registers (Pharoah *et al.* 1998), 17 per cent of 1338 cases with relevant information had severe learning, manual and ambulatory disability but no sensory disability. An additional 5 per cent had a severe visual disability and 1 per cent a hearing but no visual disability. Two children had all five functional disabilities.

The likelihood and severity of associated disabilities increases with increasing extent and severity of motor impairment. Severe or profound intellectual impairment (IQ <35) occurred in 4.4 per cent of those with mild, but 52 per cent of those with severe motor impairment among individuals on the Western Australian Cerebral Palsy register born between 1975 and 1990. In the same cohort, seizures were an ongoing problem in 20 per cent of those with mild and 60 per cent of those with severe motor impairment. Three per cent of mild and 24 per cent of severely motor impaired cases were blind, and 0.3 per cent and 3.7 per cent respectively were deaf.

All registers report significant proportions of major additional impairments as well as an excessive number of minor visual impairments such as refractive errors and strabismus. Poor proprioception (an inability to localize body parts without looking) is seldom included in the differential description because it is difficult to measure and easy to confuse with intellectual or motor impairment. However, it probably occurs frequently in association with motor impairment and may confer significant disability.

As with the motor impairment, the reproducibility of descriptions of associated impairments between observers and over time will depend on the development of standardized methods and formats. The difficulty of developing such methods is exacerbated firstly by the changing clinical description both in the short and long term and secondly by the presence of multiple impairments. Tests of cognitive ability, for example, frequently depend on normal motor, visual and/or auditory function.

Completeness and quality of recording

For research and comparative purposes it is very important to achieve an accurate, complete and standardized description of every case with cerebral palsy and, ideally, to update this at regular intervals. The account given above makes it clear that this is not a trivial exercise. The success with which it is achieved depends on whether the case descriptions are obtained from routine clinical notes or as part of a research or audit exercise. In the latter case, resources are specifically earmarked for the purpose, and quality can be checked regularly. Where the descriptions are derived from routine clinical care, their quality will vary with the motivation of the clinician and their consistency with the number of clinicians involved. For the whole of Western Australia, for many years, only a small number of clinicians were responsible for the assessment of children with cerebral palsy, and they met regularly to discuss the recording of descriptions, particularly of unusual cases. As a result, their clinical descriptions were increasingly consistent and reliable. Elsewhere, such as in the UK, a large and changeable body of clinicians may be responsible for the care of affected children in a given area, and completeness, consistency and repeatability may not be achievable, even where researchers are employed to abstract clinical records. These problems are difficult to surmount, and the production of high data quality usually requires extra resources.

Aetiological classifications

Most workers distinguish postneonatal from other causes because a recognized causal event following previously normal development is usually a prerequisite for a postneonatally acquired categorization (see Chapter 11). Many workers also distinguish antenatal from perinatal causes, but our ability to unequivocally recognize perinatal causes has been questioned (Bax and Nelson 1993, Blair 1993, MacLennan *et al.* 1995). While most studies agree that there is a group for whom aetiology is a complete mystery, the *causes* that are reported should in many instances more properly be labelled as *risk factors*. For example, preterm birth and intrauterine growth restriction are associated with cerebral palsy, but the causal pathways and biological mechanisms by which the cerebral damage is associated with these risk factors is not yet well understood (see Chapters 7, 8).

There are only a small number of correlations between causes and specific clinical descriptions. Prenatal maternal iodine deficiency is associated with spastic diplegia in association with deaf-mutism and severe intellectual deficit (Pharoah *et al.* 1971).

Choreoathetosis often accompanied by deafness follows kernicterus usually due to blood group incompatibility. Very preterm birth complicated by periventricular haemorrhage is associated with spastic diplegia and normal cognitive function. The occurrence of motor impairment with other congenital anomalies is occasionally identified as a chromosomal, metabolic or other genetically transmitted defect. A severe late intrapartum hypoxic insult to term, normally grown babies followed by a mild or moderate neonatal encephalopathy has been associated by Rosenbloom (1994) with dyskinesia but normal cognition.

It is not clear how specific these clinical signs are to their associated cause. The dramatic decline in rates of choreoathetosis following the routine administration of Anti-D to Rhesus negative mothers following delivery of their first child suggests that this, at least, is a reasonably specific association. However, most attempts to associate particular descriptions of the motor impairment to recognized antecedents have been somewhat disappointing. For instance, only 10 of 115 Mersey born children with dyskinesia reported by Rosenbloom had experienced the hypoxic insult and sequelae, and it is not certain how many infants with similar perinatal findings were normal or developed other types of cerebral palsy (Miller 1994). Similarly the association between ataxia and family history observed in Sweden (Gustavson *et al.* 1969) has not been replicated elsewhere (Miller 1988).

As will be suggested in the following chapters, a significant proportion of cerebral palsy may be of multifactorial aetiology. There are probably very many aetiological paths each followed by only a small number of cases, which greatly complicates attempts to create an aetiological classification.

Pathological classifications
For many decades researchers have used pathological classifications based on the naked eye and microscopic appearance of the brain. Patterns of damage were described in these terms by Wigglesworth in the previous book (Wigglesworth 1984). The introduction of brain imaging, using a variety of different modalities, raises new issues of repeatability for the interpretation of images derived by different modalities, on different equipment for a given modality and between different observers using the same equipment. Inter- and intraobserver variation can be reduced by using standardized protocols and training (Pinto-Martin *et al.* 1995). The question of what appearances are compatible with clinical normality is crucial. Normal control data have been reported for preterm infants (Stewart and Kirkbride 1996), but so far only for a very small number of term infants (Mercuri *et al.* 1998). As yet the sensitivity and specificity of many reported abnormal findings are not known.

However, cerebral imaging holds great promise. When imaging technology is sufficiently developed it may provide the basis for a pathological classification that will be more successful at creating clinically and prognostically homogeneous groups.

4
HOW COMMON ARE THE CEREBRAL PALSIES?

Several workers throughout the last half century have tried to answer this question, and their answers need careful interpretation. This chapter describes the problems with measuring the occurrence of the cerebral palsies and how they have been addressed. These issues need to be considered when interpreting 'How common are the cerebral palsies?' from published data. The literature on cerebral palsy occurrence is described, comparing frequencies over time, between places and by several factors of interest.

Measures of 'how common?': prevalence, incidence, and something in-between
Prevalence is defined as the proportion of a given population experiencing a condition at a given time, and is measured as an aid to planning service provision. Incidence is the rate at which a condition arises in a population and is measured by those interested in aetiology and prevention. For an irreversible condition, such as cerebral palsy, the difference between the incidence and prevalence is dependent on the difference in mortality rates between those with the condition and the population from which they arise. Table 4.1 summarizes the definitions and attributes of prevalence and incidence.

PREVALENCE
Once criteria for numerator and denominator populations have been defined, the calculation of prevalence is relatively straightforward, although it can be very labour intensive because of the large sample size required for stable estimates. For example, a 1988 survey of childhood disability in the USA interviewed caregivers of more than 17,000 non-institutionalized children under the age of 18 years and identified 34 cases of cerebral palsy. The standard error of the overall rate exceeded 20 per cent, while those of any subgroup exceeded 30 per cent (Newacheck and Taylor 1992). In addition, the exclusion of institutionalized children may have affected prevalence estimates of cerebral palsy, particularly of severely and multiply disabled children. This may partly account for the 45 per cent decrease in prevalence noted for those of 10–17 years of age, compared with younger children, since older children with severe disability are more likely to be institutionalized, as they become larger and physically more difficult to care for, thus being excluded from the prevalence estimate. This explanation is supported by the observations of 1978 prevalence estimates by Haerer *et al.* (1984). They included institutionalized persons and found 50 possible or definite cases out of 23,842 inhabitants of Copiah County, Mississippi, who had cerebral palsy recognized before the age of 2 years. Although mortality might be expected to be higher in this earlier study they found only a 33 per cent decrease in prevalence in 6- to 19-year-olds compared with 0- to 5-year-olds.

TABLE 4.1
Cerebral palsy—measures of occurrence

	Prevalence	*Incidence*
Definition	Existing/current cases in a population	New cases arising in a population
Used for	Planning of services	Aetiological studies
Relationship	Prevalence is incidence minus mortality and migration	
How measured	Surveys to identify cases as a proportion of specific population	• Follow up a birth cohort • Register cases of cerebral palsy and relate these to their birth cohorts
Problems with measure	Very large surveys required to establish precise estimates	• True incidence of brain defect/damage causing (likely to cause) cerebral palsy is not measurable • Delay in ascertainment (months or years from cerebral defect) • Cases lost due to deaths, out migration and other losses from birth cohorts

Since the 1960s epidemiologists have been primarily concerned with aetiology and the impact of changes in perinatal care, therefore registers were established in order to estimate incidence. Prevalence can be estimated from incidence if mortality rates are also known. The few published reports of mortality in people with cerebral palsy show the anticipated associations of increased mortality rates with increasing extent and severity of motor impairment and with increasing number of other additional impairments. When comparing mortality rates, the profile of severity of impairment must therefore always be considered.

Accurate data on mortality exist only for childhood as no cohorts have large enough numbers who have attained older ages to allow for stable estimates (Evans *et al.* 1985, Hutton *et al.* 1994, Crichton *et al.* 1995). Furthermore the pattern of mortality amongst earlier born cohorts may not be predictive for later born cohorts as this pattern has changed so dramatically over time. For example, in two of the surveys of one week of British births, nine (23 per cent) of the 40 cases of cerebral palsy born in 1958 but none of the 33 cases born in 1970 had died by the age of 10 years (Emond *et al.* 1989). Cerebral palsy is not a fatal condition but predisposes to several possible causes of death. Duration of survival, particularly of the severely impaired, is highly dependent on the quality of care available.
• With the closure of institutions and the increase in home care, the survival of children increased considerably.
• Before the introduction of antibiotics, few people with significant cerebral palsy survived early childhood particularly if they had (as many do) an impaired ability to cough, because they were then vulnerable to respiratory infections.
• Feeding difficulties, which occur frequently with severe and extensive motor impairment (Reilly and Poblete 1996), resulted in severe undernutrition before nasogastric tube feeding and gastrostomy were practised.

23

- The will to live in the severely motor disabled is likely to be enhanced when computer technology can circumvent communication difficulties and enable them to contribute more effectively to society.

Such social and technological advances have enabled a cohort of people with severe motor impairment to survive into middle life for the first time in history, and the ultimate extent of their survival is therefore not yet knowable. Observations of cohorts since World War II suggest that, while the cerebral lesion in cerebral palsy is not progressive, chronic motor impairment predisposes to early physical deterioration. The increasing survival of people with cerebral palsy has significant implications for the provision of services and gives rise to urgent questions about the correlates of physical deterioration in the motor impaired. For planning such services, traditional prevalence data for cohorts of adults with cerebral palsy, stratified by functional abilities, are required (Grant *et al.* 1989).

The majority of registers follow registrants only until the clinical description is considered secure. In most this is taken as age 5 years (Oxford, England; Mersey, England; Victoria, Australia; South Australia; Western Australia), in Sweden as 4 years, and it seldom exceeds 8 years. However, since population surveys are difficult and expensive, cerebral palsy registers provide an attractive alternative for estimating adult prevalence data. Either registrants can be followed indefinitely (as the Victorian Register hopes to do) or the registers may be linked to statutory collections of death certificates, as is done with individuals with cerebral palsy included on the registers in SE and NE Thames, Mersey, South Australia and Western Australia.

INCIDENCE

The essential criterion defining cerebral palsy combines two concepts, (i) a cerebral defect or lesion that results in (ii) a defect in movement or posture (see Chapter 2). Incidence may arguably be considered either as the rate at which those defects in movement and posture arise or the rate at which the cerebral defects and lesions arise. These incidences would be the same if the resultant motor defect were immediately apparent, or if there were no loss to follow-up between acquisition of the lesion and recognition of the defect. However, neither condition applies.

Figure 4.1 shows that ante- or perinatally acquired cerebral palsy is first recognized within the first year of life in the majority of severe cases but in only 50 per cent of mild or minimal cases. While permanent motor impairment is suspected at birth in some cases, the definitive description must wait until the motor signs of cerebral palsy are observable. There is always a time delay between acquisition of the cerebral lesion and ascertainment of its effect on motor ability, during which the individual may die. The true incidence will therefore differ according to whether cerebral palsy is defined by acquisition of the lesion or by expression of the motor impairment. Practically, it can only be confirmed that a lesion causing a motor defect is present if the child survives long enough to demonstrate it, because our understanding of neuropathological imaging and prognosis is inadequate. Nonetheless, for reasons associated with interpreting the epidemiology of cerebral palsy in terms of pregnancy outcomes, discussed below, the underlying incidence has been considered to be that of the brain lesion rather than its motor expression (Pharoah 1995), except for post-

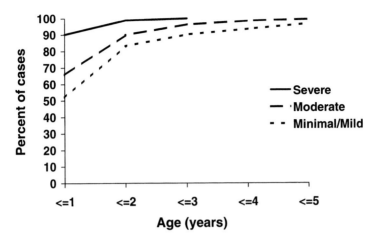

Fig. 4.1. Age at which cerebral palsy (excluding cases due to postneonatal causes) is first recognized, by severity of motor impairment (Western Australian Cerebral Palsy register, unpublished data).

neonatally acquired cases. Infants dying of a postneonatally acquired cerebral lesion that would result in motor impairment in the event of survival are not, of course, classified as having postneonatally acquired cerebral palsy, although an increase in rate of postneonatally acquired cerebral palsy could follow the increased survival of brain damaged children.

The incidence of cerebral palsy as defined by the brain lesion is not measurable. The frequency of recognized motor impairment will be less than the incidence of the relevant cerebral lesions, since early death occurs more frequently among those with brain damage than among those without. Measuring the incidence of recognized motor impairment measures the *prevalence* of the cerebral lesion since it excludes those dying before recognition.

SOMETHING IN-BETWEEN

Several measures have been proposed in the search for the most useful measure of frequency of motor impairment for aetiological study. To calculate a prevalence, both numerator and denominator are derived from the same (living) population in terms of geography and time. The terms 'birth prevalence' (Alberman 1984), 'birth cohort prevalence' (Sola and Piecuch 1994), 'crude prevalence' (Hagberg *et al.* 1996) and the more lengthy but informative 'prevalence at a given age per 1000 live births' (Paneth and Kiely 1984) have been used but are not traditional prevalence estimates because the numerator and denominator are not ascertained at the same time. The presence of the motor impairment (defining the numerator) cannot adequately be determined at birth, hence birth refers only to the denominator. Cases can be included in the numerator only when the child is old enough for the motor defect to be recognized. As mentioned earlier, the age at which this developmental stage is attained varies between months of age in severe cases and years in milder cases. Furthermore, observations that early motor delay and even frank impairments may resolve or change (Nelson and Ellenberg 1982, Stanley 1982) argue for delaying ascertainment of cases. If cases are

25

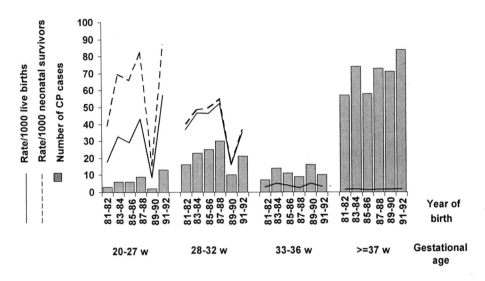

Fig. 4.2. Cerebral palsy numbers and rates (excluding cases due to postneonatal causes) by gestational age in Western Australia, 1981–1992.

ascertained in childhood, recognition will be more complete but the numerator and, to a very much lesser extent, the denominator will be depleted by intervening deaths as mortality among infants with cerebral damage is higher than among unimpaired infants. On account of these problems, the numerators for frequency measures in aetiological studies are usually cumulative numerators obtained by counting all children recognized as having cerebral palsy up to the age of final follow-up. Most registers include all children once the impairment has been recognized, irrespective of how long they survive after recognition.

Denominators
Defining the appropriate denominator for a numerator that is cumulative is problematical. It should consist of the population at risk of being recognized as having such a motor impairment, but integrating over time the number of unimpaired survivors at the moment of recognition of each case is difficult and approximations are made. In developed countries, early childhood (postneonatal) mortality among the unimpaired is extremely low, therefore using the population of neonatal survivors as the denominator is a reasonable approximation for a cumulative prevalence over the period from one month to several years. In practice, live birth data are more easily available than 1 month survivor data and much of the literature quotes rates of recognized motor impairment per 1000 live births. This ignores the neonatal mortality rate, which may be negligible for mature births but is significant for very preterm births. In many instances, population data on neonatal survivors may not be available, so comparisons using live births as denominator need to be made. Figure 4.2 uses Western Australian data to demonstrate the difference in estimated rates of cerebral palsy between using live births and using neonatal survivors as the denominators. Above 32 weeks the

26

effect is imperceptible; between 28 and 32 weeks there is a small but measurable difference in rates; but below 28 weeks using neonatal survivors as the denominator doubles the estimated rate relative to using live births as the denominator. The use of live births as the denominator artefactually decreases the apparent rate of cerebral palsy by including in the denominator neonatal deaths that are not at risk of developing cerebral palsy, although they may have cerebral defects that would manifest as cerebral palsy had they survived. Use of live births as the denominator may be partly responsible for the opinion that infants born at around 30 weeks of gestation (where neonatal mortality is now low) are at higher risk of cerebral palsy than are infants born earlier (for whom neonatal mortality is higher). Figure 4.2 shows that in Western Australia, if live births are used as the denominator, infants born at 28–32 weeks gestation are at higher risk of motor defect than earlier born infants, but the difference is much less pronounced if neonatal survivors are used as the denominator.

It is therefore important to note definitions of denominators for rates of cerebral palsy, particularly for infants born preterm or those categorized by birthweight. While rate per 1000 neonatal survivors and per 1000 live births are usually used now, rate per 1000 total births has been used in the past. This last includes stillbirths, and it is then also important to note the gestational age criterion for a birth (*e.g.* as greater than 20, 22 or 28 weeks).

Numerators
AGE FOR INCLUSION AS CEREBRAL PALSY
The definition of cerebral palsy does not specify a minimum age at which a case can be reliably considered to have cerebral palsy. Different data sets use different age limits for inclusion of cases in the cerebral palsy group as discussed in Chapter 2. This applies both to the age at which a birth cohort is considered accurately and completely ascertained, and the age to which a case must survive in order to be included. Once a motor defect is recognized it should be verified that it is neither progressive nor resolving before it is called cerebral palsy. Time is the best test, short of a reliable diagnosis which excludes cerebral palsy, *e.g.* confirmation of a progressive condition such as carbohydrate-deficient glycoprotein syndrome by metabolic testing. However, time is sometimes unavailable since mortality among children with cerebral palsy, though decreasing, considerably exceeds that of the rest of the population cohort. Some research workers stipulate a minimum age for inclusion of cases who die, such as 2 years in Western Sweden and 3 years in the California study. Others, such as Western Australia, accept all cases reliably described as cerebral palsy where early death occurs, regardless of age or how long the motor disorder has been recognized. Thus, there is no universally agreed upon age for inclusion of cases.

CAUSE AND AGE AT ACQUISITION
As discussed in Chapter 2, there are also differences between registers in the collection of postneonatally acquired cases: (1) whether this group is included at all, and (2) the maximum age at acquisition of the brain damage. Postneonatal causes (head injury, cerebral infection, etc.) are almost always well understood, and it is therefore reasonable to exclude them from studies of antenatal or perinatal aetiology or from statistics pertaining to outcomes of

pregnancy and neonatal care. However, these cases are frequently, but less reasonably, excluded from rates of cerebral palsy reported for general purposes, as are some cases due to known prenatal causes such as cytomegalovirus or chromosomal defects.

TYPE OF MOTOR IMPAIRMENT
Numerators may be qualified by aspects of motor impairment, most often by severity of disability, but also by type. While spasticity is the most common type, numerators limited to spasticity exclude about 15 per cent of cerebral palsy cases (in developed countries), and conclusions drawn from such samples cannot be assumed to apply to those with other forms of cerebral palsy.

SOURCES OF ASCERTAINMENT
In general, cases ascertained from individual medical centres cannot be assumed to be representative of the total population, unless they are referral centres for geographically defined areas and all cases meeting the defining criteria for the numerator will present at that establishment. Such samples are usually confined to more disabling forms of cerebral palsy. Only geographically defined sources of cases can represent total populations, and then the methods of ascertaining cases must be critically appraised. Milder cases and cases without easily recognized disability will almost certainly be under-ascertained without routine neurological examinations for the entire population such as is achieved in follow-up studies of very preterm infants.

SAMPLE SIZE
As cerebral palsy is relatively rare, very large denominators are required to generate enough cases for stable estimates of frequency, and estimates may vary widely from year to year by chance alone. This problem is frequently addressed by combining birth cohorts to increase the size of the denominator. This may be done either by grouping birth years (for N/n estimates of frequency where N is the number of birth year cohorts and n is the number of birth years in each group) or by moving averages (the middle birth year increases by 1 for each estimate, for N–n+1 estimates). The selection of birth year groupings using the former method can greatly affect conclusions, a problem largely avoided by using the second method. However, both methods reduce the chance of recognizing any associations between cerebral palsy occurrence and timed environmental events that could be of aetiological significance, such as the rapid introduction of prenatal, obstetric or neonatal care techniques.

It is important to compare criteria defining numerators and denominators when comparing rates of cerebral palsy estimated by different workers. The only truly comparable rates are likely to be those estimated by the same workers using constant methods over time.

Comparisons of occurrence of cerebral palsy
The longest standing collections meeting these requirements date back only to 1954 (Southwestern Sweden) and 1956 (Western Australia). Thus estimates of changes in frequency before the mid-1950s must be speculative.

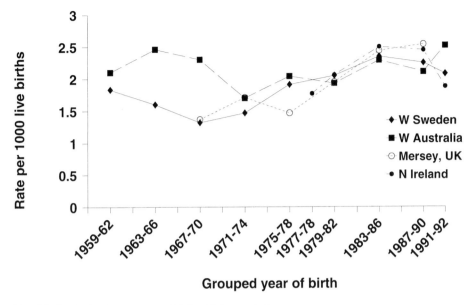

Fig. 4.3. Cerebral palsy rates per 1000 live births (excluding cases due to postneonatal causes) in four populations during the years 1959–1992 (except Mersey, 1967–1989).

DEVELOPED COUNTRIES

Figure 4.3 shows reported prevalences of cerebral palsy (excluding postneonatally acquired cases) between 1959 and 1992 obtained in four geographically defined locations that have used constant methods within each location for more than a decade of birth cohorts.

The 1960s to 1980s saw impressive declines in perinatal mortality in all the locations represented, as well as changes in obstetric and neonatal medical care practices such as the introduction of electronic fetal monitoring and neonatal intensive care. Nonetheless, there are no obvious patterns in overall cerebral palsy prevalence reproduced within each geographically defined area, even if the time axis is shifted to accommodate differences in timing of the introduction of such practices. Rates of overall cerebral palsy have remained around 2–2.5 per 1000 live births; fluctuations are common dipping down to 1.5 in Sweden, Western Australia and Mersey in 1970 and rising again throughout the 1980s. The marked changes only really appear when the rates are stratified by gestational age and birthweight (see below), which reflect the changes in preterm and very preterm survival. The availability of data on all births with some perinatal characteristics to which cerebral palsy and other registers can be linked (see Appendix) certainly enhances our capacity to obtain and interpret trends as the rates can be stratified by perinatal characteristics (Pharoah *et al.* 1997a, Stanley *et al.* 1997, Robertson *et al.* 1998).

In addition, these estimates have been derived after the introduction of antibiotics and comparatively safe caesarean delivery, in Western developed countries that probably have relatively homogeneous populations. There are no reliable estimates of trends in frequency of cerebral palsy before the 1950s, though it is plausible that they may have been higher and similar to what is currently observed in developing countries.

DEVELOPING COUNTRIES

There are grounds to believe that rates may vary with social and medical practices and that rates and profiles of aetiologies in developing countries may differ from those in more developed countries. There are no population based birth prevalence data from developing countries. Prevalence in a Turkish county has been estimated using house to house survey data as 5.6 per 1000 children below 6 years of age (95% confidence interval 3.5–7.7) (Okan et al. 1995) and for rural Kashmir as 1.46 (1.0–1.9) per 1000 children below 14 years (Razdan *et al.* 1994). Comparison with estimates in Figure 4.3 is difficult because the severity criteria required for a diagnosis of cerebral palsy are not reported and because the mortality of children with cerebral palsy is likely to differ considerably as a result of the medical and social care available so that little can be inferred about birth prevalence from these estimates. Most published evidence concerning the frequency of cerebral palsy in developing countries uses data from hospital paediatric neurology clinics. All these studies attribute a greater proportion of cerebral palsy to intrapartum asphyxia—48 per cent in Riyadh, Saudi Arabia (Taha and Mahdi 1984); 28 per cent in Al-Khobar, Saudi Arabia (Al-Rajeh *et al.* 1991); 43 per cent in Nigeria (Sathiakumar and Yakubu 1987); 43.8 per cent in India (Srivastava *et al.* 1992); and 32 per cent in Istanbul, Turkey (Özmen *et al.* 1993)—with a much higher proportion of cases being described as quadriplegic. This may be a result of considering only cases from specialized treatment centres, which are likely to treat the more severe cases, since cases attributed to birth asphyxia tend to be the more severely impaired. In the Western Australian study of moderate and severe spastic quadriplegia, 24 per cent were considered possibly or very likely to have been caused by intrapartum events (Stanley *et al.* 1993), compared with 8 per cent of the total population with spasticity (Blair and Stanley 1988). However, most of the proportions estimated in developing countries are well above the 24 per cent attributed to intrapartum events in Western Australian moderate and severe cases, suggesting that the proportion attributable to intrapartum asphyxia may be higher in developing countries, as are the proportions due to kernicterus (Duggan and Ogala 1982) and postneonatal events (see Chapter 11).

Studies from predominantly Muslim communities emphasize the role of consanguineous marriage (Al-Rajeh *et al.* 1991). Studies of Pakistani Muslim families living in Britain show that while the rate of cerebral palsy may (Sinha *et al.* 1997) or may not (Bundey 1997) be higher overall, the risk of cerebral palsy among offspring of consanguineous marriages is very much increased, with a rate of almost 1 per cent (Bundey 1997).

GENDER

Males are over-represented in all case series of cerebral palsy. Data from the Western Australian Register pertaining to 1975–1992 birth cohorts suggest that the male excess decreased temporarily in the mid-1980s. The ongoing Swedish series did not report gender ratios before 1983, but also found a lower male ratio in the mid-1980s (0.9:1 for 1983–86) (Hagberg *et al.* 1993) than in subsequent years (1.1:1 for 1987–90) (Hagberg *et al.* 1996).

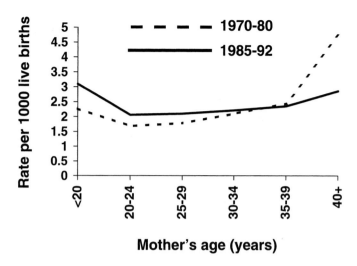

Fig. 4.4. Cerebral palsy rates (excluding cases due to postneonatal causes) by mother's age in Western Australia 1970–1980 and 1985–1992.

The excess risk of cerebral palsy for Californian males born 1983–1985 was confined to births of <1000 g (Cummins *et al.* 1993), suggesting that any decrease in male ratio is not likely to be associated with the trend toward increasing prematurity.

MATERNAL AGE AT DELIVERY

The maternal age profile of all births has changed significantly in developed countries: in Western Australia the proportion of live births to mothers aged 30 years or more increased from 19.5 per cent (1970–80) to 33.4 per cent (1985–92) (F. Stanley and L. Watson, unpublished data). There is a U-shaped curve of risk of cerebral palsy by maternal age at delivery, with the lowest risk being seen in 20- to 34-year-old mothers, rising for mothers of <20 years and >34 years of age (Fig. 4.4). Figure 4.4 also shows that the risk of cerebral palsy in births to young mothers has increased, whilst that for older mothers has fallen between 1970–80 and 1985–92. This is likely to represent more socioeconomic adversity in those mothers who continue to give birth in their teens. The lower risk in older women more recently is encouraging as this group includes those with infertility and medical problems which may *increase* the risk of poor outcome. Thus whilst there are now more older mothers, their social and other advantages must be making up for any adverse effects, in terms of cerebral palsy. The rates exclude those due to postneonatal causes (discussed in Chapter 11).

MATERNAL PARITY

In Western Australian births 1980–92, the risk of cerebral palsy was higher for first births at 2.3 per 1000 live births (95% CI 2.0–2.6) than for second or third births where the central estimate of the rate is 2.04 per 1000 live births. Rates increased with births of higher parity to 2.9 (2.3–3.5) per 1000 live births for parities of four or more, but none of the differences

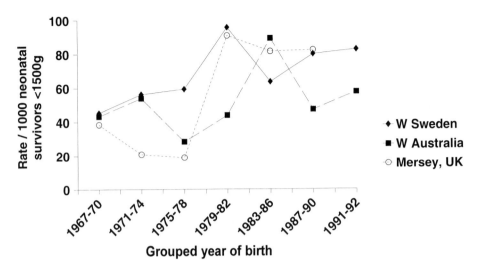

Fig. 4.5. Very low birthweight (<1500 g) cerebral palsy rates per 1000 neonatal survivors (excluding cases due to postneonatal causes) in three populations (Sweden 1967–1990, Australia 1967–1992, Mersey 1967–1989).

reach statistical significance. There have been no trends over time in risk of cerebral palsy with parity.

BIRTHWEIGHT

Cerebral palsy risk increases with decreasing birthweight (Stanley and Watson 1992, Hagberg *et al.* 1993, Pharoah *et al.* 1997b). However, birthweight is dependent on both gestational age at delivery and the rate of intrauterine growth; therefore these two risk factors must be studied independently of each other in order to separate their effects. Nevertheless, because birthweight can be measured more accurately and is more widely available than gestational age, it has long been used as a surrogate for maturity (see Chapter 8 for a discussion on this). Birthweight-specific rates have enabled the observation of trends in tiny babies before accurate population gestational age data were available (1973 in Sweden, 1980 in Western Australia) as well as comparisons between populations, and will continue to be used by centres that do not have access to population gestational age data (see Appendix). Most population based registers showed increases in cerebral palsy rates in very low birthweight infants in the 1980s. Figure 4.5 shows rising rates of cerebral palsy per 1000 neonatal survivors in <1500 g infants in Western Australia, Western Sweden and the the Mersey region between 1967 and 1992. Most of these increases in <1500 g cerebral palsy rates occurred before 1985, but the rates have remained high. Neonatal survival of babies <1500 g increased steadily throughout the 1970s and 1980s (Fig. 4.6).

At the time of writing, only one population study has recorded a fall in the cerebral palsy rates per 1000 neonatal survivors, from 128.6 in 1970–79 to 63.8 in 1980–89 in births 500–1499 g in the county of Vestfold, Norway (Meberg and Broch 1995). O'Shea *et al.* (1998c)

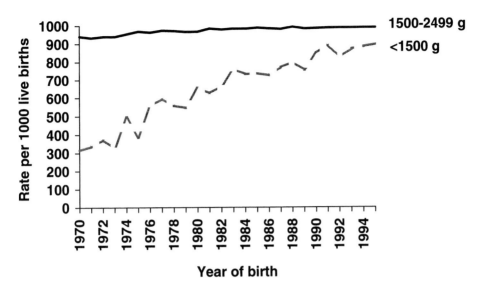

Fig. 4.6. Low birthweight neonatal survivor rates in Western Australia, 1970–1995.

reported 1-year survivor cerebral palsy rates in the north-west of North Carolina in 500–1500 g birthweight infants born 1982–94 that peaked in 1984–86 at 123.0, falling to 66.0 in 1992–94. Rates of <1500 g cerebral palsy in Slovenia 1987–90, when neonatal survivor data became available, showed a nonsignificant decline from 62.3 to 51.9 per 1000 in the short time period between 1987/88 and 1989/90 (Kavcic and Perat 1998) similar to the recent trends shown in Figure 4.5. We must continue to monitor such rates from as many registers as possible to describe trends.

Escobar *et al.* (1991) attempted to ascertain the level of disabilities among very low birthweight survivors of neonatal intensive care, including only published studies which, by certain criteria, would provide unbiased data on cohorts of these infants. They identified only 7538 survivors from 85 study cohorts born 1960 to 1986, of whom 6399 were evaluated as to cerebral palsy status. The overall rate of cerebral palsy in <1500 g infants was 77 per 1000; from 1960–77 it was 60 (95% CI 49–85) and for 1978–86 it was 80 (95% CI 57–101) with no significant trends over time. The authors lamented that the data base was small in comparison to the huge numbers of follow-up studies published from individual units which did not meet the criteria for their meta-analysis; there was no agreement on denominators nor on what constitutes an abnormal outcome; follow-up was mostly only to 3 years; there was little improvement over time; and there was considerable variation in cerebral palsy rates between studies.

Similar methodological criticisms were expressed by Lorenz *et al.* (1998) in their meta-analysis of all published studies of mortality and disabilities in extremely preterm (≤26 weeks gestation) or extremely low birthweight (≤800 g) infants. There was substantial variation in mortality and in cerebral palsy rates over the birth cohorts from 1970 to 1994, some of

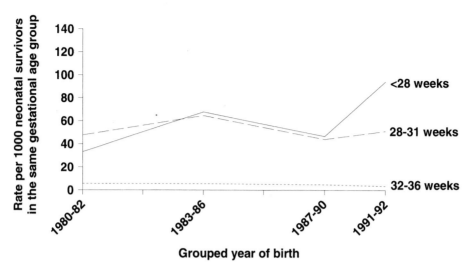

Fig. 4.7. Preterm cerebral palsy rates per 1000 neonatal survivors (excluding cases due to postneonatal causes) in Western Australia, 1980–1992.

which probably reflects the criteria for cerebral palsy ascertainment. Cerebral palsy rates were higher with higher levels of survival, the rates of both increasing over time. Variation in occurrence of cerebral palsy was also likely due to social and selective differences in cohorts, their management and follow-up. Overall nearly 50 per cent of extremely low birthweight infants survived (range 0–90%), and 7.5 per cent (75 per 1000) of the survivors had cerebral palsy (range 0–50%), a similar figure to the 8.0 per cent (80 per 1000) reported by Escobar *et al.* (1991) in very low birthweight (≤1500 g) infants. However, if survival continues to increase at these very low birthweight and early gestations, increases in cerebral palsy are likely.

GESTATIONAL AGE AT DELIVERY

The risk of cerebral palsy increases with decreasing gestation at delivery, especially when neonatal survivors are used as the denominator (see Fig. 4.2). Figure 4.2 also shows that whilst the risk is higher in early gestations, most children with cerebral palsy are born at term. Observations similar to these are found in all other case series (Hagberg *et al.* 1996, Topp *et al.* 1997c). The risk of cerebral palsy for very preterm births may be of the order of 100 times that for term births even before any other variables are taken into account. This relative risk exceeds that of any other factor; length of gestation at delivery is the strongest determinant of cerebral palsy (see Chapter 7).

Falling rates of neonatal mortality are mainly due to the increasing survival of very preterm infants resulting from the care afforded by neonatal intensive care units (NICUs). The improving outcome for very preterm deliveries (shown for <1500 g infants in Figure 4.6) has encouraged both earlier delivery for complications of pregnancy such as preeclampsia,

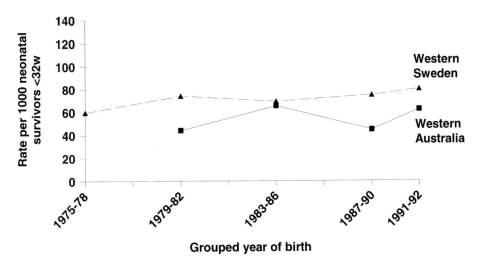

Fig. 4.8. Very preterm (<32 weeks) cerebral palsy rates (excluding cases due to postneonatal causes) in Western Sweden (1975–1992) and Western Australia (1980–1992).

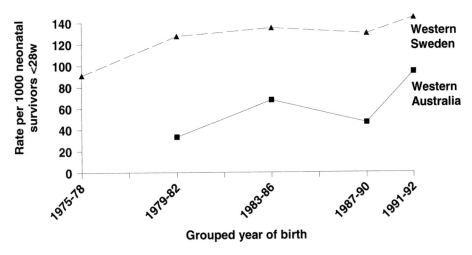

Fig. 4.9. Extremely preterm (<28 weeks) cerebral palsy rates (excluding cases due to postneonatal causes) in Western Sweden (1975–1992) and Western Australia (1980–1992).

and active resuscitation of the newborn at progressively earlier gestational ages at delivery. The increasing proportion of extremely preterm and low birthweight survivors (Fig. 4.6) has had a considerable effect on the distribution of gestational age at delivery of children with cerebral palsy. Before 1980 in Western Australia only one tenth of children with cerebral palsy were born before 32 weeks of gestation; this proportion has risen to one fifth or one quarter.

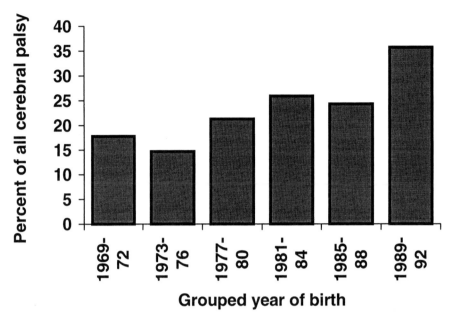

Fig. 4.10. Percentage of all cerebral palsy (excluding cases due to postneonatal causes) with severe motor impairment in Western Australia, 1969–1992.

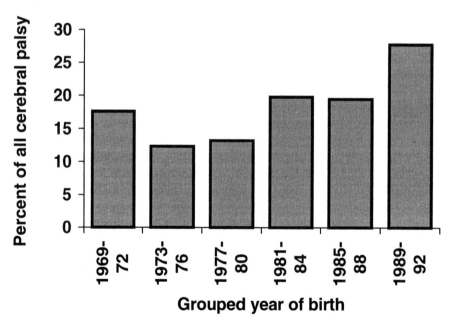

Fig. 4.11. Percentage of all cerebral palsy (excluding cases due to postneonatal causes) with severe motor impairment and IQ <70 in Western Australia, 1969–1992.

Trends in cerebral palsy rates by gestational age are only available for year of birth cohorts from the late 1970s and for only a few centres because of the difficulties of obtaining trustworthy gestational age data on all live births. As antenatal dating ultrasound becomes more widely used, better gestational age data will become available.

The trends in cerebral palsy in infants born preterm (<37 weeks) in Western Australia from 1980 to 1992 inclusive are shown in Figure 4.7. Above 31 weeks the rates changed little—from around 5.5 per 1000 neonatal survivors in 1980–82 to 3.5 in 1991–92. In those born between 28 and 31 weeks inclusive, the rates were 47.6, 64.6, 44.0 and 51.0 per 1000 in each grouped time period. The most marked change was in those born before 28 weeks: from 33.1 in 1980–82 the rate closely followed that for later born infants until the most recent time period, when it rose to 94.2 per 1000.

Only Western Sweden provides gestational age specific rates over time as a comparison (Figs. 4.8, 4.9). All infants under 32 weeks were grouped together: the rates rose steadily from around 60 per 1000 nenonatal survivors in 1975–78 to around 75.0 in 1987–90, similar to the Australian rates. Under 28 weeks, the rates were considerably higher in Sweden than in Western Australia: around 90 per 1000 in 1975–78 and rising steadily to peak at 135.0 in 1983–86 and remaining high. Thus the general trends increased in both places. Reasons for the higher rates in Sweden than in Australia are not known. For a more detailed discussion of causal pathways in very preterm infants see Chapter 7.

Escobar *et al.* (1991) and Lorenz *et al.* (1998) have reviewed the literature concerning changes in occurrence of cerebral palsy in very preterm infants following changes in neonatal management practices. The data pertain to selected populations from individual NICUs (see p. 33). Major problems in interpreting such data arise from changes in survival rates which are not always given, from the common practice of using birthweight as a proxy for gestational age which makes comparisons difficult, from other changes in the population such as antenatal and postnatal referral policy and its effectiveness, and from co-interventions which are poorly described.

From these limited assessments of cerebral palsy in very preterm survivors, the role of NICUs is hard to determine. The cerebral palsy registers become of crucial importance in providing data on these outcomes; they are also limited, however, in evaluating the NICU package or individual aspects of NICUs which may be of benefit, harm or no use (see also Chapter 12). Better (population) data should be available to evaluate care, plan for services and counsel anxious parents.

SEVERITY OF DISABILITY

The proportion of all cerebral palsy cases with severe motor impairment in Western Australia has been steadily rising (Fig. 4.10). In 1969–72 about 15–20 per cent were assessed as severe, rising to 35 per cent in 1989–97. Many of these children also had significant intellectual disability, and the increase appears to have been in those with severe and multiple disabilities (Fig. 4.11). When stratified by term and preterm births, the increase in severe cerebral palsy in the 1980s is primarily attributable to term births (Fig. 4.12). The fall in those classified as severe among preterm infants between 1969 and 1980 is unexplained. Increases in severity have also been observed in other registries.

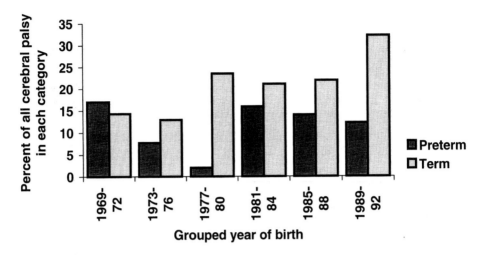

Fig. 4.12. Percentage of all cerebral palsy (excluding cases due to postneonatal causes) with severe motor impairment and IQ <70 born preterm and term in Western Australia, 1969–1992.

In Sweden, between 1971 and 1990 (Hagberg *et al.* 1996), the proportions of preterm cases not walking and with intellectual disability increased significantly, coinciding with increases in hydrocephalus in these survivors. The functional severity of disability in <1500g infants who developed cerebral palsy in the Mersey (UK) region increased in the 1980s (Pharoah *et al.* 1996). In Oxford the proportion of cases not walking by the age of 5 years increased from 28.4 per cent in 1984 to 45.7 per cent in 1992 (Johnson *et al.* 1998b). In the Denmark register data, increases were observed in the proportions of preterm cases who could not walk and who had learning disability and epilepsy between 1971 and 1982 (Topp *et al.* 1997).

Thus, not only did the occurrence of cerebral palsy in cohorts of preterm and very low-birth weight infants rise with their increased survival, but the infants who survived with cerebral palsy were more severely affected. Again, register data will be eagerly sought to ascertain future patterns of severity.

ADEQUACY OF INTRAUTERINE GROWTH
In contrast to the enormous relative risks of extremely preterm birth, poor intrauterine growth confers relative increased risks of cerebral palsy of the order of 10 or at most 20 (Blair and Stanley 1990, Uvebrant and Hagberg 1992), which are highest in the moderately preterm (see Chapter 8). Restricted intrauterine growth is therefore a major risk factor for cerebral palsy but not in very preterm infants (Murphy *et al.* 1995, Topp *et al.* 1996), perhaps because survival of very preterm infants who are also significantly growth restricted is rare. The risk of cerebral palsy is inversely related to the adequacy of intrauterine growth, as measured by the ratio of birthweight to the birthweight expected for that gestational age and allowing for the nonpathological determinants of birthweight. This risk may increase

38

exponentially with decreasing ratios below 0.85 (where 0.85 represents approximately the 10th birthweight percentile) (Blair *et al.* 1990) (see Chapter 8 for detailed discussion).

When control for maturity is desirable in epidemiological studies of cerebral palsy, it is important to control for gestational age rather than birthweight to avoid bias, because cerebral palsy is associated with poor intrauterine growth (Blair 1996a). Failure to do so can give rise to erroneous conclusions, particularly since gestational age is a more potent risk factor for cerebral palsy than is intrauterine growth restriction. We know of no data on trends over time of cerebral palsy in infants classified as growth restricted.

SOCIAL CLASS

Few published papers have examined the effect of social class on the frequency of congenital cerebral palsy, although such an association might be anticipated since social class is associated with both preterm birth and intrauterine growth restriction. Dowding and Barry (1990) showed a clear trend to increasing rates of congenital cerebral palsy with decreasing social class as estimated by father's occupation. The trend was primarily due to spastic diplegia, and, to a lesser extent, hemiplegia, but was also concentrated among children of >2500 g birthweight. The severity of disability was greater for children of semi- or unskilled parents and for unmarried mothers, who, in Ireland at that time, represented the most socially disadvantaged. Dolk *et al.* (1996) have looked at the association between cerebral palsy and social class separately in term and preterm infants and found the association exclusively in preterm infants.

Conclusions

It is interesting to contemplate whether the variety in cerebral palsy rates is due to differences in methodologies—of how and when they are defined and counted, who is excluded, what denominators are used, or the different causal patterns. We have suggested ways of counting the cerebral palsies and calculating rates for the variety of uses for which epidemiological data may be necessary.

Cerebral palsy rates differ between areas and over time, particularly in cohorts with different neonatal survival rates such as very preterm babies who have received different intensitities of neonatal care. The extent to which such variations reflect different causes is best approached by thinking of the various causal pathways to cerebral damage.

5
CAUSAL PATHWAYS TO THE CEREBRAL PALSIES: A NEW AETIOLOGICAL MODEL

> *"In a commonplace perspective that suits epidemiology, a cause is something that makes a difference. Thus, causes include all determinants of an outcome, and they may either be* active agents *or* static conditions. *Implicit in this concept of determinants is a model of multiple causes."*
> (Susser 1989)

> *"Risks are not causes."* (Ounsted 1987)

This chapter describes the concept of causal pathways, their importance to the cerebral palsies, and the challenges to elucidating such pathways, and suggests ways in which they may be handled. Known and possible pathways to the cerebral palsies consistent with associations recognized from epidemiological studies are described in Chapters 6, 7, 8 and 9.

Traditional models of causation

Our challenge in epidemiology is to assess whether observed associations between exposures (see Glossary) to possible causal agents and a given disease are causal. In other words, does the exposure makes a difference to the manifestation of the disease (Susser 1989)? The scientific method of investigating causality is to observe the effects of the exposure under a systematically planned series of experimental conditions. In epidemiological research in humans it is often not ethical to carry out such experiments. Instead we must observe naturally occurring events, over which we may have little control. Under these conditions, noncausal associations may arise, either systematically or by chance, particularly when only few observations are available. Stating an explicit hypothesis to be tested before conducting such an observational study (see Glossary) enhances its scientific rigour and reduces the likelihood of chance findings. Another method of increasing scientific rigour is to observe the frequency of the disease after avoiding exposure to the putative cause. A decrease would provide strong evidence of causality, but an initial hypothesis is required even in situations where it is possible and ethical to conduct such an experiment (Black 1996).

In his classic textbook, Bradford Hill emphasized the value of the characteristics shown in Table 5.1 when attempting to decide whether an association may be causal (Hill and Hill 1991).

In addition to these characteristics, associations should be measured in large enough samples so that the possibility of chance associations being observed is negligible (statistical significance).

TABLE 5.1
Criteria suggesting that an association is causal*

1. *Strong.* High relative risks or odds ratios.
2. *Consistent.* Cohorts from different geographic populations or time periods show the same patterns of causal associations.
3. *Specific.* The disease occurs only following exposure to the putative cause and not to other exposures and the exposure is followed by one specific disease, rather than by many diseases.
4. *Time sequence.* The putative cause precedes the outcome.
5. *Dose dependent, or with a biological gradient.* The degree of association increases with increasing intensity of exposure.
6. *Biological plausibility.* A biologically plausible mechanism for the causal association exists.
7. *Coherence of evidence.* The proposed mechanism is consistent with current biological wisdom.

*Adapted from Hill and Hill (1991).

These characteristics (often called the Bradford Hill criteria) and the analytical methods to measure the associations, such as multivariate analyses, are largely based on *single and sufficient* or, less often, *multiple independent* causal models.

Causal pathways

A causal pathway is a sequence of events or conditions culminating in the outcome or disease of interest, in which the effect of any step is dependent on the presence of other steps (Blair and Stanley 1993a). There are two types of relationships between factors on a causal pathway:

(a) The steps (A,B) on the pathway are causally independent, and the next step on the path follows the coincidence of both factors: $A + B \rightarrow C$ (*e.g.* the coincidence of a Rh+ mother and Rh– father is necessary for there to be a Rhesus-incompatible fetus).

(b) The earlier step (A) causes or predisposes to a later step (B) which causes or predisposes to the next step (or disease): $A \rightarrow B \rightarrow C$ (*e.g.* a multiple gestation may lead to very preterm birth, which may be responsible for neonatal cerebral damage).

If all factors on a causal pathway are included as separate independent factors in a multivariate analysis, their combined effect is divided between each factor. In the search for a single cause, factors may be excluded from the analytical model, and only the exposure with the strongest association will be identified. This strategy can be very misleading, particularly if early signs of disease are included as exposures, such as neonatal cranial ultrasound abnormalities or neonatal encephalopathy. In multivariate analysis such outcomes are likely to demonstrate the strongest association with cerebral palsy, and weaker associations with real, and perhaps more preventable, causes may be ignored.

Figure 5.1 illustrates a known and now successfully prevented causal pathway and the importance of understanding the chain of events when devising preventive strategies. The syndrome of choreoathetosis and deafness due to kernicterus following Rhesus incompatibility

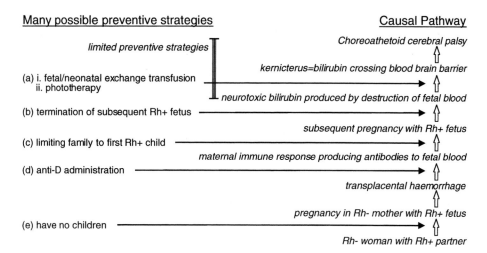

Fig. 5.1. The causal pathway to choreoathetoid cerebral palsy, and suggested preventive strategies. (Adapted from Blair and Stanley 1993a.)

between mother and child in a second or later pregnancy used to be a common form of cerebral palsy and still is in developing countries. Cerebral damage occurs at the final step and thus kernicterus could be considered as the sole sufficient cause. However, this focuses preventive efforts only on reducing kernicterus, using either exchange transfusion or phototherapy. By elucidating the whole causal pathway, the choice of preventive strategies (a–e) is increased, enabling the most effective to be selected. Where strategy 'd' is routinely implemented, the frequency of choreoathetosis with deafness has dropped dramatically (Stanley and Alberman 1984). If the causal pathway had not been investigated we could still be doing costly exchange transfusions to prevent brain damage in affected infants with the real possibility that the intervention may be too late. Thinking in causal sequences opens up more opportunities for prevention and avoids concentrating on limited time periods when the optimal time for successful prevention may have passed.

The causal pathways model of causation has developed from the recent appreciation of the aetiological heterogeneity of the cerebral palsies. This model is proving fruitful in the search for plausible mechanisms—for example of how preterm birth might be associated with the cerebral palsies (Leviton 1993)—by suggesting that some specific causes of preterm birth may be more damaging to the infant brain than others. Studies using the causal pathways model include those focusing on possible antenatal causes (Nelson and Ellenberg 1986a, Nelson 1991, Stanley 1994c), on multiple causes (Leviton 1987, Blair and Stanley 1993a,b), and on antenatal factors which may render the fetus vulnerable to subsequent intrapartum damage (Berg 1988). Another important research area relates to the position on a causal path of signs of birth asphyxia, which in some cases may be early markers of cerebral palsy resulting from earlier, rather than intrapartum, damage (Ellenberg and Nelson 1988, Kuban and Leviton 1994, Stanley and Blair 1994).

Recent research has implicated antenatal factors as antecedents for many adult diseases (Stanley 1997, Stephan and Murray 1997, Godfrey 1998, Newnham 1998, Susser *et al*. 1998), so developing methods of identifying multifactorial causal pathways that commence antenatally may be important not only for the cerebral palsies but for many other conditions as well.

Varying causal models and the Bradford Hill criteria

The appropriateness of inferring causality from the Bradford Hill criteria and the methods of assessing association need to be reconsidered where models of causation other than those with a single sufficient cause are possible. Such alternative models include:
(a) causal pathways where factors are caused or influenced by earlier factors;
(b) a pathway in which a factor requires additional, independent exposures in order to constitute a cause;
(c) the outcome has several distinct causes; or
(d) several different adverse outcomes are possible following the exposure.

In addition, recognition of causality is complicated if factors considered as a single 'exposure' are heterogeneous with some on causal pathways and others not. Some antecedent exposures, such as preterm birth and intrauterine growth restriction, may have several quite distinct possible causes, not all of which are associated with cerebral palsy.

Many of the situations described above apply to the cerebral palsies. A good example of the situation described in (a) above is choreoathetosis secondary to kernicterus. A recognized risk factor, namely a mother being Rhesus negative, would only lead to exposure to kernicterus if a number of conditions predating the affected pregnancy were met. Thus the father and at least one fetus from a previous pregnancy would need to be Rhesus positive, and a transplacental haemorrhage would have had to have occurred in that previous pregnancy to lead to maternal isoimmunization.

Similarly, the situations described in (b), (c) and (d) also occur in cerebral palsy. Many different causes of cerebral palsy have been recognized, such as toxic exposures, Rhesus incompatability, certain genetically inherited conditions and postneonatal cerebral infections. On the other hand, fetal viral infections, preterm birth, cord prolapse or trauma may result in an array of other physical or developmental problems, or in death, before the recognition of cerebral palsy.

How does the possibility of these alternative models affect the Bradford Hill criteria for inferring causality?

The *strength of association* with an individual factor will be diminished if there is more than one independently sufficient cause. Moreover, some genetic defects are sufficient causes but are responsible for only a small proportion of cases. The strength of association with an individual factor will also be diminished if it is a necessary but not a sufficient cause of the disease and if its cofactors on the causal path are also included in the analysis. The strength of the observed association will also be diminished if a significant fraction of individuals damaged by a specific causal path die before their cerebral palsy can be recognized.

Moreover, in any epidemiological study, but particularly in observational studies, strong associations do not necessarily signify causation. They could be confounders, epiphenomena (see Glossary) or early signs of the disease. If this is the case, prevention of the associated factor alone will not prevent the disease because it is not a step on a causal pathway to that disease. Examples of such associations are shown in Chapters 7, 8 and 9.

The presence of *consistency of association* between populations reduces the possibility that the associations have arisen by chance. However, given the multifactorial nature of the cerebral palsies, aetiological patterns may vary between geographical populations and between different birth cohorts. This is certainly true between wealthy and poor nations and between different cultures. For example, where consanguineous marriages are common or communities are inbred, genetically inherited conditions are responsible for a higher proportion of cerebral palsy. Methylmercury exposures and endemic cretinism are also very localized in time and geographical location. Whilst multicentre studies may be recommended to solve problems of sample size, they may not be a means of achieving statistical significance for individual factors if aetiological patterns vary significantly between the centres.

The presence of multiple causes and exposures, and the possibility that a single cause may lead to different outcomes, render *specificity of association* untenable as a necessary criterion for identifying cause in the cerebral palsies. Thus maternal smoking in pregnancy, which causes intrauterine growth restriction, possibly through a variety of different mechanisms, may also lead to a range of other poor outcomes. Likewise, maternal iodine deficiency is associated with a range of neurological outcomes in the child which include death and cognitive problems as well as cerebral palsy, albeit from the same underlying mechanism.

Time sequence is a most necessary though not sufficient criterion. Intuitively one would expect this to be easily verified. However, it is difficult to make observations on the fetus during pregnancy and to be sure of the timing of antenatal exposures. We cannot always know which risk factor comes first: for example, does intrauterine growth restriction come before cerebral damage or after it?

Dose dependency is a compelling criterion when present but can only be invoked for quantifiable exposures. Even theoretically quantifiable exposures, such as intrapartum hypoxia, are not easily measured. Furthermore, absence of a dose response in quantifiable factors does not rule out the possibility of causality if the cause is multifactorial or if the pattern of association is threshold or otherwise nonlinear.

Given our propensity for pattern recognition, *biological plausibility* will always be found compelling. However, if we are ignorant, which is often the case with respect to cerebral palsy aetiology, we must be prepared to alter our theories if warranted by robust observations. The erratic use of biological plausibility in causal inference is reviewed by Weed and Hursting (1998) and mentioned again in Chapter 14.

Statistical significance and power are important, and whilst cerebral palsy is the most common motor disorder in childhood, it occurs only in about 2.5 per 1000 live births. The commonest causes may account for as much as 10 per cent, but other causes account for much less. Thus it is very difficult to amass sample sizes sufficient to attain statistical significance without multicentre studies.

TABLE 5.2
Epidemiological challenges to identifying causal pathways to the cerebral palsies

Challenges	Possible solutions
1. Amass sufficient subjects with homogeneous disease	1. Conduct retrospective multicentre studies, with reliable methods of describing the component diseases, or at least excluding these with completely understood aetiologies
2. Differentiate the component diseases included under the rubric of cerebral palsy	2. Distinguish different syndromes by recognizing specific patterns of brain damage using *in vivo* imaging
3. Delayed recognition (years after birth)	3. Cerebral imaging may allow earlier recognition of cerebral palsy
4. Retrospectively obtain good quality antenatal exposure data	4. (a) Earlier disease recognition to collect better exposure data (closer to the time of action of the exposure) (b) Better markers for exposures by collaborating with basic and clinical sciences: • DNA and other biomarkers, • Neuroimaging • Placental and other pathological diagnoses

Identifying causal factors within alternative models of causation

The possibility of alternative models of causation makes it harder to recognize potentially causal factors. Each factor must be considered on its own merits. It is important to question whether a factor may be on a pathway and not always to assume a single sufficient cause or multiple independent causes. The possibility must be explored of each exposure being: (a) a component of a multi-factorial cause (*i.e.* on a causal pathway); (b) a rare cause; (c) the cause of an identifiable type of cerebral palsy; or (d) a cause of early death as well as cerebral palsy. This requires a better understanding of the disease process and challenges us to collect better exposure data and carefully consider study design. How we may do this is suggested in Chapter 14.

EPIDEMIOLOGICAL METHODS

Table 5.2 lists the major challenges to improving aetiological research in the cerebral palsies. While cerebral palsy occurs in about 2.5 per 1000 live births, the component diseases grouped under the cerebral palsy rubric occur much more rarely. This rarity means they are seldom observed as outcomes in intervention studies and makes cohort studies impractical, leaving the less scientifically rigorous retrospective study designs with multicentre recruitment as more attainable alternatives. Multicentre studies require interobserver agreement concerning disease identification, but the different component diseases are not always easily identified. Attempts on the basis of currently available clinical description have met with limited success. This may be because our clinical descriptions are inadequate or because the brain has a limited repertoire of responses to insult, and which response occurs is determined by factors such as the timing of the insult in addition to its cause. It is logical that similar cerebral damage will result in similar abnormal outcomes regardless of cause. For example, spastic

45

hemiplegia resulting from a cerebrovascular accident may be clinically indistinguishable from that due to skull trauma.

Clinical manifestation is therefore neither sensitive nor specific and is only available once the child is several years old and past the duration of follow-up of most intervention studies. Abnormalities seen on cerebral imaging *may* not only correlate more sensitively and specifically with aetiology but would be available much earlier. Earlier disease recognition would allow for shorter follow-up in intervention studies and earlier exposure data collection in retrospective studies. The inaccessibility of the fetus complicates the identification and measurement of antepartum and intrapartum exposures. Many significant brain damaging events or situations in pregnancy may go completely unrecognized or unrecorded, such as placental bleeding or infarcts, transient drops in maternal blood pressure, and exposure to a teratogen or an infection. Better markers of antenatal exposures need to be developed in collaboration with basic and clinical scientists (see Table 5.2 and Chapter 14).

ANALYTICAL METHODS

In view of the multiplicity of possible causal models, the criteria for causal inference must be considered somewhat differently.

Strength of association can only be a requirement of causality for a multicausal disease if the contributing causes can be considered separately. Strong associations will be diluted if heterogeneous groups are combined. However, splitting the cerebral palsy group into its various causes requires that the cerebral palsy syndromes be recognizable (see above).

Using multivariate analysis, the extent to which the strength of association of a particular exposure with the outcome is altered by the inclusion and exclusion of other exposures, or on defining a new variable for exposures which occur together, can help to identify steps on causal pathways (Blair and Stanley 1993a; and Appendix 2 of Blair and Stanley 1993b). For example, exposures which show strong associations with disease only when they occur in combination can be identified and may represent steps on the same causal pathway.

The *power* of any study must be carefully considered before setting criteria of statistical significance on which to reject the possibility of a causal role. Given our ignorance, it is currently more important not to reject hypotheses that may be causal than to accept any that may not be causal.

Consistency should be sought by testing biologically plausible *a priori* hypotheses in independent data sets. Consistency should always be sought, since if found, it reduces the possibility than an association is due to chance. However, the likelihood of population specific causes must be borne in mind.

It is vital to be aware of the variety of aetiological models that are possible and to avoid relying only on one-step multivariate regression analyses. Development of appropriate bio-statistical methods aimed at identifying interrelationships between exposure variables has already begun.

Time sequence is the only logically necessary (though not sufficient) criterion for inferring the direction of causation between two variables. Consideration of the time ordering of exposures was pioneered by Nelson *et al.* (1986) in their multivariate analysis of data from the NCPP (see Glossary) to determine the antecedents of cerebral palsy. In that analysis, exposure variables were categorized in stages as: (1) before conception; (2) in pregnancy; (3) during labour and delivery; (4) immediately postpartum; and (5) the nursery period. Analysis proceeded in stages commencing with the earliest (before conception). Factors that were found to increase, by at least 5 per cent, the predictive ability of a model limited to variables included in the stage in question and earlier stages were retained in subsequent models which added factors from later stages. There was no attempt to order variables within each stage, and the rationale behind the allocation of stage was not always clear. For example, maternal learning disability seems obviously a 'before pregnancy' variable, but it is less obvious why gestational age <33 weeks should be classified as a 'labour and delivery' variable or major non-CNS malformation as a 'nursery period' variable (this is the stage at which they are recognized). However, the principle of reducing the likelihood that early manifestations of cerebral palsy might overshadow earlier and possibly causal factors by forcing the entry/retention of earlier factors was clearly demonstrated in this landmark paper.

Leviton *et al.* (1991) reported a similar time-ordered analysis in which earlier occurring covariates of the outcome (early germinal matrix haemorrhage) could not be displaced by later occurring covariates. In a subsequent time-ordered analysis (Leviton *et al.* 1993) inferences were made by examining the effect on the estimated association of one variable of including and excluding another variable and of acknowledging the possibility of inter-dependence of variables by either combining highly correlated variables or choosing that with the strongest association with the outcome. Strategies of this type were also utilized independently in the time-ordered analysis of a case–control study of subjects with spastic cerebral palsy born 1975–80 in Western Australia (Appendix 2 of Blair and Stanley 1993b).

Conclusion

The search for causes in the cerebral palsies is littered with examples of lumping together diverse diseases, of failing to consider interactions between exposures and of concentrating unduly on the intrapartum period. The way forward in the epidemiology and prevention of many developmental disorders requires more sophisticated attempts to elucidate cause while maintaining an open mind about the several possible models of causation. It is an area in which the work has only recently commenced and will require the thoughtful cooperation of basic and clinical scientists, epidemiologists and biostatisticians.

6
CAUSAL PATHWAYS INITIATED PRECONCEPTIONALLY OR IN EARLY PREGNANCY

"Whether or not a disorder is of prenatal origin is not always clear. The same type of manifestation may take origin either before conception, during pregnancy, or after birth . . .

"The environment provided for the developing organism by the pregnant woman goes beyond her own physiological and anatomical attributes. All external influences that impinge on her, and that through her may impinge on the developing organism, are part of this environment . . ."

Kline *et al.* (1989)

Development of the motor cortex in the human fetus

NORMAL DEVELOPMENT

Brain development has been described as "exquisitely integrated and mutually interdependent, especially during early development, when timings of multiple events have to occur in sharply limited periods for functional links to develop between neurons and for the formation of functional circuits to occur" (Morgane *et al.* 1992). With motor function we are most interested in the development and maturation of the motor cortex, the basal ganglia, the cerebellum, and their interconnecting pathways.

The cerebral grey matter undergoes a complex but ordered developmental process beginning with the production of neuronal and glial precursors in the germinal zones lining the lateral and third ventricles, followed by migration of neurons out to their final destinations (Barkovich *et al.* 1992). As shown in Figure 6.1, in the first 20 weeks of embryonic and fetal life the glia and neurons form and migrate out to their final destinations, creating the various structures of the brain. After 20 weeks, rapid growth in all structures results in a dramatic increase in brain size and weight. Myelination and synaptogenesis commence at 20 weeks to form the circuits and connections necessary for successful brain function and continue for a considerable time after birth. By about 36 weeks the cortex, cerebellum and basal ganglia are formed but are still immature.

Thus motor competence at birth is limited in the human neonate. The voluntary control of movement develops and matures during a prolonged period up to puberty (Bruce and Rawson 1994)—hence the delays already alluded to in diagnosing cerebral palsy syndromes, because we must wait for the development of the motor system before abnormalities of movement, posture and gait can be demonstrated. However, many involuntary and reflex

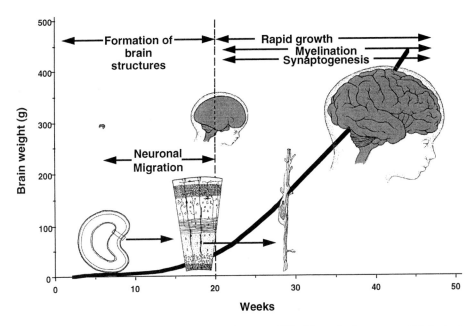

Fig. 6.1. Brain development during gestation and early postnatal life. (Illustration by courtesy of M. Squiers.)

functions are developed early, in order to ensure that the newborn baby can breathe, suck, swallow, and respond to noxious stimuli. These essential functions for immediate neonatal life depend upon normal brainstem and spinal cord pathways. Fetuses without such capacities do not survive for long.

Motor pathways initiated *in utero* form the basis on which postnatal experiences build systems for mature and coordinated motor function. It thus follows that any disturbance that interferes with these early connections could result in a cascade of deficits which impede development of more advanced motor circuits.

How well matched is our knowledge of antenatal exposures and factors with that pertaining to the timing and vulnerability of fetal brain development? Does a specific motor disorder result from interference with neurogenesis, or with migration, cell to cell connections or myelination?

ABNORMAL DEVELOPMENT

Interruption of normal processes of neuronal generation and migration result in brain malformations and variable degrees of neurological dysfunction including the motor system (Barth 1987; Barkovich *et al.* 1992, 1996; Evrard *et al.* 1997). Some influences may interrupt circuits, creating significant functional deficit, but leave the brain with a grossly normal appearance.

Damaging influences, then, depend on timing as much as the events. Some may be less likely to cause permanent sequelae if they occur early, when the developing brain still has the capacity to replace cells and create functioning pathways (Lebeer 1998)—for example, term infants appear more vulnerable to hypoxia than those born preterm (Blair and Stanley 1993a, Mallard *et al.* 1994, Carr 1996). Timing also has implications for which areas of the brain are most susceptible to hypoxia. Vascular accidents are more likely to affect those areas with vulnerable blood supply, but there is considerable controversy about 'watershed areas' and whether they actually exist. Some insults, such as rubella and CMV infection, prevent the formation of brain structures if exposure is sufficiently early, but are relatively innocuous to the fetal brain if they occur in later pregnancy (Gilbert 1996). Other exposures, such as methylmercury, are toxic to neurons throughout gestation and beyond (Stanley and Alberman 1984, Stanley 1997). It seems that the type of insult, its timing and its predilection for certain areas of the brain all determine the extent and the effects of the final damage. This is superimposed upon the programmed development of the nervous system and its capacity to accommodate and regenerate.

Situations or events which interfere with migrating and differentiating motor cortex, basal ganglia or cerebellum could be the expression of abnormal genes, hostile fetal environments resulting from maternal disease, toxicity, infections or trauma, or interference with blood supply. The challenge is to identify them and their causal pathways, traces of which may have disappeared by the time the child is recognized as having cerebral palsy.

Neuronal migration disorders
The neuropathology of the various migration disorders has been described using high quality neuroimaging techniques as well as post mortem examination findings and clinical patterns (Barth 1987, Barkovich *et al.* 1992, Evrard *et al.* 1997). They include lissencephaly types I and II (agyria and pachygyria); polymicrogyrias; schizencephaly syndromes; and the grey matter heterotopias. The site and severity of the lesions determine the type, site and severity of the motor disorder. Grey matter heterotopias are collections of normal neurons in abnormal locations secondary to an arrest of radial migration. They may be of particular relevance to the cerebral palsies if they involve specific motor regions. They have been implicated more in children with epilepsy than in those with cerebral palsy, but this may be because children with epilepsy are more likely to undergo brain imaging to decide whether they may be candidates for surgery. Some infants with abnormal cerebral development appear neurologically depressed at birth and exhibit neonatal encephalopathy and can be (mis)diagnosed as having birth asphyxia and hypoxic–ischaemic encephalopathy (Paneth and Stark 1983, Barth 1984, Dobyns *et al.* 1992). Until recently, very few children with cerebral palsy had proper neuroimaging examinations, and thus it is possible that abnormal cerebral development may be missed amongst cases of unexplained cerebral palsy or even amongst individuals with cerebral palsy attributed to birth asphyxia (Nelson and Grether 1998). In summary, the extent of the contribution of these syndromes to the cerebral palsies is not yet known (Badawi *et al.* 1998b). This must await wider use of neuroimaging techniques that are accurate at diagnosing these lesions, as well as better ascertainment of genetic and family history, toxic environmental and personal exposures which may not be recorded in medical records. Methods of selecting and measuring exposures are discussed in Chapters 5 and 14.

TABLE 6.1
Periconceptional and early antenatal causes of the cerebral palsies

Type of factor	Description	Timing
Maternal	Genetic, family history (*e.g.* epilepsy)	Periconceptional
	Infertility, related problems	Periconceptional
Fetal malformation syndromes	Known and unknown genetic or teratogenic influences	Periconceptional and early gestation
Infections	TORCH, other organisms	Early gestation
Deficiences	Iodine	Early-mid gestation
	Thyroid hormone	?Throughout gestation
Toxic	Methylmercury	Throughout gestation
	Alcohol	Early–mid gestation
	Carbon monoxide poisoning	Throughout gestation
Vascular	Hypoxia, ischaemia, thrombotic disorders (*e.g.* maternal)	?Mid–late gestation

From Barth (1984), Grant *et al.* (1992), Grant and Barkovich (1997) and Stanley (1997).

A comment on magnetic resonance imaging
Recently a spate of papers have been published on magnetic resonance imaging (MRI) in cerebral palsy cases (Krägeloh-Mann *et al.* 1994, 1995; de Vries *et al.* 1993; Sugimoto *et al.* 1995; Barkovich *et al.* 1996; Grant and Barkovich 1997). MRI is easier to interpret than ultrasound scanning and can be performed after closure of the fontanelle. It can define the anatomical extent of involvement and often provides some information about both the aetiology and the timing of the cerebral insult, even when it is done several years after birth. While it is an exciting new tool for epidemiological research in cerebral palsy, studies are needed to test the accuracy of interpretations by comparing them with neuropathology found at autopsy. In addition both intra- and interobserver reliability studies must be done to test whether assessments of diagnosis and timing of damage from images are reproducible between and within observers. Only then we can we use them as Grant and Barkovich (1997) suggest: "To further elucidate the various causes and identify prognostic factors in cerebral palsy, correlation of MR findings with the clinical history is required."

Causal pathways initiated before conception or in early pregnancy

Table 6.1 lists the periconceptional and early antenatal causes of the migration disorders and other syndromes which are most likely to be associated with the cerebral palsies (Barth 1984, Barkovich *et al.* 1992, Grant and Barkovich 1997, Stanley 1997). The list includes both familial and fetal genetic causes; teratogens causing fetal malformation syndromes including congenital infections (TORCH, others); iodine deficiency; toxic exposures and antenatal vascular events causing hypoxia/ischaemia.

FAMILY HISTORY AND GENETIC FACTORS
It is clear that the cerebral palsies can recur in families but mostly without clear patterns

of monogenic inheritance (Stanley and Alberman 1984, Wild and Rosenbloom 1986, Hughes and Newton 1992). Several studies have shown a significant contribution to cerebral palsy from familial factors in small isolated populations or populations in which consanguinous marriage is relatively common (Gustavson *et al.* 1969, Al-Rajeh *et al.* 1991, Morton *et al.* 1991, Bundey 1997, Sinha *et al.* 1997). Familial factors appear less important where consanguinous marriage is rare (Miller 1988; Petterson *et al.* 1993b; Palmer *et al.* 1994, 1995), although some studies report more relatives with cerebral palsy, intellectual deficit or seizures in the families of children with cerebral palsy compared with controls (Monreal 1985). Recent family history data concerning persons with epilepsy (Ottman *et al.* 1996) suggested a shared genetic susceptibility to congenital epilepsy and congenital cerebral palsy, but numbers were extremely small. An increased risk of athetoid/dystonic and hemiplegic cerebral palsy with advanced paternal age suggests that perhaps some of these cases may arise from fresh dominant mutations (Fletcher and Foley 1993). Only three of 74 Western Australian family pedigrees of a total population of children with spastic quadriplegia demonstrated recurrent similar phenotypes or genetic syndromes (Petterson *et al.* 1993b). However, rates of both fetal and neonatal loss were higher in families of all cerebral palsy types than in the families of controls matched on year of birth, gestation or birthweight. A family history of preterm births or being small for gestational age affected the risk of cerebral palsy primarily by influencing the risk of preterm birth or being small for gestation in the index pregnancy (Palmer *et al.* 1994). Thus family history no doubt encompasses a range of influences including direct and less direct genetic effects and interpregnancy or even intergenerational environmental effects. Any of these may lie on a causal pathway.

A few studies with proven zygosity suggest a higher concordance of cerebral palsy in monozygotic than in dizygotic pairs (Grether *et al.* 1993, Weig *et al.* 1995). However, most large studies of twins do not have accurate zygosity. Studies of like sexed twins (a proportion of whom will be monozygotic) show no difference in cerebral palsy risk to that seen in twins of differing gender (Grether *et al.* 1993, Petterson *et al.* 1993a). However, numbers in these studies were also small. Any increased risk of cerebral palsy in monozygotic twins may result from shared placental vasculature as well as from other indirect genetic and malformation factors, and not necessarily mean an increase in genetic causes. However, current opinion is shifting to pregnancy complications as more important than genetic factors in the aetiology of cerebral palsy in multiple births. This may be as a result of the marked increase in multiple births seen following infertility treatments, since these are more likely to result in dizygotic than in monozygotic multiples and to be complicated for reasons unrelated to direct genetic risk. Chapter 10 describes the risk factors for cerebral palsy in multiple births.

Maternal mental retardation, motor deficit in an older sibling, maternal seizures and more than two prior fetal deaths were all associated with cerebral palsy in the NCPP (see Glossary) (Nelson and Ellenberg 1986a). Even when all later occurring important risk factors for cerebral palsy were included in the model, maternal mental retardation and motor deficit in a sibling remained important and significant predictors, although they did not account for many cases.

The Western Australian Maternal and Child Health Data Base (Stanley 1992, Stanley *et al.* 1997) (see Appendix) links perinatal factors to later mortality and morbidity for the whole population of births. Linkage to registers of birth defects, mental illness, intellectual disability and cerebral palsy enables us to identify and study their frequency and the characteristics of sibships (see Glossary) and families in which these neurodevelopmental problems might cluster. A study documenting the characteristics of families with developmental disorders is currently underway to measure the contribution of familial factors to cerebral palsy in this population, which is anticipated to be at low risk of genetic contributions to cerebral palsy as consanguinous marriage is very rare. Of greater interest and relevance are data about clustering of defects in families resulting from causal pathways including familial environments or maternal diseases such as endocrine or thrombotic disorders.

INFERTILITY AND OTHER REPRODUCTIVE DISORDERS

There are some suggestions that delayed onset of menses, irregular menstruation or long intermenstrual intervals and infertility may be related to cerebral palsy risk (Nelson and Ellenberg 1986a). It may be that these result from factors which disturb effective placentation or intrauterine competence or from undiagnosed minimal chromosomal anomalies such as translocations. They may be significant influences in the current group of idiopathic intrauterine growth restricted or very preterm births. Large population data bases that are linked to create sibships will be essential to describe these patterns and risks, about which we know little.

FETAL MALFORMATION SYNDROMES

As might be anticipated, there are more CNS anomalies among cerebral palsy cases than in the rest of the population. However, they also have more malformations outside the CNS (Monreal 1985, Holmes and Hassanein 1988; Miller 1988, 1989, 1991; Coorssen *et al.* 1991; Hughes and Newton 1992; Fletcher and Foley 1993; Palmer *et al.* 1995). In our Western Australian series, 63 of 215 children (29.3 per cent) with moderate or severe cerebral palsy were reported to have a congenital malformation compared with 4.9 per cent of both the control group and the normal population (Palmer *et al.* 1995). Of these 63 cases, 34 did and 29 (almost half) did not have a cerebral malformation. Since only a proportion of children with cerebral palsy have brain imaging, the proportion with CNS anomalies is likely to be significantly underestimated. In the same Western Australian series of moderate/severe cerebral palsy cases, 15 per cent had other neurological problems compared with only 0.5 per cent of controls, suggesting that had MRI been available, a congenital malformation may have been diagnosed. In common with other population studies the Western Australian Register shows that 30 per cent of people with cerebral palsy have ongoing epilepsy (see Chapter 3), which in some cases may have resulted from the same cause as the cerebral palsy (Ottman *et al.* 1996).

Primary malformations, of either the brain or other organs, are known to be due to teratogens causing structural malformations by interrupting embryogenesis at critical periods in early pregnancy. Thus associated defects in children with cerebral palsy suggest that an exposure occurring early in pregnancy may be responsible for both the malformation and the cerebral palsy (Coorssen *et al.* 1991). However, it may be that not all apparently primary structural malformations do result from interrupted embryogenesis. Table 6.2 lists some of

TABLE 6.2
Syndromes associated with neuronal migration disorders, which may be described as cerebral palsy

Metabolic	*Chromosomal*
Zellweger syndrome	Trisomies 13, 18
Glutaric aciduria type II	Deletion 4p, 17p13 (Miller–Dieker syndrome)
Gangliosidosis	
	Neuromuscular
Neurocutaneous	Walker–Warburg syndrome
Neurofibromatosis type I	Myotonic dystrophy
Encephalocranial cutaneous lipomatosis	
Tuberous sclerosis	*Other CNS dysplasias*
Epidermal naevus syndrome	Aicardi syndrome
	Joubert syndrome
	Hemimegalencephaly
Multiple congenital anomalies	Atelencephaly
Smith–Lemli–Opitz syndrome	Congenital rubella syndrome
Potter syndrome	Fetal CMV infection
Cornelia de Lange syndrome	Fetal iodine deficiency
Oculo-renal-cerebellar syndrome	Fetal methylmercury poisoning

the known syndromes found in association with the migration disorders and which may also have motor disability. Barth (1984) calls these defects prenatal clastic encephalopathies rather than migration disorders and stresses that they can mimic primary malformation syndromes even though many result from later destructive lesions rather than from early interference during organogenesis. Thus whilst porencephaly is known to follow the destructive effects of infections, intoxications or hypoxia/ischaemia, more extensive lesions can result in hydranencephaly and other brain anomalies indistinguishable from primary defects. The proportion of cerebral palsy attributable to malformations and genetic syndromes is unknown (see Table 2.1, p. 11).

Infantile spasms share similar antenatal and perinatal risk factors with both neonatal encephalopathy and cerebral palsy (Cowan and Hudson 1991). Whilst many are of unknown aetiology, some are thought to be genetic or malformation syndromes. Can the causes of fetal malformations initiate common causal paths to neonatal encephalopathy, infantile spasms and cerebral palsy? The answer is yes: there are several rare syndromes which have all these components. A large population based case–control study of neonatal encephalopathy in Western Australia (Badawi *et al.* 1998a) is being followed up to ascertain its natural history: the proportion that end in cerebral palsy will be determined and the role of antenatal antecedents will be analysed.

Causal pathways to early antenatal/fetal vascular accidents are not well understood but are included here for completeness. Their incidence and timing are unknown. They are mentioned (Encha-Razavi 1995, Evrard *et al.* 1997, Grant and Barkovich 1997) as important causes of neuronal migration disorders.

Genetic disorders of thrombotic mechanisms are being suggested as causes of some of these vascular problems with resulting antenatal porencephaly (Thorarensen *et al.* 1997, Debus *et al.* 1998). They include thrombophilias, factor V Leiden, anticardiolipin antibodies and hyperhomocystinaemia mutations. J. Kingdom (personal communication 1998) investigated 16 women with perinatal deaths following severe growth restriction under 30 weeks: seven were found to have abnormal thrombotic function, either genetic (*e.g.* mutations) or acquired. There may be 'environmental' triggers for all of them, and pregnancy itself may be a trigger.

Many exposures occurring in early or mid-trimester, such as those described below, may contribute to causal pathways to cerebral palsy and/or epilepsy.

Pathways involving pregnancy exposures
CONGENITAL INFECTIONS AS TERATOGENS

The group of organisms best known to be involved in early damage to the human fetal CNS are collectively known as the TORCH group, which are vertically transmitted viral infections. These are *to*xoplasmosis, *r*ubella, *c*ytomegalovirus (CMV) and *h*erpes simplex virus. The natural history and effect of an infection transmitted from the mother to her fetus in the first and second trimesters is quite different from those of the same infection in an infant or child. The neurological sequelae of a CNS infection depend less on the infective agent and more on the stage of development or maturation of the fetal nervous system and on the fetal immune defences at the time of the insult (Miller *et al.* 1982, Grant and Barkovich 1997). Infections occurring before the third trimester often result in cerebral malformation with little or no reactive change, whereas those occurring late in gestation commonly result in destructive lesions (Barkovich *et al.* 1995). These infections are often asymptomatic in the mother but have devastating long term effects on the child (Gilbert 1996) including early death, visual and hearing defects, learning disability and, sometimes, cerebral palsy. Such infections may persist into the postnatal period and may lead to further damage. With the exception of rubella, few can be prevented cost-effectively. Recent reviews (Bale and Murph 1992, Miller *et al.* 1993, Gilbert 1996, Grant *et al.* 1997) describe the changing epidemiology of congenital infections over the last 20 years.

Maternal rubella vaccination has led to falls in congenital rubella, leaving CMV infection as the most important congenital infection in terms of neurological sequelae including cerebral palsy, sensorineural deafness and learning disability. Yow and Demmler (1992) estimated that around 800,000 babies born in the USA between 1971 and 1991 were infected *in utero* with CMV. Recent unpublished data from three hospitals the UK in which babies were screened for evidence of congenital CMV infection suggest that perhaps 0.3 per cent of all births may be infected *in utero*, although this risk varies with maternal age and social circumstances, the highest risk being in teenage, unmarried mothers (S. Logan, personal communication 1998). Black mothers also are at increased risk, although this may be due in part to their age and socioeconomic conditions (Preece *et al.* 1986). Another report suggests that the risk of intrauterine transmission may be increased in the presence of reproductive tract infections in pregnancy, including bacterial vaginosis, trichomoniasis and gonorrhoea (Fowler and Pass 1991).

With CMV, fetal damage is more likely and more severe with primary maternal infection occurring in the first or second trimesters of pregnancy. It is uncertain what proportion of infected children will be symptomatic, since symptoms can develop at birth or later. Nor

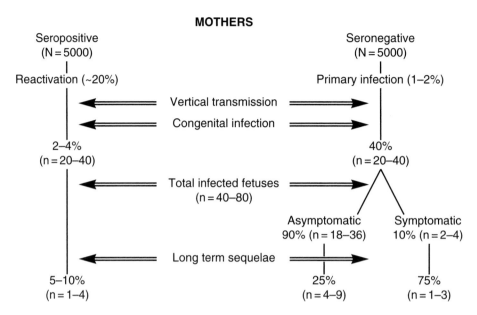

Fig. 6.2. Maternal and fetal cytomegalovirus infection: outcomes based on best estimates (adapted from Gilbert 1996).

are there enough good data to suggest whether this risk is greater in mothers who have their primary infection during pregnancy, or whether it is important when in pregnancy such an infection first occurred. Figure 6.2 (Gilbert 1996) suggests that very few (1–2 per cent) seronegative pregnant women have a primary infection; 40 per cent of these are estimated to have an infected fetus. Overall the risk of infection is 0.4–0.8 per cent, fairly close to the 0.3 per cent reported above from the UK study (p. 55). These children have a high risk of sequelae (including cerebral palsy), particularly if symptomatic at birth. There are few data sets which allow accurate estimates of how many infected children are likely to develop cerebral palsy. The UK study quoted above followed up 102 out of 103 babies who screened positive for CMV and found four cases of cerebral palsy, suggesting a rate of about 4 per cent (S. Logan, personal communication 1998). If the risk of transmission to the fetus is 0.4 per cent of all pregnancies it can be calculated that the risk of cerebral palsy attributable to CMV is somewhere between 5 and 10 per cent, depending on the estimated population prevalence of cerebral palsy. However, this proportion seems to be considerably higher than that clinically attributed to CMV. In Western Australia the proportion due to CMV is about 1.7 per cent of all cerebral palsy. Data from the cerebral palsy register set up in the North-East Thames region of England, excluding postneonatal and mild cases, revealed four cases out of 584 attributed to CMV(Williams and Alberman 1998). This suggests that CMV is underascertained in retrospectively reported cerebral palsy.

Many other microorganisms, including syphilis, varicella, parvovirus and HIV, are recognized as capable of infecting the human fetus, sometimes with devasting effects.

TABLE 6.3
The iodine deficiency disorders

Fetus	Abortion
	Stillbirth
	Brain damage—cretinism
Neonate	Neonatal goitre
	Brain damage—congenital hypothyroidism
Child	Goitre
	Thyroid deficiency (fatigue)
	Impaired school performance
	Retarded physical development
Adult	Goitre and complications
	Thyroid deficiency
	Impaired mental function

*Adapted from Hetzel *et al.* (1997).

However, few appear to act early in pregnancy, none occur frequently and none have been associated specifically with cerebral palsy (Bale and Murph 1992).

IODINE DEFICIENCY

Iodine deficiency can result in many pathological outcomes with severe adverse effects on the fetus, neonate, child and adolescent as well as the adult (Table 6.3) (Hetzel *et al.* 1987, 1997; DeLong *et al.* 1989; Hetzel 1994b). With deficiency in early pregnancy there is a spectrum of disorders from death through clinical endemic cretinism (spastic diplegia and deaf mutism) to more subtle deficits of motor and cognitive performance (DeLong 1987, Hetzel 1994, Pharoah and Connolly 1995). Endemic cretinism has a strong association with low maternal thyroid hormone levels (T_4 but not T_3) in pregnancy (Pharoah *et al.* 1981, 1984; Pharoah and Connolly 1989) and with severe periconceptional iodine deficiency. Maternal T_4 crosses the placenta and is crucial for neuronal migration and early neuronal integrity (Pharoah *et al.* 1989, Pharoah and Connolly 1995) as the fetal thyroid does not make any thyroid hormone until late in the first trimester. Later in pregnancy fetal deficiency results in the very different picture of congenital hypothyroidism which is reversible if diagnosed at birth, hence the rationale for neonatal screening (Pharoah and Connolly 1995).

The population at risk of iodine deficiency due to low iodine levels in soil is increasing. In 1993 the World Health Organization estimated that 1.6 billion people were at risk of iodine deficiency (Hetzel *et al.* 1997), up from 1 billion in 1990. Of these, 2 per cent (or 320 million) may have preventable brain damage and an estimated 5.7 million have overt cretinism (Hetzel 1994a, Hetzel and Pandav 1996), making it the most common cause of preventable brain damage in the world. Endemic cretinism tends to occur in areas in which iodine deficiency is sufficiently severe to cause goitre in about 30 per cent of the population (Hetzel *et al.* 1987). It is still found in southern and eastern European countries and is common in Asia, Africa and Latin America (Hetzel *et al.* 1997). As shown in Figure 6.3, cretinism represents the tip of the iceberg with far larger proportions suffering from either

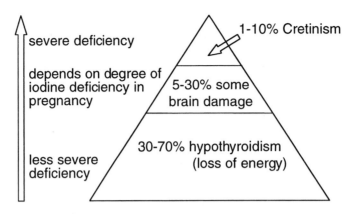

Fig. 6.3. The iodine deficiency disorder 'iceberg' (adapted from Hetzel and Pandav 1996).

subclinical cretinism (Hetzel 1994b, Hetzel and Pandav 1996) or hypothyroidism which results in loss of energy, mental torpor and apathy.

THYROID HORMONE ABNORMALITIES
Abnormal maternal thyroid function in pregnancy may also play a role in cerebral palsy in developed countries. While it is found in only 1–2 per cent of cases of cerebral palsy, several epidemiological studies have suggested that maternal thyroid disease is a risk factor for both cerebral palsy (Nelson and Ellenberg 1986, Blair and Stanley 1993a) and neonatal encephalopathy (Adamson *et al.* 1995, Badawi *et al.* 1998a). "If circulating T_4 is crucial to the normal maturation of the fetal nervous system, any process which interferes with fetal neural cell access to T_4, whether it be failure of maternal hormone production, ineffective placental transport, abnormal hormone receptivity at cellular level or other such mechanism, may result in cerebral palsy" (Pharoah and Connolly 1995). Abnormalities of thyroid hormone, particularly deficiency of T_4, interferes with neuronal cell differentiation, migration and gene expression (Bernal and Nunez 1995). T_3 may have a role in programmed neuronal cell death. Elucidation of causal pathways awaits further studies (necessarily multicentre) of neurological outcomes in fetuses exposed to maternal thyroid disease.

TOXICITY
Methylmercury
The neurotoxicity of fetal exposure to methylmercury was described in the previous book (Stanley and Alberman 1984). To our knowledge no further outbreaks of cerebral palsy following methylmercury poisoning have been reported, and the lesson may have been learned. There are continuing concerns about mercury in various occupations or in dental amalgam but there is no evidence associating these exposures with cerebral palsy. We must nonetheless continue to be vigilant about environmental exposures and not ignore the lessons from Minamata (Stanley 1997).

Alcohol

Women who drink excessively during pregnancy are at an increased risk of their infants being affected by fetal alcohol syndrome (Olegård *et al.* 1979). While the major problems of these children are severe intrauterine growth restriction, microcephaly, facial dysmorphisms and intellectual deficits, in Olegård's series around 8 per cent also had cerebral palsy. Alcohol appears to interfere with neuronal migration and thus is listed as a cause in these early pregnancy pathways (Jones and Smith 1975, Clarren *et al.* 1978, Evrard *et al.* 1997).

Most studies of cerebral palsy and other neurodevelopmental problems rely on obtaining evidence of exposure from medical records in retrospective case–control studies. Alcohol exposure is poorly recorded in most antenatal medical records (Walpole *et al.* 1990, 1991b; Delgado-Rodriguez *et al.* 1995), and even direct questioning of mothers via questionnaires or interviews is likely to underascertain exposure. Thus the proportion of children with cerebral damage associated with excessive maternal alcohol ingestion may be greater than is currently reported. It has been suggested to be a most important preventable cause of learning disability in developed countries and this may also be true for cerebral palsy.

Summary and conclusions

Collectively, the genetic, familial, periconceptional and early pregnancy factors which may be on pathways to cerebral damage and motor disability are many, although individual factors occur rarely in developed countries. Cerebral anomalies such as neuronal migration disorders are likely to be unrecognized in many individuals with cerebral palsy as they may not have had the appropriate diagnostic tests. The most important preventable cause of cerebral palsy worldwide is endemic cretinism due to severe maternal iodine deficiency in early pregnancy. Maternal reproductive or endocrine dysfunction appears to be related to cerebral palsy, which suggests a process of considerable duration rather than a cataclysmic event. Possibilities for prevention are described in Chapter 12. How such factors may influence further pathways, such as those involving preterm birth, fetal growth restriction or birth asphyxia, is discussed in the following chapters.

7
PATHWAYS TO CEREBRAL PALSY INVOLVING VERY PRETERM BIRTH

> "It is nevertheless apparent that cerebral palsy is a widespread problem among VLBW and immature infants who graduate from modern intensive care units. . . {We} speculate that there may be a high rate of fetal aberration associated with the abnormal event of premature birth and that although modern perinatal care has a large impact on mortality there may be little influence on the occurrence of cerebral palsy. To accept this view absolves the perinatologists of blame but is anathema to those striving to improve outcome by ever more strenuous efforts to optimize care."
> (Kitchen *et al.* 1987)

At the time the previous book (Stanley and Alberman 1984) was written, almost all population samples in the literature of neurodevelopmental outcomes were described in terms of birth-weight. This was in spite of the knowledge that both gestational age at delivery and adequate intrauterine growth make independent contributions to weight at birth and also to outcome. Since 1984, due to a better appreciation of the difficulties of interpreting observations of samples defined only by birthweight (Blair 1996c), more studies have separated the individual effects of gestational age (being born early) from those resulting from poor intrauterine growth (being smaller than expected). Unfortunately many studies still use birthweight as a proxy for gestational age.

What is very preterm birth?
Very preterm birth (VPTB) needs to be defined as there is variation in how it is used in the literature. The World Health Organization suggests it refer to births before 32 completed weeks of gestation (see Chiswick 1986). This criterion has a biological rationale pertinent to cerebral palsy aetiology in that the risk of germinal matrix haemorrhage is high before 32 weeks and declines thereafter as the germinal matrix involutes (see Glossary).

Extremely preterm birth (EPTB) is a subset of very preterm birth which is also variably defined in the literature. The World Health Organization suggests a cut-off at <28 weeks. The biological rationale could be that it represents the age of initiation of neuronal myelination or the ability to mount a glial response (scarring) to neuronal damage. However, neither of these processes has a clear-cut age of initiation or of recognition on ultrasound imaging, though they begin to be observable around the 28th postmenstrual week.

Is cerebral palsy associated with VPTB?
VPTB is the strongest predictor of later cerebral palsy, and the risk increases as gestational

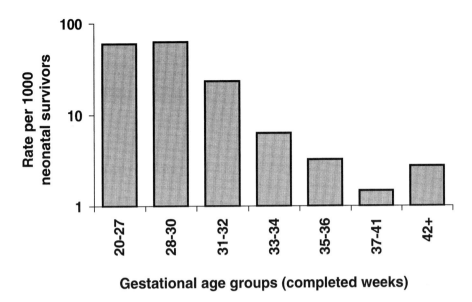

Fig. 7.1. Gestational-age-specific cerebral palsy rates (log scale) in Western Australia, 1980–1992 combined (L. Watson and F. Stanley, unpublished data—excludes cases due to postneonatal causes).

age at delivery decreases (Fig. 7.1). The rate of cerebral palsy amongst neonatal survivors born below 33 weeks is up to 30 times higher than among those born at term (Stanley 1992, Kuban and Leviton 1994). Of all children registered with the Western Australian Cerebral Palsy Register born 1986–1992, 34.7 per cent were born before 37 weeks and 24.8 per cent were born before 33 weeks, compared with 7.5 and 1.3 per cent respectively of all neonatal survivors in the same birth cohorts. The increase in birth prevalence of cerebral palsy in preterm and low birthweight infants throughout the 1980s, coincident with the marked falls in neonatal mortality, was described in Chapter 4.

As the data showing increases in birth prevalence of preterm and low birthweight infants with cerebral palsy were published throughout the late 1980s and early 1990s (Hagberg *et al.* 1989b, 1993, 1996; Pharoah 1990, 1993, 1995; Pharoah *et al.* 1990, 1996, 1997b; Stanley 1992, 1994b,c; Stanley and Watson 1992, Kuban and Leviton 1994, Stanley and Blair 1994), the debate centred around two possible explanations. The first was that the increase in preterm cerebral palsy reflected an increased survival of very preterm infants whose brains were already damaged at birth by a range of antenatal factors (Paneth *et al.* 1993, Pharoah *et al.* 1997b). The alternative explanation, perhaps more commonly held amongst neonatologists caring for these new survivors, was an increase in incidence, due to their vulnerability to the postnatal complications peculiar to very preterm birth (Stanley 1992, 1994b,c; Hagberg and Hagberg 1993; Stanley and Blair 1994; Pharoah 1995; Hagberg *et al.* 1996; Pharoah *et al.* 1996).

These two interpretations have different implications for both care and prevention. If the cerebral damage is effected antenatally it has been argued that no increase in quality or

$$\text{Rate CP} = \frac{\text{CP cases}}{\text{Neonatal survivors}}$$

A. If damage occurs antenatally:

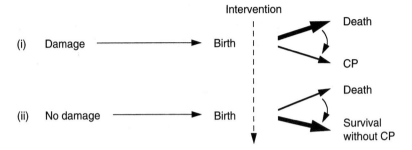

If more survive without CP than with it, and it is primarily damaged babies who die, then the rate of CP will increase as death rates fall.

B. If damage occurs postnatally:

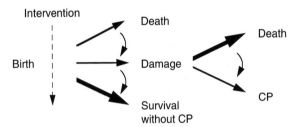

Change in rate of CP will depend on balance of death and survival with and without CP.

Fig. 7.2. Assessments of the effects of timing of cerebral damage in very preterm infants from changes in rates of cerebral palsy and mortality observed following neonatal intensive care (curved arrows denote effect of intervention).

quantity of neonatal care can affect outcome. If the cerebral damage is effected postnatally, it could be argued that no effort should be spared in improving neonatal intensive care to prevent and/or treat the postnatal complications of very preterm delivery (Kitchen *et al.* 1987), and in pursuing policies that might decrease the rate of preterm birth.

Figure 7.2A shows that if damage occurs antenatally, the change in rate of cerebral palsy effected by neonatal interventions will reflect the difference in proportional change in mortality in damaged and undamaged babies. Interventions will only decrease the rate of cerebral palsy if they allow a greater proportion of undamaged than of damaged babies to survive. However, if the risk of death is greater in brain damaged babies, more of them are available to be rescued from death by new therapies (Paneth *et al.* 1994). Any intervention reducing mortality is therefore more likely to allow a greater proportion of damaged babies to survive, so cerebral palsy rates may well increase. If the damage is effected postnatally the changes in cerebral palsy rates following neonatal interventions that decrease perinatal mortality will depend on the balance of proportions between those who die and those surviving with or without cerebral palsy (Fig. 7.2B). They may not be associated with reduced cerebral palsy rates because the *new survivors* may be more vulnerable than previous survivors to the postnatal brain damage associated with preterm birth, particularly for example if they are of lower gestational age.

The observed increase in cerebral palsy rates following increased use of neonatal intensive care, and the resulting decrease in neonatal mortality could therefore have occurred whether the cerebral damage was effected ante- or postnatally. By themselves, therefore, changes in very preterm cerebral palsy rates do not help us to differentiate between the two possible scenarios.

These arguments, however, considered only two possibilities: that the cerebral damage responsible for cerebral palsy in very preterm infants is acquired either *always* antenatally or *always* postnatally. It is quite likely that the damage occurs antenatally in some infants, perinatally in others, and postnatally in yet others. And there may be some in whom damage occurs in more than one time period, for example an infant damaged antenatally may also be further damaged postnatally. Cerebral palsy rates in very preterm infants would tend to vary widely as the introduction of various management interventions tip the balances between death, intact survival and survival with impairment. Whilst attributing some of the considerable heterogeneity in levels of cerebral palsy in very low birthweight cohorts to variable methods of definition and ascertainment (Escobar *et al.* 1991), some of this variability may also reflect the oscillating balances suggested in Figure 7.2.

Pragmatically, we would like to reduce the rate of survival with cerebral palsy. It is therefore frustrating that so few randomized trials of perinatal interventions for very preterm babies have followed their subjects to an age at which cerebral palsy can be reliably recognized. We know disappointingly little about which individual interventions affect the rates of long term disability. Moreover, any beneficial effects on mortality can mean that it becomes unethical to repeat such trials in order to measure longer term outcomes (see Chapter 12). All efforts should therefore be made *now* to ascertain long term outcomes for subjects of current and past randomized controlled trials of perinatal interventions, and long term follow-up of future trials should be mandatory.

Specific Cerebral Palsy Syndromes and Preterm Birth

Figure 7.3 shows the risk of different subtypes of cerebral palsy by gestational age at delivery, using Western Australian Cerebral Palsy Register data for 1980–1992 birth cohorts. Both hemiplegic and diplegic spastic types showed much stronger associations with very preterm birth than did the other cerebral palsy types. While 24.8 per cent of all children with cerebral palsy were born before 33 weeks gestation, over 40 per cent of those with spastic diplegia were born before 33 weeks, compared with 25.2 per cent with spastic hemiplegia, 15.6 per

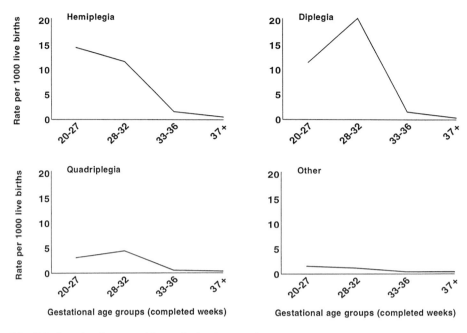

Fig. 7.3. Gestational-age-specific cerebral palsy rates by predominant cerebral palsy type, Western Australia 1980–92 combined (L. Watson and F. Stanley, unpublished data—excludes cases due to postneonatal causes).

cent with quadriplegia and 4.8 per cent with other types of cerebral palsy. Therefore very preterm infants are at particular risk of specific patterns of cerebral palsy.

Is very preterm birth an epiphenomenon in some pathways to cerebral palsy? Is it a necessary factor on other causal pathways to cerebral palsy?

As early as the mid-1980s, Nelson and Ellenberg questioned the assumption that decreasing the rate of low birthweight would necessarily decrease the rate of cerebral palsy, based on their analysis of data from the National Collaborative Perinatal Project (Nelson and Ellenberg 1985a, 1986). Interventions aimed at reducing the occurrence of very preterm birth can only influence cerebral palsy rates if very preterm birth is on a causal pathway to cerebral palsy.

Obviously any activity which results in a reduced rate of very preterm delivery should be pursued. However, until the relationship between very preterm birth and cerebral palsy is understood, it would be premature to promise that cerebral palsy rates will fall if very preterm birth rates fall. If most cerebral damage occurs antenatally, merely delaying delivery would have little effect on the rate of cerebral palsy. Antenatal pathways to preterm birth and to cerebral palsy may be different, and as suggested earlier it is unlikely that all cerebral palsy in very preterm infants occurs due to postnatal complications (Paneth *et al.* 1993; Gaffney *et al.* 1994b; Spinillo *et al.* 1995; Stanley 1995; Murphy *et al.* 1996a,b; Morikawa *et al.* 1997).

White matter cerebral damage, very preterm birth and cerebral palsy

While germinal matrix/intraventricular haemorrhage is the single most common brain pathology seen in the very preterm infant, white matter damage is the most important antecedent of cerebral palsy in these infants (Levene 1990, Leviton and Paneth 1990, Levene *et al.* 1992, Paneth *et al.* 1994, Weindling 1995). Over the last few years there has been a considerable literature on the clinical, pathological and epidemiological aspects of cerebral injury in very preterm infants, which has been helped enormously by the widespread use of neonatal cranial ultrasound (Leviton and Paneth 1990, Kuban and Leviton 1994, Paneth *et al.* 1994, Dammann and Leviton 1997b, Dammann *et al.* 1997, Govaert and de Vries 1997).

Two systematic studies of neonatal cranial ultrasound imaging from the USA use samples defined by birthweight, but a third study from Holland is defined by gestational age. The New Jersey Brain Haemorrhage study considered 1105 infants born in the mid-1980s with birthweights in the range 510–2000 g and so far have published follow-up to 6 years (Paneth *et al.* 1994, Whitaker *et al.* 1996). The second US study—of 1605 infants born in the 1990s with weights between 500 and 1500 g—does not yet have follow-up data concerning cerebral palsy (A. Leviton, personal communication 1998). The Dutch cohort study at a regional neonatal intensive care unit is ongoing and had collected data on 1332 infants born at ≤34 weeks gestation by January 1996 (de Vries *et al.* 1998a); however, little has yet been published on long-term outcomes.

Interpretation of cranial ultrasound images is not easy, and an important contribution of these cohort studies has been to measure the reproducibility of interpretation of images between observers and of accuracy of interpretation by comparison with autopsy investigations where these were available. The New Jersey study found that while interobserver agreement on the existence of cerebral haemorrhage was fair (between two observers) and specificity was high, the sensitivity was only a little greater than 50 per cent: almost half the haemorrhages seen at autopsy were missed on ultrasound. The good interobserver reliability suggests that haemorrhages that were missed may have been harder to recognize; for example, they may have been smaller or less accessible to ultrasound scanning. This is supported by the much lower incidence of false negative ultrasound scans found for more severe white matter lesions in the neuropathological study of 83 infants born before 32 weeks (Murphy *et al.* 1996b). Only two of 30 cases with white matter damage at autopsy had been considered to have normal ultrasound scans, and conversely only one of 21 cases with no white matter lesions was considered to have a parenchymal lesion on ultrasound scan.

Among the 777 survivors of the New Jersey study followed to 2 years, 664 did not have a recognized ultrasound abnormality, and of these 34 (5.1 per cent) had nondisabling cerebral palsy and none had disabling cerebral palsy (Pinto-Martin *et al.* 1995). Autopsy validation is of course not possible in survivors, and it may be that a proportion of these 34 cases had had small unrecognized cerebral haemorrhages, particularly since their disability was mild.

Germinal matrix haemorrhage or intraventricular haemorrhage (IVH) is reported in about 20–40 per cent of very low birthweight infants (Paneth *et al.* 1993, Berger *et al.* 1997, Govaert and de Vries 1997), though the poor sensitivity of ultrasound scanning and the inclusion

TABLE 7.1
Rate of cerebral palsy in very preterm/very low birthweight survivors following cranial ultrasound abnormalities

Abnormality	Pooled prevalence studies before 1993*			Prevalence in New Jersey Brain Haemorrhage Study**				Prevalence in Dutch cohort study of infants ≤34w GA***		
	N	CP	(%)	N	CP	(%)	DCP¹	N	CP	DCP¹
None	—	—	—	664	34	(5.1)	0	—	—	—
Isolated GM/IVH²	378	18	(4.8)	108	17	(15.7)	12	—	—	—
Ventricular enlargement	392	190	(48.5)	63	41	(65.1)	33	26	3	—
Parenchymal involvement	358	212	(59.2)					30	20	—
Middle cerebral artery infarcts	—	—	—	—	—	—	—	16	4	1

¹DCP = disabling cerebral palsy.
²GM/IVH = germinal matrix/intraventricular haemorrhage
*Paneth et al. (1994).
**Pinto-Martin et al. (1995).
***de Vries et al. (1997, 1998a,b).

of more mature infants (above 32 weeks) in samples defined by birthweight means that this may underestimate the rate in infants born before 32 weeks. Table 7.1 shows that pooling several small studies published in 1992 or before revealed only 18 cases of cerebral palsy (4.8 per cent) among 378 infants with recognized isolated germinal matrix/intraventricular haemorrhage (Paneth *et al.* 1994). However, the New Jersey Study found that among 108 cases with isolated IVH, 15.7 per cent had cerebral palsy which was disabling in 12 cases and nondisabling in a further five cases.

As the cerebral palsy was disabling in the majority of cases in the New Jersey cohort it seems unlikely that underascertainment would account for such a large discrepancy. A more likely explanation is that since this cohort was born more recently, its survivors would have a lower mean gestational age, and infants who would previously have died as a result of their haemorrhage, now survived with disability.

A higher proportion of cerebral palsy was found in children with cerebral haemorrhage with ventricular enlargement, of whom 48 per cent (Leviton *et al.* 1993) developed cerebral palsy in studies conducted prior to 1992, whereas only three of 26 survivors in the Dutch cohort study with a large IVH (defined as distending the ventricle and filling it by more than half in the acute phase) went on to have cerebral palsy (de Vries *et al.* 1998b). The risk of cerebral palsy does not seem to be reduced by interventions which reduce the fluid in the ventricles by shunting or fluid taps (Ventriculomegaly Trial Group 1990). This suggests that the enlargement may be the result of preexisting damage which caused a decrease in periventricular tissue, rather than causing the damage itself by tissue compression. This possibility is supported by the observations that ventriculomegaly need not be accompanied by raised intracranial pressure, nor is haemorrhage a necessary precursor. Ventriculomegaly can result from the ventricles enlarging to fill the void left by a reduction in white matter volume from any cause (Leviton and Gilles 1996).

Early studies suggested that parenchymal echolucencies carried a higher risk of cerebral palsy, around 60 per cent, comparable with the 20 cases seen among 30 survivors in the Dutch study (Table 7.1). The New Jersey study combined ventricular enlargement with parenchymal echolucencies and echodensities and found that 65 per cent developed cerebral palsy: 33 with disabling and only eight with nondisabling cerebral palsy (Mittendorf 1994, Whitaker et al. 1996).

Table 7.1 indicates that infarcts in the vascular distribution of the middle cerebral artery, a pattern more commonly reported in term newborns, also occur in infants born preterm (de Vries *et al.* 1997). Six infants demonstrated this pattern at ≤32 weeks, the earliest being born at 27 weeks. Although only two of these six children were considered to be developing normally, only one with athetoid cerebral palsy and a bleed diagnosed at 30 weeks was categorized as having as cerebral palsy. A further 10 children had their bleed in the 33rd or 34th week: none had normal development, two died, and three with hemiplegia were described as having cerebral palsy.

Table 7.1 suggests a steep increase in risk of cerebral palsy from the lowest rates with isolated germinal matrix/intraventricular haemorrhage, increasing with ventricular enlargement, to the highest rates with parenchymal echolucencies. It is possible that the risk associated with isolated IVH has increased over time; however, differences within categories

TABLE 7.2
Echolucent parenchymal lesions on cranial ultrasound scans: proportions of very
preterm children with cerebral palsy*

Study	Lesions	Survivors N	Survivors with CP
de Vries *et al.* (1985)	Extensive PVL	10	10
Bozynski *et al.* (1985)	PVL	4	4
Smith, Y. (1985)	PVL	16	14
Weindling *et al.* (1985a)	PV cysts	8	8
Graziani *et al.* (1986)	Large PV cysts/porencephaly	15	12
Cooke (1987)	Porencephalic cysts	32	22
Fawer *et al.* (1987)	Extensive PVL	11	8
Graham *et al.* (1987)	Cystic PVL	13	8
	Multiple cysts	8	7
Stewart *et al.* (1987)	Cysts	10	8
Total		127	101 (80%)

*Adapted from Leviton and Paneth (1990).

between different studies may arise because categorization methods are not standardized. While there was no disabling cerebral palsy without recognized ultrasound abnormalities, about 80 per cent of the cerebral palsy following both ventricular enlargement without cystic changes and parenchymal echolucent lesions was disabling. It is reassuring that the majority (60–80 per cent) of very preterm infants did not have ultrasound abnormalities, and without ultrasound abnormalities no cerebral palsy was disabling.

Parenchymal echolucency, also called cystic changes or periventricular leukomalacia (PVL) as determined by cranial ultrasound, is the strongest predictor of cerebral palsy in very preterm infants. In some reported studies all surviving children with cystic lesions developed cerebral palsy, as shown in Table 7.2. While PVL may undoubtedly be considered the *cause* of the motor impairment, it may be more useful to consider it as the *outcome* (the pathology underlying the disordered motor function), unless effective preventive strategies exist which avoid the motor dysfunction following the development of the PVL (see Chapter 13). In the absence of such strategies, effective interventions must be developed aimed at preventing the PVL. In order to achieve this we need to understand which antecedents are specific to these lesions (its causal pathways).

Table 7.3 lists the risk factors found to be associated with ultrasound-diagnosed PVL in preterm infants (Kuban and Leviton 1994). As low gestational age at delivery is strongly associated with both PVL and cerebral palsy, it is not clear whether the postnatal factors listed here are on the causal pathways to PVL and cerebral palsy or whether they are merely epiphenomena or other independent outcomes of very preterm delivery. Inflammatory antenatal events occurring close to delivery are strongly associated with PVL and are very likely to be on causal paths to cerebral palsy (Kuban and Leviton 1994). In contrast, chronic fetal distress such as severe growth restriction or pre-eclampsia are reported to decrease the risk of intraventricular haemorrhage in cohorts of very low birthweight infants (Kuban *et al.* 1992, Perlman *et al.* 1997) but not in a study of very preterm infants dying perinatally,

TABLE 7.3
**Risk factors associated with PVL (as
diagnosed by neonatal cranial ultrasound)***

Pregnancy
Placental vascular anastomosis
Twin gestation
Antepartum haemorrhage

Labour and delivery
Inflammation umbilical cord/membranes

Postnatal period
Low gestational age
Acidosis, low Apgar scores
Intracranial haemorrhage
Hypotension
Mechanical ventilation
Patent ductus arteriosus
Sepsis
Necrotizing enterocolitis

*Adapted from Kuban and Leviton (1994).

where both restricted growth and pre-eclampsia were associated with white matter changes (Murphy *et al.* 1996b). White matter damage superimposed on chronic distress may be more likely to be fatal than white matter damage in a very preterm infant without chronic compromise. However, it is not known the extent to which these associations are real, given that the populations studied were sometimes defined by birthweight rather than gestational age cut-offs, and hence their mixture of prematurity and chronic compromise may vary considerably.

Can ultrasound cranial imaging early in neonatal life help to determine whether the increase in preterm cerebral palsy is due to increased survival of already damaged infants or whether the brain damage was initiated after birth?

Table 7.4 shows the timing of onset in the 976 subjects in the New Jersey study of infants ≤2000g birthweight for those infants in whom observers agreed as to timing. One quarter had their cerebral haemorrhage recognized within seven days of birth, of which 44 per cent (95% CI 38–50%) were present at the first opportunity to scan, usually on day 1 (Paneth *et al.* 1993). Govaert and de Vries (1997) state that 30–40 per cent of liveborn infants with birthweights <1500g will have a cerebral haemorrhage, occurring within 48 hours in 75 per cent and within 72 hours in 90 per cent. This proportion is higher than in the New Jersey study, probably reflecting the lower birthweight criterion (<1500g rather than ≤2000g) which would exclude many of the more mature infants. However, a positive first scan does not necessarily imply an antenatal event as the first scans often occurred too long after delivery to exclude the possibility of intrapartum or very early postnatal damage.

PVL does not appear on the ultrasound image at the time the sequence of brain damage is initiated but takes between one and three weeks to develop. In contrast, haemorrhage appears on the ultrasound image within seconds or minutes (Govaert and de Vries 1997).

TABLE 7.4
Timing of GMH/IVH[1] (ascertained by neonatal cranial ultrasound[2]) in 976 infants
≤2000g[3] with confirmed time of onset

Ultrasound scan	Scanning interval		Incidence of GMH/IVH occurring in interval from last scan	
	Mean (±SD)	Range	Cases/number scanned	%
1st scan	4.9h (±2.2)	0–12h	108/906	11.9
2nd scan	25h (±4.8)	13–48h	67/817	8.2
3rd scan	7.2d (±0.8)	5–10d	69/721	9.6
All			244/976	25.0

Of all lesions (244), 1082 (44 per cent) were present on first scan.
[1]GMH/IVH = Germinal matrix haemorrhage/intraventricular haemorrhage
[2]Only infants with interobserver consensus were included.
[3]From New Jersey Brain Haemorrhage Study (Paneth *et al.* 1993).

There is frequently a progression from haemorrhagic (echodense) images to cystic changes (echolucent), during which images may pass through an isodense period and be harder to interpret accurately. Therefore the events from which to best infer timing in survivors are the initial appearance of haemorrhage which follows immediately after the initiation of the sequence, and PVL which occurs one to three weeks after the initiation of the sequence of cerebral damage. De Vries *et al.* (1998b) devised criteria to recognize supposed haemorrhagic and/or ischaemic lesions of antenatal onset from very early scanning. Of 1332 infants born before 34 weeks gestation, they could be confident of an antenatal initiation of cerebral damage in only 24 cases. A further 25 cases may have had an antenatal initiation but did not meet the study's strict criteria. Therefore, if these criteria are valid, between 1.8 and 3.7 per cent of infants born before 34 weeks had an antenatal initiation of cerebral damage. The outcomes in this group were very poor with no normal survivors: of the 24 with definite antenatal onset 17 died, five had cerebral palsy and two had other neurological deficits. Of the 25 possible cases, 11 died and nine had cerebral palsy. Thus while cerebral damage commenced antenatally in only a small proportion of very preterm births, it accounted for at least five of the 68 cases (7.3 per cent) of cerebral palsy seen in the entire cohort and possibly as many as 14 (20 per cent).

In the necropsy study of Murphy *et al.* (1996b), cellular indicators of timing were also available. Of the 39 cases with white matter damage, they felt confident in classifying 12 as antenatal and 12 as postnatal, while in 15 they could not differentiate with confidence. Thus there is much imprecision in the reported proportion of white matter damage in very preterm infants that occurs before birth, but more appears to occur postnatally. Antenatal damage may carry a higher risk of impaired survival than postnatal damage. It must always be remembered that white matter damage does not always follow germinal matrix/intraventricular haemorrhage and that ultrasound appearances do not necessarily provide accurate timing of the initiation of the lesion (A. Leviton, personal communication 1998). Clearly, also, to ensure elucidation of the risks of cerebral palsy following very preterm delivery and white matter damage, the proportion that die (as suggested in Fig. 7.2) is a crucial aspect of data collection in any study.

Parenchymal echolucencies in very preterm infants are so often followed by cerebral palsy (see Table 7.2) that it has been suggested and used as a proxy measure of cerebral palsy in these infants (Leviton and Paneth 1990). Studies of the neonatal period using outcome measures much closer in time to exposures are attractive as they are more likely to uncover causal pathways than studies of cerebral palsy, which can only be ascertained with certainty years after birth. However, such proxy end-points can provide only part of the picture. Only 41 of all 113 cases of cerebral palsy (36 per cent), or 33 of 70 disabling cases of cerebral palsy (37 per cent) in the New Jersey study had white matter damage or ventricular enlargement recognized on ultrasound, and of 63 survivors with PVL or ventricular enlargement only 41 (65 per cent) had cerebral palsy. Children with cerebral palsy resulting from PVL differ both in aetiology and outcome from the majority without PVL, and the latter would be missed by using PVL as a surrogate end-point. Olsén et al. (1997) described MRI findings in 42 8-year-old children who had been born preterm (<37 weeks) with birthweights less than 1750 g and 43 control children born at term and weighing 2500 g and over. The children were all from a 1-year birth cohort of 9479 infants born in northern Finland from 1 January 1985 to 30 June 1986. All children were traced, and neurological status at 8 years was correlated with MRI findings. Of all preterm children (N=41), 13 had PVL, including all four with cerebral palsy, three of 12 with minor neurodevelopmental problems and six of 24 without neurological problems. No control children had PVL. While this study is small, it suggests that not all PVL (detected by MRI) will result in cerebral palsy in preterm infants.

A most useful epidemiological study of this subject would be a total population cohort of very preterm infants defined by *gestational age at delivery* and not by birthweight. Complete antenatal and perinatal data would be collected, and frequent serial cerebral imaging would commence as soon as possible after birth. All deaths would be autopsied to assess local, current validity of image interpretation, and follow-up would include ascertainment of cerebral palsy with full clinical and MRI examinations. Such a study would allow confirmation of the timing of initial haemorrhage and proper assessment of how the neonatal lesions related to death and to cerebral palsy, and how later MRI images related to neonatal pathology as assessed by neonatal ultrasound scans. The Dutch study may meet this description, and the current trials investigating the effects of magnesium sulphate on rates of cerebral palsy would be ideal for such cohort analysis (Crowther et al. 1997).

How could very preterm birth be associated with cerebral palsy?
Figure 7.4 shows three possible pathways whereby cerebral palsy may be associated with very preterm delivery. Path A suggests that an antenatal factor (or factors) could cause both cerebral palsy and preterm delivery independently; the latter would then be an epiphenomenon and not on the causal path to cerebral palsy. Examples may be ascending bacterial infection, placental abruption, twin–twin transfusion syndrome, cofetal death or endocrine disturbance. Path B suggests that preterm infants may be more vulnerable than term infants to physiological disturbances such as hypoxia/acidosis, hypoglycaemia, cerebral blood flow disturbance

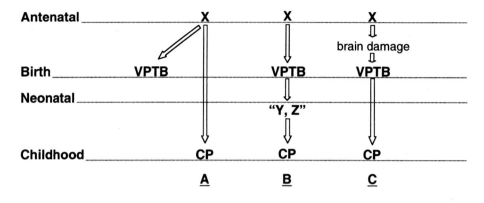

X = antenatal events (s)   "Y, Z" = neonatal complications

Fig. 7.4. How could very preterm birth be associated with cerebral palsy?

and circulatory problems resulting in cerebral haemorrhage or infarcts, hypothyroxinaemia, sepsis and shock occurring during or after delivery. There may also be extrinsic factors that magnify the vulnerability resulting from preterm birth, such as being born in a level 1 centre without a neonatal intensive care unit, or hypothermia. Path C suggests that early damage to the cerebral motor cortex leads to preterm delivery; that is, the affected fetus triggers its own early delivery. There is no known example of Path C but the possibility is suggested by the increased rate of miscarriage of abnormal embryos and fetuses with chromosomal anomalies (Alberman and Creasy 1977, Kline et al. 1989, Jacobs 1990) and is included for completeness. In all recognized pathways, then, the initiating step is the cause of the very preterm birth.

What are the pathways to very preterm birth?
Several workers (Savitz *et al.* 1991, Ananth *et al.* 1997, Läärä *et al.* 1997, Berkowitz *et al.* 1998) have categorized preterm births as (a) the result of idiopathic preterm labour, (b) following premature rupture of membranes, or (c) electively induced for medical reasons, primarily pre-eclampsia, maternal haemorrhage and fetal distress. However, Klebanoff and Shiono (1995) point out that the three types often have similar risk factors and this categorization does not clearly distinguish aetiologically distinct and mutually exclusive syndromes. Nonetheless, Ananth *et al.* (1997) report that some underlying causes are associated with both the distribution of these categories and the gestation of the very preterm delivery. For example, of infants born before 33 weeks of gestation, 50 per cent of those whose mothers had mild pre-eclampsia and 94 per cent of those with severe pre-eclampsia were delivered as a result of medical intervention, compared with only 12 per cent of those born before 33 weeks due to other causes. If the underlying cause is associated with gestational age at delivery it is very likely to be associated with the risk of cerebral palsy, whether or not there are any cause-specific risks.

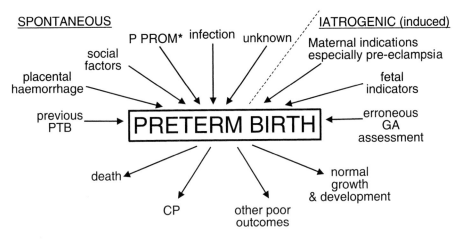

SPONTANEOUS   IATROGENIC (induced)

P PROM* infection unknown   Maternal indications
social   especially pre-eclampsia
factors
placental   fetal
haemorrhage   indicators

previous   **PRETERM BIRTH**   erroneous
PTB   GA
                                           assessment

death   normal
                                  growth
                             & development
CP   other poor
            outcomes

* prolonged premature rupture of membranes

Fig. 7.5. Causes of preterm birth: which are on a causal pathway to cerebral palsy?

Figure 7.5 shows the antecedents of very preterm birth. They are not mutually exclusive; for example, social factors and previous preterm birth may occur together. Some such as placental haemorrhage or prolonged premature rupture of membranes may result in very preterm delivery because of medical intervention, although they are listed as 'spontaneous'.

Which particular pathways to very preterm birth are more strongly associated with cerebral palsy than others?

Table 7.5, from the study of cerebral palsy in infants delivered before 32 weeks gestation in Oxford (Murphy et al. 1995), shows the distribution of risk factors in survivors with and without cerebral palsy. These antenatal complications are not mutually exclusive, and it may be that some combinations of risk factors are more strongly associated with cerebral palsy than are individual components of the combination. Chorioamnionitis is the most strongly associated risk factor (odds ratio 4.2) but was present in only 10 of the 59 cases, only five of which could be attributed to it if it were the single sufficient cause. In contrast, prolonged rupture of membranes and maternal genital tract infection are less strongly associated with cerebral palsy but occurred more frequently, and 26 per cent and 18 per cent of cases may be attributed to each factor respectively (if single sufficient causes). While it is biologically plausible that chorioamnionitis might be associated with other maternal genital tract infection, adjustment for signs of other infection did not greatly reduce the strength of its association with cerebral palsy. More research with better methods of diagnosing genital tract infection and inflammatory responses is required to tease out these causal sequences. A smaller study of infants born before 30 weeks gestation (Gray *et al.* 1997) agreed that membrane rupture and antepartum haemorrhage were the most common precursors of very preterm birth, closely followed by pre-eclampsia, but no precursors were more strongly associated with adverse neurological outcome than the others.

TABLE 7.5
Antenatal complications in cases with cerebral palsy and controls, all born before 32 weeks gestation, from same regional cohort*

Antenatal complication	Cases (N=59)		Controls (N=244)		OR[2] (95% CI)	PAR[1]
	N	(%)	N	(%)		%
Rupture of membranes >24 h	25	(42)	64	(27)	2.3 (1.2–4.2)	26.0
Chorioamnionitis	10	(17)	8	(3)	4.2 (1.4–12.0)	8.8
Maternal infection	22	(37)	40	(17)	2.3 (1.2–4.5)	18.1
Abruptio placentae[3]	16	(27)	35	(15)	1.5 (0.7–3.0)	7.0
Pre-eclampsia	6	(10)	56	(24)	0.4 (0.2–0.9)	—

[1]PAR = population attributable risk (see Glossary).
[2]OR = odds ratio (see Glossary).
[3]Severe (≥200 mL) haemorrhage after 20 weeks gestation with evidence of placental bleed at delivery.
*Adapted from Murphy *et al.* (1995).

The epidemiological evidence as to whether each antecedent of preterm birth shown in Figure 7.5 is likely to be on a causal path to cerebral palsy is now reviewed.

UNEXPLAINED
The existence of unexplained onset of early labour demonstrates our limited understanding of the pathways to very preterm delivery. As more research is done investigating the various causal paths to preterm delivery (Di Renzo *et al.* 1998), we hope that a greater proportion will be explained and that we gain a better understanding of which paths may also lead to cerebral palsy.

PREVIOUS PRETERM BIRTH
While a preterm birth in a previous pregnancy is a strong risk factor for preterm birth in the current pregnancy, it confers no explanation if the previous preterm birth is not explained; it only indicates that the underlying mechanism persists from one pregnancy to the next. A previous preterm birth is not associated with any additional risk of cerebral palsy over and above the risk associated with the gestation of the index delivery (Nelson and Ellenberg 1985b, Palmer *et al.* 1994).

SOCIAL FACTORS
Dolk *et al.* (1996) have analysed cerebral palsy risk by social class and found an association only in infants born at term. An earlier study, also from Ireland, showed that the risk of cerebral palsy was associated with social class only for infants with birthweight >2500 g (Dowding and Barry 1990). This suggests that social class does not increase risk of cerebral palsy via its important influence on very preterm delivery.

PLACENTAL HAEMORRHAGE
Antepartum haemorrhage or evidence of it having occurred (finding a retroplacental clot at delivery) is variably defined and recorded but in the Western Australian data base occurs

in about 3.8 per cent of all births and 27.1 per cent of very preterm births (unpublished data). Few researchers have used their data to address the question of whether haemorrhage resulting in very early delivery puts the child at increased risk of cerebral palsy over and above the risk from early gestation alone.

Antepartum haemorrhage has been associated with mortality, cerebral palsy (Nelson and Ellenberg 1984, 1985a, 1986a; O'Shea *et al.* 1998a) and white matter damage in preterm infants as assessed by ultrasound in some (Weindling *et al.* 1985b, Calvert *et al.* 1987, Leviton and Paneth 1990, Gibbs and Weindling 1994, Zupan *et al.* 1996) but not in all studies (Trounce *et al.* 1988). Most studies are compatible with the interpretation that antepartum haemorrhage increases risk of cerebral palsy by increasing risk of preterm birth but is not associated with further risk once gestation of delivery has been controlled (Nelson and Ellenberg 1985b, Murphy *et al.* 1995, Topp *et al.* 1997a, O'Shea *et al.* 1998a).

Vaginal bleeding at the time of admission was a risk factor for cerebral palsy in children who weighed <1500g at birth, and the odds ratio rose from 2.9 (CI 1.1–7.4) to 19 (CI 1.9–97) in the small number born at more than 29 weeks gestation (Grether *et al.* 1996). Otherwise, neither abruption nor placenta praevia was associated with an increased risk of cerebral palsy. Placental abruption, with its dramatic effects on placental blood flow, would intuitively be more likely than placenta praevia to be associated with cerebral palsy. However, placenta praevia is associated with higher rates of many adverse factors such as history of miscarriage, advanced maternal age and parity, impaired fertility, smoking and fetal malformations (Nelson 1994). Thus any of these may confound the association between cerebral palsy and haemorrhage, or alternatively haemorrhage may not be on a causal pathway to cerebral palsy but be an epiphenomenon.

INFECTION

Irrespective of whether white matter damage is initiated ante- or postnatally, there is now considerable epidemiological evidence (*e.g.* Murphy *et al.* 1995; see Table 7.5) that cerebral palsy in very preterm infants is associated with perinatal infection. This new and promising hypothesis generated from epidemiological studies of the cerebral palsies is considered here in some detail as it well illustrates the importance of thinking in causal pathways.

Epidemiological observational studies have related markers of maternal infection to cerebral palsy (Table 7.6) (den Ouden *et al.* 1990; Murphy *et al.* 1995, 1997; Grether *et al.* 1996; Murphy 1996; Dammann and Leviton 1997a,b; Nelson and Grether 1997; O'Shea *et al.* 1997, 1998). Maternal infection has also been associated with preterm birth and PVL in clinical (Romero *et al.* 1994, Foulon *et al.* 1995, Mercer *et al.* 1997) and biochemical studies (Adinolfi 1993, Leviton 1993, Yoon *et al.* 1997), but the following overview concentrates on the epidemiological evidence.

Figure 7.6 shows possible pathways involving ascending infection and cerebral palsy. Path A suggests that ascending infection results in intrauterine infection which may release a cascade of cytokines and initiate preterm birth. The immature neonatal brain is then at increased risk of postnatally acquired white matter damage. Path B suggests that cerebral damage may result directly from the infection *in utero* without any signs of white matter damage.

75

TABLE 7.6

Associations between markers[1] of perinatal infection and cerebral palsy in singleton VLBW[2] cases and controls and by clinical subtype*

	Controls (N = 124)		All CP cases (N = 62)			Spastic diplegia (N = 24)		Quadri/hemiplegia (N = 22)	
	N	(%)	N	(%)	OR[3] (95% CI)	N	OR (95% CI)	N	OR (95% CI)
Clinical chorioamnionitis	11	(10)	12	(23)	2.6 (1.0–6.5)	7	3.2 (1.1–9.7)	4	1.8 (0.5–6.6)
Maternal antibiotics	22	(21)	20	(38)	2.2 (1.0–4.7)	13	4.3 (1.7–11.0)	5	1.0 (0.3–3.0)
Uterine tenderness	5	(5)	7	(13)	2.6 (0.8–9.3)	4	3.6 (0.8–15.1)	3	2.3 (0.5–11.3)
Maternal fever	14	(13)	15	(28)	2.6 (1.1–6.0)	9	3.9 (1.4–10.9)	6	2.2 (0.7–7.0)
Neonatal sepsis	6	(6)	9	(17)	2.9 (0.9–8.9)	3	2.1 (0.5–9.3)	5	3.7 (1.0–14.2)

[1]These markers of perinatal infection are, naturally, not mutually exclusive.
[2]VLBW = very low birthweight: 500–1500 g without major congenital anomaly; all inborn at a major level III centre.
[3]OR = Odds ratios, adjusted for gestational age.
*Adapted from O'Shea et al. (1998b).

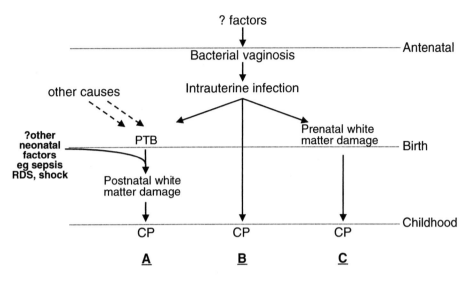

Fig. 7.6. Possible pathways involving genital bacterial infection and cerebral palsy in very preterm infants. (Adapted from Dammann and Leviton 1997a.)

Path C suggests that the infection directly causes white matter damage *in utero*. There could also be a combination of paths C and A with infection causing either fetal damage or compromise and preterm birth, with neonatal complications exacerbating the situation causing further damage. In paths B and C preterm birth is an epiphenomenon and not on the causal pathway. Only in path A would the prevention of the preterm birth prevent the cerebral palsy; that due to paths B and C can only be prevented by avoiding the brain damaging effects of infection before birth occurs. We do not yet know what proportion follows each pathway, and in many relevant studies subjects are either confined to preterm births or described by birthweight rather than gestational age, making it difficult to assess the contribution of very preterm birth to the overall picture.

Evidence for the existence of path B comes from a case–control study from California (Eschenbach 1997, Grether and Nelson 1997). These children were all of normal birthweight, and those with known antenatal causes of brain pathology (such as structural malformations) were excluded. Markers of maternal infection in labour were all strongly associated with unexplained spastic cerebral palsy. This suggests that a pathway from infection to cerebral palsy need not involve preterm birth and its complications to result in brain damage.

Data from the American National Collaborative Perinatal Project (NCPP) (Nelson and Ellenberg 1985b) showed a relative risk of cerebral palsy of 3.4 with chorioamnionitis in infants of <2500 g birthweight who may have been either preterm or growth restricted. Chorioamnionitis was present in less than 3 per cent of all NCPP births and in about 20 per cent of infants weighing <1501 g, almost all of whom would have been very preterm. Chorioamnionitis also contributed to the risk of cerebral palsy over and above its risk to low birthweight.

O'Shea *et al.* (1998b) analysed associations between markers of perinatal infection and cerebral palsy in singletons of <1500 g birthweight by subtype of cerebral palsy. Markers of infection other than postnatal sepsis were more common in cases of diplegia than of hemiplegia or quadriplegia. The association with chorioamnionitis and diplegia persisted when adjustment was made for maternal magnesium sulphate and betamethasone receipt, method of delivery, acidosis on initial neonatal blood gas analysis, systolic blood pressure level and the diagnosis of major neonatal neurosonographic abnormality (Table 7.6).

Analyses from Oxford in infants born before 32 weeks gestation (Murphy *et al.* 1995, Murphy 1996) were consistent with those from California in infants of <1500 g (Grether and Nelson 1996, Grether *et al.* 1996) in that both found strong associations between cerebral palsy and signs of infection, particularly chorioamnionitis. The lack of standardized criteria for chorioamnionitis is demonstrated by the great difference in prevalences reported in these two studies. Thus while both find significant associations with chorioamnionitis followed by neonatal seizures, this accounted for all the association with cerebral palsy and chorioamnionitis in the US study but only a part of that seen in the UK study. The explanation for the discrepancy is likely to lie in differences in the range of disease attracting the description of chorioamnionitis. If there is a wide range of disease severity and cerebral palsy is only associated with the severe end of the spectrum, the effect will be diluted if a much larger number of subjects with milder disease are included in the analysis. Neonatal seizures, like PVL, may be considered to be the outcome if, after their occurrence, interventions to prevent cerebral palsy are not possible. In these reported cases neonatal seizures may only reflect the severity of insult inflicted by the infection and not have any independent causal role.

The US study also underlined the risk associated with presentation and delivery at a level one facility rather than a tertiary institution, particularly if delivery occurred within three hours of admission, but provides no indication of which pathological maternal or fetal characteristics were associated with place of delivery. Presumably it was not chorioamnionitis since this was only a risk factor for cerebral palsy if there was an admission-to-delivery interval of more than five hours. Rupture of membranes may have been associated since this was only a risk factor if it occurred within two hours of admission in the presence of preterm labour which would have constituted a contraindication for transport. This suggests that membrane rupture and chorioamnionitis were on independent causal pathways. No bivariate exposure analyses including chorioamnionitis were reported by the UK study, except that with neonatal seizures. Careful bivariate analyses of this type, with variables chosen on the grounds of both biological plausibility and epidemiological observations, are important in the generation of aetiological hypotheses. Since these are hypotheses to be further tested in other data sets, it is completely appropriate to conduct exploratory studies and test multiple associations (Blair and Stanley 1993b). Thus it seems that both chorioamnionitis and other maternal genital tract infections are associated with very preterm cerebral palsy: they may be on independent pathways, but we need hypotheses to suggest which preventable risk factors, either antenatal or factors such as timing or place of delivery, are associated with them.

The group of neuroepidemiologists and neonatologists in Boston have suggested some hypotheses which are to be tested in their new study (ELGAN: extremely low gestational age newborn—A. Leviton, personal communication 1998). They are postulating that infants of low gestational age have less capacity to respond to certain challenges because they have inadequate amounts of developmentally regulated proteins, such as surfactant and other protectors which may block, ameliorate or enhance responses to a variety of adverse situations. Such situations may arise as a result of ascending infection (which may also have triggered the early delivery) and may result in a fetal inflammatory response (measured chemically by cytokine levels or histologically as vasculitis of the umbilical cord). They suggest that the resulting outcomes, such as white matter damage or hyaline membrane disease or no disease, may depend not only on a balance between the potentially damaging influences but also on the capacity of the infant to mount a protective response to them. This capacity includes both "disease promoters and response modifers" (A. Leviton, personal communication 1998). A range of factors in addition to gestational immaturity are likely to influence this capacity.

Once hypotheses like these concerning causal pathways are generated, collaborations between biochemical, microbiological and radiological sciences and clinical epidemiology will be needed to test them.

Multiple Births

Causal pathways to cerebral palsy involving multiple birth are considered in chapter 10.

Rupture of Membranes (ROM)

There are no standardized criteria for this variable. The acronym (ROM) is usually preceded by a P (PROM), but the P may represent *preterm* (before 37 weeks), *pre-labour* (before the onset of contractions), *premature* (representing either of the above), or *prolonged*, referring to the duration between membrane rupture and delivery and often defined as >24 hours, but sometimes as >12 hours. The information enabling a standardized interpretation between studies is not always reported: for example, if PROM is defined as rupture >24 hours before delivery, it may be that rupture mostly preceded contractions: if the period is only >12 hours, this assumption is not so secure. It is not possible to infer duration of rupture from a prelabour criterion.

The role of very premature membrane rupture, whether pre-labour and/or prolonged, in the aetiology of cerebral palsy in very preterm births is not clear from the sparse epidemiological evidence available.

In Finland, Kurki *et al.* (1992) conducted a prospective intervention study of the effect of penicillin in 221 women with membrane rupture before 37 weeks of gestation for whom the mean gestation at delivery was 32.9 weeks. Of the 202 infants available for follow-up at 6 years, they observed that cerebral palsy occurred more often (8/43) among those with a recognized duration of membrane rupture of less than five hours (none of whom had evidence of infection or received penicillin), than among those with rupture of longer durations (14h–56d) (7/159). This result could not be attributed to differences in infection rates, which were higher with ruptures of longer durations, nor in gestational age, as mean gestations at delivery were the same in the short and the long duration of rupture groups and, of course, the mean gestation at rupture was slightly higher in the short duration group. The curious absence of any recognized duration of membrane rupture between five hours and 14 hours strongly suggests at least two disease processes. For example, ruptures recognized within five hours of delivery are more likely to have occurred in association with labour.

Spinillo *et al.* (1995) conducted a retrospective case–control study in Pavia, Italy of deliveries at or before 34 weeks of gestation, comparing those with rupture of membranes of more than 12 hours duration with those without. Of all 342 singleton deliveries occurring at or before 34 weeks of gestation, 9 per cent had ruptured membranes for more than 48 hours. The risk of cerebral palsy was highest (8/30) in this group, whereas for those with shorter duration of membrane rupture the risk of cerebral palsy (8/110) did not differ from that for those without membrane rupture (10/120).

In a retrospective case–control study of children with cerebral palsy born at or before 32 weeks gestation in Oxford, UK, Murphy *et al.* (1995) defined PROM as membrane rupture of >24 hours and found it to be present in 25 of the 59 cases of cerebral palsy compared with only 64 of 234 controls, giving an odds ratio of 2.3 (95% CI 1.2–4.2). The duration of rupture was not explored in greater detail.

In a cohort study of 189 infants born before 30 weeks gestation in a regional perinatal centre in Brisbane, Australia, Gray *et al.* (1997) observed that prelabour rupture of membranes occurred in one-third of these very preterm births, and in the same proportion (8/24) of those with subsequent neurodevelopmental disability. Duration of membrane rupture was not explored.

Membrane rupture is likely to have more than one aetiology, and membrane rupture with differing aetiologies may not be associated with the same risks of cerebral palsy (Fig. 7.7). The apparently conflicting epidemiological observations could arise if the distribution of aetiologies varied between populations in different geographical locations or varied with gestational age at delivery. The study samples above were defined by different gestational criteria, and while each included a range of preterm gestational ages at delivery, none of the published reports explore the effect on risk of cerebral palsy of gestational age at either membrane rupture or delivery, no doubt on account of the small numbers of cerebral palsy outcomes in each study. An effect of gestational age at delivery on the association between prolonged (>24 hours) membrane rupture and cerebral palsy is suggested at later gestations in the Western Australian case–control study of spastic cerebral palsy. In that study there was a strong association between prolonged rupture and cerebral palsy in cases born before 37 weeks compared with their birthweight-matched controls (odds ratio = 3.32, CI 1.6–7.1) (Blair and Stanley 1993a), but not in cases born at term (odds ratio = 1.15, CI 0.4–3.6). However, the birthweight matching creates the possibility of residual confounding by gestational age at delivery and/or intrauterine growth in the preterm but not in the term infants (Blair 1996c).

All the above studies compare the risk of cerebral palsy in infants with very preterm PROM with infants delivered without PROM at similar gestations. If some aetiology or aetiologies of membrane rupture *initiate* events leading to the very preterm birth, then the appropriate comparison group from which to estimate the contribution of very preterm membrane rupture to cerebral palsy would be term infants.

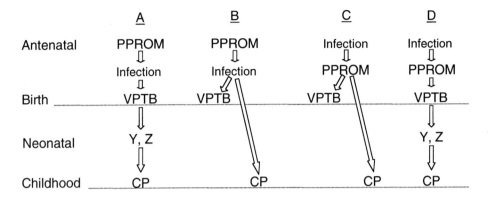

	A	B	C	D
Antenatal	PPROM ⇕ Infection ⇕	PPROM ⇕ Infection	Infection ⇕ PPROM	Infection ⇕ PPROM ⇕
Birth	VPTB	VPTB	VPTB	VPTB
Neonatal	Y, Z			Y, Z
Childhood	CP	CP	CP	CP

Y, Z = neonatal complications

Fig. 7.7. Hypothetical sequences involving very preterm birth, prolonged rupture of membranes and cerebral palsy.

INDUCED DELIVERY

The main reason for inducing preterm and very preterm delivery for maternal causes is pre-eclampsia, and for fetal causes is growth restriction, both of which are described in Chapter 8.

Pathways involving postnatal complications of very preterm birth

Pathway B in Figure 7.4 suggests that some very preterm infants develop complications of their immaturity, and these cause irreversible brain damage and cerebral palsy. Postnatal factors known to be associated with both preterm birth and cerebral palsy but which are unlikely to be markers of prior causes or early measures of the outcome include patent ductus arteriosus, hypotension, blood transfusion, prolonged mechanical ventilation, pneumothorax, sepsis, shock, hyponatraemia, total parenteral nutrition, hypoglycaemia and low serum thyroxine (Lucas *et al.* 1988, Cooke 1990, Levene 1992, Reuss *et al.* 1993, Cooke 1994, Spinillo *et al.* 1995, Grether *et al.* 1996, Reuss *et al.* 1996, Murphy *et al.* 1997).

While some of these may merely be indicators of severity of morbidity (as has been suggested for hypothyroxinaemia) rather than causes of cerebral palsy in themselves, others are plausibly factors which interfere with cerebral blood flow (Leviton and Paneth 1990) or result in brain damage from infection or inflammation. Thus these postnatal complications may well be on causal pathways to white matter damage, the majority of which is initiated postnatally.

Conclusions

Many different pathways result in very preterm birth, but they vary in their contribution to cerebral palsy. Children with cerebral palsy who were born preterm may have acquired their cerebral lesions either pre-, peri- or postnatally. We need further epidemiological and other studies to ascertain these many pathways. These pathways will suggest opportunities for prevention, both primary prevention of the cause of very preterm delivery and strategies to minimize damage once very preterm delivery has occurred (see Chapter 12). The epidemiological challenges include obtaining good quality data, often from retrospective review of obstetric and neonatal records, standardizing criteria to enable pooling of data, and finding 'gold standards' against which other markers of exposures can be tested. Studies need to be large enough to be enable bivariate analyses, to see how coexistence of factors affects their association with cerebral palsy as an aid to generating hypotheses for causal pathways. In addition, we need to describe quantitatively the cerebral palsies of very preterm infants in terms of cerebral pathology as ascertained by cerebral imaging, and to further encourage multidisciplinary studies of white matter damage in cohorts of preterm infants.

8
PATHWAYS TO CEREBRAL PALSY INVOLVING INTRAUTERINE GROWTH RESTRICTION

"On Being the Right Size" J.B.S. Haldane (J.M. Smith 1985)

Is cerebral palsy associated with intrauterine growth restriction?
Babies born small for their gestational age (SGA)are at increased risk of cerebral palsy. SGA babies include both those who have achieved their full growth potential but are at the lower end of the normal distribution and those who might have grown faster had it not been for suboptimal genetic and/or environmental factors. Intrauterine growth restriction suggests that the fetus has not grown as fast as it ought to have, and it is this (or its sequelae) which is most likely associated with risk of subsequent neurological deficits. However, it can be difficult to distinguish between slow, normal and pathological restriction of growth. Most epidemiologists studying this question define a 'small for gestational age' group according to statistical criteria defined by birthweight and gestational age and use it as a surrogate for intrauterine growth restriction. It is the aim of this chapter to explore and elucidate further the relationships between cerebral palsy and intrauterine growth, seeking methods which will better delineate the difference between normal and abnormal growth.

THE EFFECT OF SLOW FETAL GROWTH AT DIFFERENT GESTATIONS ON CEREBRAL PALSY
Figure 8.1 illustrates the relationship between risk of spastic cerebral palsy and birthweight centile at different grouped gestational ages (Blair and Stanley 1990). The most marked gradient of risk with decreasing birthweight centile is after 33 weeks gestation, suggesting that those at highest risk were those with the most long-standing growth restriction (Blair and Stanley 1992). Compatible findings have been described from six case–control studies (Kyllerman *et al.* 1982, Uvebrant and Hagberg 1992, Spinillo *et al.* 1993, Murphy *et al.* 1995, Palmer *et al.* 1995, Topp *et al.* 1996).

Further evidence of the excess of neurological problems in this group comes from cohort studies of infants classified as small for gestational age born mostly at term, although these do not usually have sufficient power to provide definitive answers in relation to rare outcomes such as cerebral palsy (Fitzhardinge and Steven 1972, Rubin *et al.* 1973, Neligan *et al.* 1976, Parkinson *et al.* 1981, Low *et al.* 1982, Dowding and Barry 1990, Hawdon *et al.* 1990, Kjellmer *et al.* 1997). Such studies have demonstrated that while most of these infants are not impaired, more have major disability—particularly cerebral palsy—than those

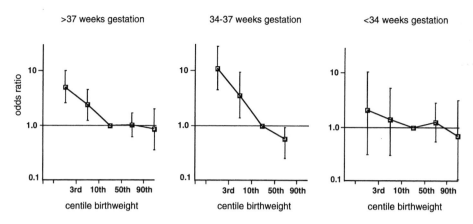

Fig. 8.1. Odds ratios and 95% confidence intervals for spastic cerebral palsy by percentile birthweight category and gestational age at delivery. (Reproduced by permission from Blair and Stanley 1990.)

not small for their gestational age. An excess of cognitive defects and behavioural disturbances has also been observed (Henderson-Smart 1995, Blair 1999). Only two cohort studies of unselected populations of infants born around term have published data on cerebral palsy and fetal growth. In the US National Collaborative Perinatal Project there was a significantly increased risk of cerebral palsy in both White and Black children born small for gestational age at term, that is with birthweights for gestational age below the fifth centile (Ellenberg and Nelson 1979). White children classified as small for gestational age had double the expected rate of cerebral palsy and Black children nearly three times the rate. The data from the much smaller Finnish study (Rantakallio 1985) shows that half of the cases of cerebral palsy born between 34 and 37 weeks were below 10th percentile birthweight, as were nine of the 34 cases born at term, but none of the three born before 34 weeks (P. Rantakallio, personal communication 1998). All data are therefore compatible with an increased risk of cerebral palsy in small for gestational age infants born at term or moderately preterm. The few data pertaining to very preterm infants do not suggest that being small for gestational age increases their risk of cerebral palsy.

What is intrauterine growth restriction and how is it best assessed for epidemiological studies?
SMALL FOR GESTATIONAL AGE AND GROWTH RESTRICTION

As implied above, satisfactory epidemiological criteria do not yet exist to reliably measure growth restriction, which is still defined conceptually (Pollack and Divon 1992, Blair 1999). Without routinely available serial intrauterine measures of growth, epidemiologists have to estimate degree of intrauterine growth anomalies by the extent to which birthweight for gestational age deviates from that expected. Accurate gestational age is crucial in distinguishing the small preterm from the small growth restricted infant; as more pregnancies have ultrasound dating, gestational age assessments will become more reliable (Kramer *et al.*

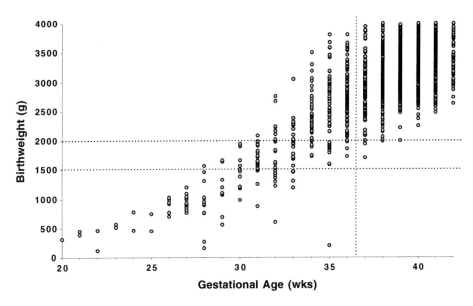

Fig. 8.2. Scattergram of birthweight by gestational age at delivery. Low birthweight cut-offs preferentially exclude preterm infants who are well grown. (Western Australian total birth cohort, February–April 1990.)

1990, Mul *et al.* 1996, Allen *et al.* 1998). Accurate measurement of birthweight poses less of a challenge. The temptation to use birthweight as a surrogate measure of gestation should be avoided because infants with very different gestational lengths and growth patterns are then grouped together, particularly at low and very low birthweights (Blair 1996c). Figure 8.2 shows a scattergram from the Western Australian Maternal and Child Health Research Data base (Stanley *et al.* 1997) of birthweights of infants at each gestational age. This demonstrates how the use of birthweight as a cut-off point unintentionally selects or excludes certain important groups of infants. Taking <1500 g or <2000 g as a cut-off excludes a considerable proportion of infants who are born before 32 weeks, and is therefore not a reliable method to identify very preterm infants.

Variations in neonatal morphology are indicative of the severity and duration of growth restriction but require accurate measures of length, head and abdominal circumferences and skinfold thickness. These are not routinely available for retrospective epidemiological study (Blair and Stanley 1992). Furthermore, their complex relationships with intrauterine growth patterns do not lend themselves to simple dichotomous classifications or linear relationships.

In contrast to intrauterine growth restriction, small for gestational age is a statistical definition (Mahadevan *et al.* 1994, Kingdom *et al.* 1999). Infants are assigned to the group 'small for gestational age' if their birthweight falls below some arbitrarily selected point on the population distribution of birthweight at the same gestational age. This assignation is regardless of the cause for the low weight. It is not synonymous with intrauterine growth restriction which is by definition pathological and varies with environmental or genetic factors

85

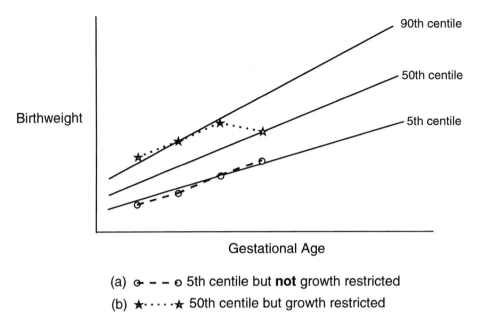

Fig. 8.3. Growth trajectories of (a) an infant who is small for gestational age but not growth restricted, and (b) an infant who is growth restricted but not small for gestational age.

that reduce fetal growth, such as pre-eclampsia, maternal smoking and fetal anomalies. An infant who is genetically destined to grow at the fifth weight percentile and achieves this, is small for gestational age but not growth restricted. Conversely, an infant destined to be at the 90th weight percentile, but due to pathological interference achieves only the 50th weight percentile, is growth restricted but will not be classified as small for gestational age. Figure 8.3 shows these two different fetal growth trajectories.

SENSITIVITY AND SPECIFICITY OF MEASURES OF SMALL FOR GESTATIONAL AGE
Samples of infants classified as small for gestational age will include a higher proportion of growth restricted babies than samples of larger babies but there will always be a balance between sensitivity (proportion of true positives) and specificity (proportion of true negatives). We could increase specificity—that is, increase the proportion of growth restricted babies included in our small for gestational age sample—by making the criteria for defining small more restrictive, for example by defining small for gestational age as <75 per cent of expected birthweight rather than <80 per cent. However, that would also decrease sensitivity by excluding more growth restricted babies from our small for gestational age sample. Intrauterine growth restriction will, of course, be highly correlated with small for gestational age but this is not necessarily adequate for individual categorization in studies of outcomes such as cerebral palsy. Ideally these would require accurate and routinely collected evidence of the presence of intrauterine growth pathology.

NONPATHOLOGICAL DETERMINANTS OF FETAL SIZE
Fetal size has many determinants in addition to duration of gestation. Plurality is clearly important and is usually taken into consideration. Other determinants such as fetal gender, maternal parity and height are often considered in deciding the cut-off for small for gestational age (Rantakallio 1985, Gardosi *et al.* 1992, Pollack and Divon 1992). If all nonpathological determinants of fetal size could be accounted for, any remaining variation would be the result of pathological determinants. We neither know nor can measure all nonpathological determinants of fetal growth, but adjusting for gender, maternal height and parity results in significant reclassification of a high risk group (Kline *et al.* 1989, Sanderson *et al.* 1994, Mongelli and Gardosi 1996, Kingdom *et al.* 1999).

PROBLEMS WITH PRETERM INFANTS
Babies born preterm tend to be smaller than fetuses of the same gestation that continue to term. This means that 'growth' charts based on liveborn populations will underestimate the degree of growth restriction in preterm infants. Growth parameters derived from serial ultrasound measurements of infants delivering at term show that weight increases linearly from about 26 weeks (Marsál *et al.* 1996) and that the familiar sigmoid curve is an artefact that occurs because infants born preterm tend to be smaller for gestational age.

PROBLEMS WITH PERCENTILES
Small for gestational age is a dichotomous variable which does not measure degree of growth restriction and so cannot be used to examine dose–response relationships. Traditionally the position on the birthweight for gestational age distribution has been indicated by percentile position (*e.g.* the 10th percentile), but this measure has several disadvantages. Firstly, percentile estimation is least accurate at the extremes, where accuracy is most important. Secondly, the percentile scale is not linear in respect to the degree of growth restriction. In the centre of the distribution large differences in percentile distribution represent small and clinically insignificant changes in birthweight, while at the extremes small differences in percentile position represent larger and clinically very significant differences in weight.

A BETTER MEASURE OF INTRAUTERINE GROWTH RESTRICTION
To obtain the best possible epidemiological measure of growth restriction, it is preferable to use the ratio of birthweight to the median birthweight for a population of the same gestational age, gender and other nonpathological determinants. This measure has been called 'birthweight ratio', 'individualized/customized birthweight ratio', or 'proportion of expected birthweight'. It is simpler to compute than the deviation from mean or median birthweight in multiples of standard deviations, and less likely than empirically derived standard deviations to be influenced by the proportions of babies with pathological intrauterine growth delivered at the extremes of gestation.

How could cerebral palsy be associated with intrauterine growth restriction?
There are several possible pathways that could explain how cerebral palsy might be related to intrauterine growth restriction (Fig. 8.4).

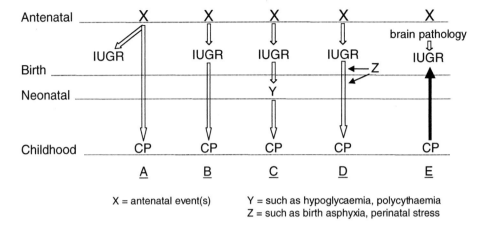

Fig. 8.4. Possible pathways to explain the association between intrauterine growth restriction and cerebral palsy.

A. Do some factors cause both cerebral palsy and poor growth, with poor growth being an epiphenomenon and not on the causal pathway?

B. Is growth restriction, irrespective of aetiology, causally linked to cerebral palsy and the more severe it is the higher is the risk of cerebral palsy?

C. Does intrauterine growth restriction cause conditions such as hypoglycaemia or polycythaemia, which may be responsible for cerebral damage?

D. Are fetuses with growth restriction, irrespective of aetiology, more vulnerable to irreversible brain damage from other factors such as birth asphyxia?

E. Do fetuses already neurologically damaged *in utero* grow poorly (that is does cerebral palsy cause poor growth)?

These questions are important not just for describing the epidemiology of the cerebral palsies but for elucidating possibilities for intervening to prevent the adverse effects, if any, of growth restriction. Clearly important for any planning of preventive action is the identification of the cause(s) represented as 'X' in Figure 8.4.

What are the causes of intrauterine growth restriction?

Growth restriction is heterogeneous with respect to aetiology, time of onset and severity (Kramer *et al.* 1990, Spinillo *et al.* 1993, Blair 1999). Some aetiologies of intrauterine growth restriction such as chromosomal and congenital anomalies are likely to have poor outcomes such as cerebral palsy but the growth restriction *per se* is not responsible for the poor outcome. Although only a small proportion of infants with intrauterine growth restriction have major congenital anomalies, these infants may account for a disproportionate number of poor outcomes; for example, only 6.9 per cent of small for gestational age infants (birthweight <2 SD below mean for gestational age and gender) studied by Ounsted *et al.* (1981) had anomalies, but they accounted for 62 per cent of the deaths.

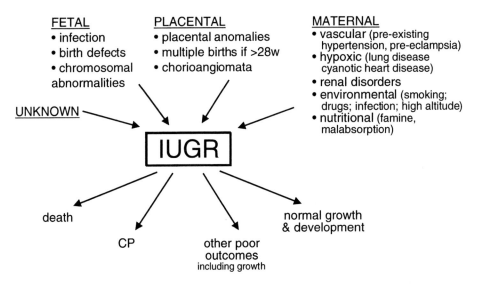

FETAL
- infection
- birth defects
- chromosomal abnormalities

PLACENTAL
- placental anomalies
- multiple births if >28w
- chorioangiomata

MATERNAL
- vascular (pre-existing hypertension, pre-eclampsia)
- hypoxic (lung disease cyanotic heart disease)
- renal disorders
- environmental (smoking; drugs; infection; high altitude)
- nutritional (famine, malabsorption)

UNKNOWN

IUGR

death

CP

other poor outcomes
including growth

normal growth & development

Fig. 8.5. The causes of intrauterine growth restriction.

Causes of intrauterine growth restriction have been divided into fetal, placental and maternal causes (Pollack and Divon 1992, Bernstein and Divon 1997, Gross 1997) (Fig. 8.5). Fetal causes include chromosomal anomalies, inborn errors of metabolism, and infections whether they are viral, bacterial or protozoal. A fetal cause is suggested by the presence of a variety of congenital malformations or dysplasias of the central nervous, cardiovascular, genitourinary, gastrointestinal or skeletal systems. Placental causes may be associated with abnormalities in cord insertion, multiple infarcts, placenta praevia, abruptio placentae, circumvallate placenta, multiple gestation and chorioangiomata, many of which will have their own antecedents. The maternal causes can be nutritional (famine, inflammatory bowel disease, other malabsorption syndromes), hypoxic (severe maternal lung or cyanotic heart disease), vascular (pre-eclampsia, chronic hypertension, other vascular problems), renal disorders, or environmental (such as smoking, drugs, infections).

Kramer (1987) conducted an epidemiologically rigorous review using a meta-analytical approach to estimate the contributions of each determinant of low birthweight in both developed and developing countries, differentiating between intrauterine growth restriction and preterm birth. For example, he reported that anaemia, protein intake and specific vitamin deficiencies were not important determinants of being small for gestational age in developed countries, but that the relevant data were not available in developing countries. However, many factors included in that meta-analysis are not pathological, and some pathological factors well known to restrict growth, such as toxaemia, hypertension and placental problems, were not considered. The methodology needs to be applied to a greater range of factors with careful consideration as to their pathological/nonpathological status, which varies between populations. For example, low maternal height, particularly in developed countries,

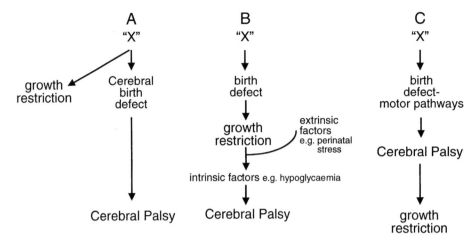

Fig. 8.6. Possible pathways that would explain an association between birth defects, intrauterine growth restriction and cerebral palsy.

may be genetically determined and not pathological, whereas in developing countries it is more likely to result from nutritional deficiencies before maternal growth is completed, and thus be a marker for this pathological determinant.

Some of these very heterogeneous causes are more likely to be directly causally related to cerebral palsy than others. Thus in order to devise preventive strategies we need to look in greater detail at pathways rather than simplistically at the association of intrauterine growth restriction and cerebral palsy.

Which causes of intrauterine growth restriction are also associated with cerebral palsy?
CHROMOSOMAL AND OTHER CONGENITAL ANOMALIES

Biologically plausible pathways by which chromosomal and other congenital anomalies may be related to growth restriction and cerebral palsy are shown in Figure 8.6. Factors such as central nervous system anomalies, other anomalies with the potential to damage the brain such as metabolic errors, maternal rubella and other infections, chromosomal defects and methylmercury exposure are known antecedents of cerebral palsy and are also associated with growth restriction. The role of the growth restriction in pathways to cerebral palsy that include these risk factors is unknown. It may be either an epiphenomenon, as suggested in Figure 8.6 pathway A, or a necessary causal link as shown in pathway B. Pathway C indicates that the motor defect could restrict growth, possibly via reduced muscle development resulting from reduced fetal movement (see p. 96). Births affected by chromosomal anomalies or by a teratogen are often excluded before analysing the small for gestational age subgroups in order to increase the aetiological homogeneity of the remainder. In a case–control study of spastic cerebral palsy, Blair and Stanley (1990) looked at the antenatal risk factors recorded for 24 cases with cerebral palsy and 96 controls who had

TABLE 8.1
Pregnancy induced hypertension and risk of cerebral palsy: odds ratios from various studies*

Study	Maternal disease	Population	Odds ratio (95% CI)
Term or predominantly term infants			
Gaffney *et al.* (1994b)	Pre-eclampsia	Term	2.0 (1.2–3.4)
	Severe pre-eclampsia	Singleton	3.7 (1.4–9.9)
Palmer *et al.* (1995)	Pre-eclampsia	All (case control)	1.2 (0.6–2.1)
Blair (1996c)	Pre-eclampsia	All (total population)	1.6 (1.1–2.5)
Nelson and Ellenberg (1986)	Severe	All	4.0 (2.0–8.1)
Preterm or low birthweight infants			
Topp *et al.* (1997a)	Pre-eclampsia	<37 weeks	0.65 (0.32–1.30)
Stanley and English (1986)	Pregnancy induced hypertension	501–2000 g	No effect
Murphy *et al.* (1995)	Pre-eclampsia	<32 weeks	0.4 (0.2–0.9)
Nelson and Grether (1995)	Pre-eclampsia	<1500 g	0.11 (0.01–2.4)
Spinillo *et al.* (1998)	Pre-eclampsia	24-33 weeks	0.16 (0.04–0.74)

*Adapted from Collins and Paneth (1998).

birthweights below the third percentile and who were born after 33 weeks gestation. None of the 24 cases had a congenital anomaly compared with nine of the 96 controls.

PLACENTAL AND UTERINE ANOMALIES
In their case–control study of spastic cerebral palsy, Blair and Stanley (1990) found that none of the 24 small for gestational age cases had placental or cord anomalies compared with four of the 96 controls, but we know of no other relevant data.

PREGNANCY-INDUCED HYPERTENSION/PRE-ECLAMPSIA
Pregnancy-induced hypertension covers a spectrum of disease and includes hypertension with or without proteinuria (pre-eclamptic toxaemia) and seizures (eclampsia). In series of term or predominantly term born infants, pre-eclampsia is associated with a modest increase in risk of cerebral palsy, and severe pre-eclampsia with a somewhat greater risk (Collins and Paneth 1998) (Table 8.1). In preterm and low birthweight infants no association of cerebral palsy with isolated hypertension, and a negative association with pre-eclampsia have been observed.

This apparently 'protective' effect of pre-eclampsia in infants born very preterm is supported by cranial ultrasound studies that showed a reduced incidence of germinal matrix and intraventricular haemorrhage in infants whose mothers had pre-eclampsia (Kuban *et al.* 1992, Perlman *et al.* 1997). However, given that pre-eclampsia is a major cause of intrauterine growth restriction, which is a most important risk factor for cerebral palsy, it appears biologically implausible that pre-eclampsia would *protect* against cerebral palsy.

In contrast to the very low birthweight cohorts, data from 83 infants born before 32 weeks gestation and dying perinatally showed a strong association between both pre-eclampsia and intrauterine growth restriction and postnatally acquired ischaemic white

TABLE 8.2

Risk of cerebral palsy by pre-eclampsia and gestational age among Western Australian neonatal survivors (NNS) born 1980–1989*

Gestation (weeks)	Pre-eclampsia		No pre-eclampsia		Odds ratio (95% CI)
	CP/NNS	CP risk[1]	CP/NNS	CP risk[1]	
20–27 weeks	0/47	0	25/435	57.47	0.2 (0.0–2.0)
28–32 weeks	13/404	32.18	89/1953	45.57	0.7 (0.4–1.3)
33–36 weeks	9/1893	4.75	51/11,689	4.36	1.1 (0.4–1.3)
≥37 weeks	30/14,700	2.04	290/198,263	1.46	1.4 (1.0–2.0)
All	52/17,044	3.04	455/212,340	2.14	1.4 (1.1–1.9)

[1]Cerebral palsy risk calculated per 1000 neonatal survivors.
*Data from the Western Australia Cerebral Palsy Register.

TABLE 8.3

Distribution of gestational age at delivery in pregnancies with and without pre-eclampsia in Western Australian neonatal survivors born 1980–1989*

Gestational age	Pre-eclampsia %	No pre-eclampsia %	Relative risk
20–27 weeks	0.3	0.2	1.37
28–32 weeks	2.4	0.9	2.57
33–36 weeks	11.1	5.5	2.02
≥37 weeks	85.9	92.9	0.93
	99.7	99.3	

*Data from the Western Australian Midwives Database.

matter damage (Murphy *et al.* 1996b). This smaller study differs from the previous reports principally in that all cases died perinatally and the lesions reported were more severe: it does however suggest the hypothesis that the reduced incidence of cerebral palsy and cerebral lesions among surviving very preterm infants who were chronically compromised (as evidenced by their growth restriction) may arise because they are more likely to die than are equally preterm infants with cerebral lesions who are not chronically compromised.

Data from the Western Australia Cerebral Palsy register and all Western Australian neonatal survivors shows that without stratification by gestational age there is a 43 per cent increase in risk of cerebral palsy with pre-eclampsia (Table 8.2). Since most children are born at term, with or without pre-eclampsia (Table 8.3), this increase is explained primarily by the 40 per cent increase in risk of cerebral palsy in term born infants whose mothers had pre-eclampsia. Moreover, pre-eclampsia leads to preterm birth, primarily as a result of elective deliveries in the interests of the mother and fetus (Savitz *et al.* 1991, Ananth *et al.* 1997).

If very preterm birth is on the causal pathway between pre-eclampsia and cerebral palsy it is not a confounder (see Glossary). In measuring the risk of cerebral palsy associated with pre-eclampsia it is therefore not appropriate to control for gestational age at delivery.

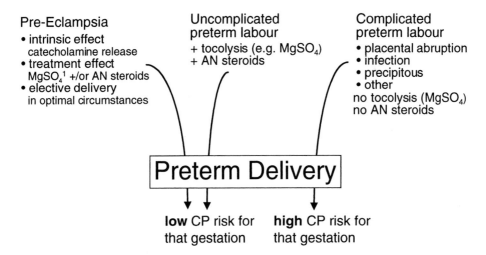

Fig. 8.7. Pathways involving preterm birth and cerebral palsy. Why does pre-eclampsia appear protective against preterm cerebral palsy?

Without adjustment for gestational age, Table 8.2 shows that pre-eclampsia is associated with a 43 per cent, statistically significant *increased* risk of cerebral palsy. Pre-eclampsia does not protect against cerebral palsy and we should not say that it does, particularly in view of possible misinterpretation by journalists and effects on litigation.

Nevertheless it is relevant to ask why very preterm infants born to mothers with pre-eclampsia are less likely to have cerebral palsy than infants of comparable maturity without such a history (Collins and Paneth 1998). Several possible explanations have been suggested:

• Pre-eclampsia may lead to a release of catecholamine which matures the fetus in much the same way as do antenatal steroids (Amiel-Tison and Pettigrew 1991).
• Chronically compromised very preterm infants sustaining postnatal cerebral damage are more likely to die than to survive with impairment (Murphy *et al.* 1996b).
• Antenatal steroids or magnesium sulphate used for prophylaxis or in the management of pre-eclampsia may be neuroprotective (Nelson and Grether 1995, Crowley 1998) (see Chapter 12).
• Elective preterm delivery is usually carried out in optimal circumstances, and caesarean section without labour may avoid inflammatory responses and other situations associated with spontaneous preterm labours, such as infections, preterm prolonged rupture of membranes and precipitate deliveries, which increase cerebral palsy risk (Fig. 8.7).

MULTIPLE BIRTHS
Growth restriction accompanying multiple birth may be associated with cerebral palsy in moderately preterm births (Blair and Stanley 1990). However, intrauterine growth restriction

may be an epiphenomenon of the multiple birth since the association between cerebral palsy and multiple birth could arise by several other mechanisms (see Chapter 10).

INFECTION

The group of congenital infections such as rubella and cytomegalovirus are discussed in Chapter 6. While these TORCH infections (see Glossary) are associated with poor intra-uterine growth, the study of Blair and Stanley (1990) did not suggest that they are important precursors in pathways including poor growth and cerebral palsy, as only one of the 24 small for gestational age cases compared with two out of 96 controls had such infections. Bacterial genital tract infections in very preterm birth pathways are discussed in Chapter 7. While they are strongly implicated in pathways to very preterm birth, there is little evidence that they contribute by restricting growth (Blair and Stanley 1990).

SOCIAL FACTORS

Pathways to growth restriction which commence with social factors include low socioeconomic status, young teenage mother, poor weight gain in pregnancy, inadequate caloric intake and smoking. There is little evidence that any of these are related to cerebral palsy via growth restriction (Lumey 1992, Susser 1994). As DeLong (1993) wrote, "Brain development in humans is remarkably resistant to permanent damage from protein-energy malnutrition." Studies of children born in Holland during the severe famine of 1944–45 show that reduced maternal caloric intake has a marked effect on fetal growth; however, the only psychological or neurological problems observed in any of these children were an increase in neural tube defects and schizophrenia in males exposed to famine *in utero* (Lumey *et al.* 1993). Although the numbers were small, no effects were seen in terms of cerebral palsy or intellectual deficits in spite of marked reductions in birthweight for gestational age, head circumference and ponderal index with second trimester exposure to famine. There was, however, a high perinatal mortality in the birth cohorts exposed to famine and there is a possibility that children who were destined to develop cerebral palsy may have died (Stanley 1997). DeLong (1993) suggested an alternative explanation: "birth weights are decreased in the offspring of mal-nourished mothers, but by a well-known (though poorly understood) adaptive mechanism, brain growth is spared while other organs and body weight and height are reduced. Maternal protein-energy malnutrition appears to produce no permanent neurological or intellectual deficit in the fetus."

Smoking is another socially related factor that restricts fetal growth, but there are few data to ascertain whether it is on any causal pathway to cerebral palsy despite accounting for one-fifth to one-third of small for gestational age births (Kramer 1987). The large Finnish birth cohort (Rantakallio *et al.* 1987) did not report whether the slight increase in disability among infants born to smokers was seen primarily in children classified as small for gestational age.

Studies by Olegård *et al.* (1979) and Holman *et al.* (1996) have associated intrauterine alcohol exposure with growth restriction as well as the cognitive impairment and congenital abnormalities known as fetal alcohol syndrome. Unfortunately, while Olegård *et al.* reported that a birthweight of more than two standard deviations below the mean for gestational age

94

was associated with later cognitive impairment in the 48 affected children, they did not report the birthweight for gestational age of the four children who had cerebral palsy.

HIGH ALTITUDE

While there is considerable evidence of growth restriction amongst those living at higher altitudes (Reed and Stanley 1977), no data exist to suggest that this is associated with cerebral palsy or other neurodevelopmental deficits.

Does intrauterine growth restriction affect the fetus directly?

Is there evidence that growth restriction, irrespective of its origin, is capable of causing neurological damage as suggested in Figure 8.4 pathway B or by direct consequences of growth restriction as suggested in pathway C? No studies have addressed this question rigorously. One of the strongest pieces of evidence would be data showing increasing risk of cerebral palsy with increasing severity of growth restriction. While this is suggested by the correlation between the rate of cerebral palsy and proportion of expected birthweight (Blair and Stanley 1990), it may be confounded if the severity of growth restriction is related to its cause.

There are plausible mechanisms whereby intrauterine growth restriction resulting from deprivation of oxygen or nutrients, from whatever cause, can result in pathology, including hypoxia, fetal heart rate abnormalities, hypoglycaemia, hypocalcaemia, polycythaemia, cerebral lesions and iatrogenic intervention leading to very preterm birth. Postnatally, hypothermia, pulmonary haemorrhage, meconium aspiration, neonatal depression and death have all been described (Allen 1984, Kramer *et al.* 1990). Blair and Stanley (1990) attributed only 4.4 per cent (95% CI 0–25 per cent) of their spastic cerebral palsy cases with birthweights below the 10th centile to hypothermia and 3.7 per cent (0–19 per cent) to hypoglycaemia. Confidence intervals were wide and compatible with a clinically significant proportion following this pathway, but the data really suggest a very modest contribution. Growth restriction may be a relatively benign cause of hypothermia and hypoglycaemia because their associations with spastic cerebral palsy were stronger in appropriately grown infants.

It is harder to find biologically plausible mechanisms by which these pathological states could be associated with restricted growth resulting from chromosomal anomalies, and subjects with chromosomal anomalies are frequently excluded from studies demonstrating these associations (Kramer *et al.* 1990). It may be that the effects of restricted growth resulting from fetal deprivation are independent of the origin of the deprivation but that these effects differ from those of growth restriction resulting from congenital anomalies. Other possible intermediate factors on causal pathways to cerebral palsy include meconium aspiration, hypocalcaemia, polycythaemia leading to cerebral lesions (Gaffney *et al.* 1994b, Burke *et al.* 1997), massive pulmonary haemorrhage and even iatrogenic very preterm birth.

Do some causal pathways from intrauterine growth restriction to cerebral palsy involve additional exposures?

This question addresses pathway D in Figure 8.4. Some researchers suggest that most of the risk of increased cerebral palsy in intrauterine growth restriction comes from an increased vulnerability of the growth restricted infant to other factors, particularly intrapartum stress (Berg 1988, 1989; Taylor and Howie 1989). The idea that the undernourished fetus with low glycogen reserves is less able to withstand the hypoxic stress of labour is plausible, and the role of intrapartum stress in small for gestational age outcomes has been investigated in several studies. Dijxhoorn *et al.* (1987) found that indicators of antepartum stress were better predictors of neonatal neurological morbidity than those of intrapartum stress and concluded that intrapartum stress did not substantially increase the risk of neurological morbidity associated with being small for gestational age. Blair and Stanley (1990) came to the same conclusion, estimating that while 22 per cent of spastic cerebral palsy cases could be attributed to being below 10th centile birthweight, only 2 per cent could be attributed to the combination of small for gestational age and intrapartum hypoxia. Uvebrant and Hagberg (1992) concluded that small for gestational age infants were at lower risk of cerebral palsy as a result of intrapartum hypoxia than were appropriate for gestational age infants. In contrast, Kyllerman (1982), Berg (1988) and Taylor and Howie (1989) found that only small for gestational age infants who exhibited signs of intrapartum stress were at increased risk of childhood neurological morbidity or dystonic cerebral palsy. However, the clinical criteria for intrapartum stress were low Apgar scores (Kyllerman 1982), requirement for resuscitation, cord knots or placenta praevia (Berg 1988), which may well be either the cause or the result of chronic stress and are not specific to intrapartum stress (Blair and Stanley 1990).

An association of intrauterine growth restriction and intrapartum stress with cerebral palsy might be explained by a reduced ability to compensate for intrapartum hypoxia and earlier decompensation. Another explanation is that the factors which purport to measure intrapartum stress, such as apnoea, cyanosis or the need for resuscitation, could be the result of abnormalities present prior to delivery (Chapter 6). Thus, rather than intrapartum stress being a cause of the damage, the clinical signs used to define it may be the first indications of prior damage (Berg 1988). If so, the intrapartum signs may in part be distinguishing the relatively normal infants with growth restriction from those who are *already* irreversibly compromised. Until we get better measures of intrapartum stress and brain damage, epidemiologists will not be able to work out these pathways satisfactorily.

Is there evidence for cerebral palsy causing growth restriction *in utero*?

The underlying mechanism being considered here, shown in Figure 8.4 pathway E and, for birth defects, Figure 8.6 pathway C, is that children whose motor centres are impaired *in utero*, regardless of cause, do not subsequently grow as quickly as normal fetuses. A reduced amount of, or less energetic, movement could cause poorer development of muscle mass. Ferrari *et al.* (1990) studied spontaneous early postnatal movements of very preterm infants with and without cerebral lesions. All but one of 29 infants with cerebral lesions (19 of whom went on to develop cerebral palsy) were classified as having abnormal general movements, but there was no difference in the quantity of movement. This is supported by antenatal observations of anencephalic fetuses (Visser *et al.* 1986). The quantity of fetal movement in anencephalic fetuses was little different to normal fetuses, but the movements were jerky, larger and more forceful, so that the greater accelerations involved might be anticipated to increase rather than decrease muscle mass development. Therefore, while growth restriction due to fetal deprivation is associated with a slight decrease in quantity of general movements (Bekedam *et al.* 1985), antenatal cerebral lesions do not appear to reduce fetal movements and lead to growth restriction by this means.

Conclusions and unanswered questions about growth restriction *in utero* and cerebral palsy

In order to devise rational strategies to prevent cerebral palsy associated with growth restriction, we need rigorous answers to the following questions:

- How much of the association between growth restriction and the cerebral palsies is related to early pregnancy factors, such as malformations or viral infections, which interfere with development of organs including the brain and for which the growth restriction is an epiphenomenon?
- Do causal pathways to cerebral palsy that include intrauterine growth restriction resulting from fetal deprivation always involve perinatal stress?
- What criteria, including cause, determine the optimal timing of delivery for the growth restricted fetus (GRIT Study Group 1996)?

In summary, growth restriction has been associated with an increase in the risk of cerebral palsy in term and moderately preterm infants, and the risk increases with degree of birthweight deficit. However, the underlying mechanisms are not clear. Since cerebral palsy is rare, the majority of small for gestational age infants do not have cerebral palsy except at the extremes of viability. It is intuitively appealing to differentiate between different aetiologies of restricted growth when studying its sequelae, and this may be appropriate for malformations and infections of the central nervous system.

As Allen (1984) stated, "the time has come for us to look beyond the SGA classification and separate this heterogeneous group into more meaningful groupings based on etiology, timing of the insult, perinatal complications, and other pertinent, and perhaps as yet unknown, characteristics."

However, different aetiologies may also be associated with differences in timing of onset and severity of restriction, timing of delivery and social factors (Nelson and Ellenberg 1986b, Blair 1999).

9
PATHWAYS TO CEREBRAL PALSY INVOLVING SIGNS OF BIRTH ASPHYXIA

At the time of writing the 1984 book, birth asphyxia was believed to be an important and obstetrically preventable cause of cerebral palsy. This belief underpinned much of the justification for the rapid expansion in the use of electronic fetal monitoring in labour and of increasing caesarean section rates (Nelson 1988; Stanley and Chalmers 1989; Niswander 1991; Stanley and Blair 1991, 1994; Nelson and Emery 1993; Stanley 1994a,b, 1995; Blair 1996b; Nelson et al. 1996). This was so firmly entrenched that researchers and clinicians were discouraged from looking at other possible causal pathways or even examining the concept of birth asphyxia. Few thought of the possibility that the clinical signs from which birth asphyxia was inferred could be part of causal pathways that commenced well before labour.

Evidence available from several epidemiological studies suggests that about 10 per cent of cerebral palsy in developed countries is now associated with intrapartum events (Nelson and Ellenberg 1986a; Blair and Stanley 1988; Nelson 1988, 1989; Nelson and Emery 1993; Kuban and Leviton 1994; Stanley 1995; Yudkin et al. 1995; Nelson et al. 1996; Roland and Hill 1997). These studies attempted to identify those cases of cerebral palsy who had observations compatible with severe intrapartum asphyxia but no obvious antenatal risk factors or antecedents likely to have caused brain damage prior to labour. Even though intrapartum factors are less important than originally thought, we must not, as Henderson-Smart (1991) wrote "[throw] the baby out with the fetal monitoring". Ten per cent is more than has been attributed to most other individual causes of cerebral palsy, and there may remain some intrapartum causes that are obstetrically preventable (Blair 1996b). The proportions attributable to intrapartum causes may be higher in developing countries and may also have been greater in the past (Little 1862, Blair 1996b) (see Chapter 4).

What is birth asphyxia?
A critical reading of the literature of birth asphyxia makes it clear that, like intrauterine growth retardation, birth asphyxia is a theoretical concept, and its existence in a patient is not easy to recognize accurately by clinical observation.

The concept of birth asphyxia is that the fetus is deprived of oxygen during the process of labour and that this hypoxia has an irreversible and detrimental effect on function. Both hypoxia and sequelae are necessary for the concept of asphyxia. The cellular and physiological responses to excessive hypoxia have been intensively investigated in animals experimentally deprived of oxygen (Gluckman and Williams 1992, Williams et al. 1993, Edwards and Mehmet 1996) and follow the sequence shown in Figure 9.1.

Birth asphyxia: Events that are clinically observable but nonspecific

| Reduced fetal growth | Fetal heart rate abnormality | Metabolic acidosis | Low Apgar scores | Abnormal conscious state | Altered muscle tone | Seizures |

Birth asphyxia: Sequence of pathogenic cellular events that are not measurable

Impaired gas exchange $\longrightarrow$ 1° energy failure $\longrightarrow$ Cytotoxic neuronal death $\longrightarrow$ 2° energy failure $\longrightarrow$ Apoptotic neuronal death

Fig. 9.1. Two concepts of 'birth asphyxia': fundamental but unmeasurable pathogenic sequence, and observable but nonspecific clinical signs. (Adapted from Blair 1993.)

Animal and some human evidence supports the concept of two phases of neuronal cell death following acute intrapartum hypoxic insult in those who are resuscitated and survive. Initial neuronal necrosis occurs during the hypoxic phase, and delayed apoptosis (programmed cell death) follows hours or even days later (Gluckman and Williams 1992, Roth *et al.* 1992, Edwards and Mehmet 1996). The delayed effects are not dependent upon continuing hypoxia nor do they seem to be related to intracellular acidosis. The severity of the permanent damage resulting in later neurological impairment appears to be correlated with the severity of this secondary phase of hypoxic reaction (Edwards *et al.* 1998). A range of mechanisms may be inducing this inappropriate apoptosis in neurons, such as interference with receptors, activation of genes and effects of tumour necrosis factor (du Plessis and Johnston 1997, Hetts 1998). Hypothermia seems to be a powerful inhibitor of apoptosis and this may have therapeutic implications (see Chapter 12).

The scientific study of birth asphyxia in the human fetus and its role in cerebral palsy is enormously challenging for many reasons (Nelson 1988, MacLennan *et al.* 1995, Goodlin 1996, Low 1997). Both the postulated exposure and the outcome are multifactorial and rare, and there are many possible confounders, but the inability to measure birth asphyxia is the most challenging of all. The variety of observations described collectively as *intrapartum fetal distress* is an attempt to describe the clinical associations of the sequence of cellular events occurring in asphyxiated fetuses during labour (Fig. 9.1). However, these clinical signs cannot yet be precisely matched to our theoretical knowledge of the cellular events, such as level of cerebral oxygenation, primary and secondary neuronal cell death and compensatory cerebral metabolism. Researchers and clinicians have therefore devised a variety of secondary measures to identify fetuses and neonates with neuronal damage that may have resulted from intrapartum hypoxia. These measures are of questionable validity. This confusion in terminology between *birth asphyxia* (theoretical concept) and *signs compatible with birth asphxia* (clinical observations) may account for much of the confusion in trying to link birth asphyxia and cerebral palsy. Intrapartum and neonatal signs compatible with but not specific to birth asphyxia include fetal distress in the intrapartum period (such as meconium stained liquor), intrapartum and immediate postnatal metabolic acidosis, neonatal encephalopathy and neonatal renal, cardiac and respiratory dysfunction.

New techniques using near infra-red (NIRS) and magnetic resonance spectroscopy (MRS) can measure fetal cerebral oxygenation during labour and may detect deranged brain energy metabolism postnatally. They suggest that normal labour and vaginal delivery induces considerable hypoxia which the healthy fetus appears to be able to withstand without lasting adverse effects (N. Robertson, personal communication 1998). These tools are still being developed but have already been used in neonates with intrapartum problems to chart the progression of brain pathology and cerebral metabolism. They have not yet contributed to epidemiological studies of either neonatal encephalopathy (see Glossary) or cerebral palsy.

Defining birth asphyxia for epidemiological studies

Before accepting a diagnosis of birth asphyxia, evidence is required of the presence of (1) hypoxia; followed by (2) decompensatory fetal response(s) indicating that the severity of hypoxia has exceeded the adaptive capacity of the fetus; (3) neonatal encephalopathy; and (4) a probable causal link between the encephalopathy and the hypoxia. This probability is enhanced if there is no evidence of a preexisting neurological deficit. Such evidence includes a history of teratogenic, infectious or other major antenatal risk factors for cerebral palsy or early imaging evidence of a long-standing lesion such as cystic changes present at birth or a neuronal migration disorder (see Chapter 6). Further evidence of birth asphyxia is the type and timing of onset of neonatal encephalopathy. That due to intrapartum asphyxia usually begins immediately, at least on the first day of life, with prolonged low Apgar scores, and differs from the encephalopathy known to be due to some other causes.

A major problem is that in the absence of direct evidence of hypoxia, its presence is sometimes inferred from the fetal or neonatal response, such as low Apgar scores, or the outcome, such as an altered conscious state (Fig. 9.1). This leads to a circular argument, when the outcome, neonatal encephalopathy, is used as evidence of exposure to intrapartum hypoxia. Several studies have actually reported positive associations between neonatal encephalopathy and hypoxia–ischaemia using such criteria (Finer *et al.* 1981, Ergander *et al.* 1983, Levene *et al.* 1985, Leviton and Nelson 1992, Badawi *et al.* 1997).

THE ROLE OF NEONATAL ENCEPHALOPATHY

The highest rate of cerebral palsy in term infants in the US National Collaborative Perinatal Project was observed in children who had all the combination of low Apgar scores, neonatal signs and neonatal seizures (Ellenberg and Nelson 1988, Nelson and Emery 1993). "Low Apgar score–abnormal signs–seizures constituted a cluster of events that served to identify, within the first days of life, a tiny subgroup of term newborn infants in whom risk for chronic motor disability was 55%, and for death or disability was 70%" (Ellenberg and Nelson 1988) (Table 9.1). Once these neonatal characteristics were taken into account, the occurrence of obstetric complications added no further predictive information, suggesting that essentially all children in whom intrapartum factors were part of the causal pathway to cerebral palsy

TABLE 9.1
**Predicted risk of cerebral palsy, percentage of population in each risk group, and
percentage of cerebral palsy contributed***

Early characteristics			Predicted risk[1] CP/1000	Children in risk group (%)	Cases of CP in risk group (%)
Low Apgar score	Neonatal signs	Neonatal seizures			
No	No	No	1.3	90.1	62.7
Yes	No	No	2.9	0.9	1.3
No	No	Yes	1.3	0.06	0.0
Yes	No	Yes	2.9	0.01	0.0
No	Yes	No	3.2	8.1	13.3
Yes	Yes	No	7.0	0.7	2.7
No	Yes	Yes	96.8	0.08	4.0
Yes	Yes	Yes	545.5	0.06	16.0

[1]Predicted risk based on multiple logistic model with Apgar score, presence or absence of neonatal
signs, and neonatal seizures, and their interactions, as predictor variables.
*Adapted by permission from Ellenberg and Nelson (1988).

were identified through manifestations of neonatal neurological abnormality. This pathway
has been confirmed in other studies (Fenichel 1983; Hey 1985; Levene *et al.* 1985, 1986;
Towbin 1986; Paneth 1993; Low *et al.* 1994; Yudkin *et al.* 1994). "In general, indicators
of birth asphyxia that do not include neurological findings are poor predictors of cerebral
palsy" (Paneth 1993).

Like all other signs compatible with intrapartum asphyxia, neonatal encephalopathy
has other possible causes (Adamson *et al.* 1995, Badawi *et al.* 1998c) and is not inevitably
followed by cerebral palsy (Robertson and Finer 1985). When studying neonatal encephalopathy it is very important not to use it as a surrogate marker for asphyxia or for later cerebral
palsy. Like cerebral palsy, encephalopathy is a heterogeneous condition (Nelson and Leviton
1991, Adamson *et al.* 1995, Badawi *et al.* 1998c) comprising many syndromes, some of
which are pathways to cerebral palsy.

Defining antecedents or causes of birth asphyxia
Certain factors which may on occasion be early signs of cerebral palsy are commonly
assumed to be antecedents or causes. These include intrapartum complications such as
abnormal fetal heart rate traces on electronic fetal monitoring; meconium stained liquor;
and malpresentation such as persistent occipitoposterior or breech regardless of method of
delivery (Nelson and Ellenberg 1986a). Other possible early signs of an antenatally
compromised fetus or of cerebral palsy, such as delay to the onset of respiration, low Apgar
scores, seizures, central apnoea or poor suck, may also be assumed to be causes. Later
neonatal factors, such as ultrasound evidence of periventricular leukomalacia (PVL) or
porencephaly, represent the pathological basis of the neurological damage which will lead
to the label of cerebral palsy, yet they have also been included as predictors of cerebral
palsy. What is needed is to understand the causal pathway to the fetal compromise and the
signs of the resulting cerebral damage (Paneth 1993, Prechtl 1997).

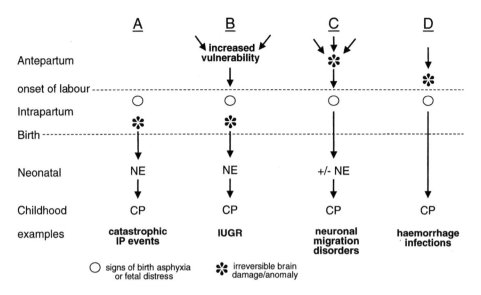

Fig. 9.2. Possible pathways to cerebral palsy with signs of birth asphyxia.

With these problems of accurately ascertaining the existence of birth asphyxia, many individuals and professional groups have recommended that the term birth asphyxia be dropped as it cannot be measured or defined clinically (Blair 1993, Nelson and Emery 1993, American College of Obstetrics and Gynecology Committee on Obstetric Practice 1994). Instead each clinical observation relevant to hypoxia, which may include a sentinel event such as uterine rupture, or to intrapartum decompensatory fetal responses, neonatal encephalopathy, neurological function before labour, or the existence of any other pertinent factors should be recorded. The best estimate of whether birth asphyxia occurred and the avoidance of circular arguments can only be made when all this evidence is available.

Karin Nelson has summarized this well: "I know of no signs of fetal compromise specific to asphyxia and few that are any good in general. Essentially all the clinical signs commonly taken to mean 'birth asphyxia', including acidosis, multiple organ failure, and encephalopathy with seizures, can arise from other disorders such as maternal infection. Misattribution is easy" (K. Nelson, personal communication 1997).

How could signs of birth asphyxia be associated with cerebral palsy?
Possible causal pathways which could involve asphyxia are shown in Figure 9.2. This figure raises a number of questions:
- Can we currently identify pathways from intrapartum asphyxia due to a catastrophic intrapartum event to cerebral palsy in fetuses who were normal before the onset of labour (pathway A in Figure 9.2)? Such events include prolapsed cord, massive intrapartum haemorrhage, uterine rupture and maternal shock, such as a cardiac arrest. What are the antecedents of these catastrophic intrapartum events? Could they be prevented?

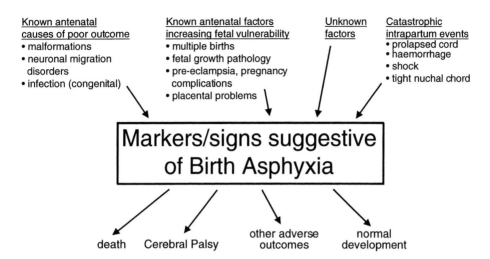

Fig. 9.3. Likely antecedents of signs of 'birth asphyxia' or intrapartum 'fetal distress'.

- Are there antenatal factors such as growth restriction, maternal disease or infection which increase the vulnerability of the fetal brain to intrapartum hypoxia (pathway B)?
- Do pathways which include signs compatible with birth asphyxia but with known prenatal brain damage always involve neonatal encephalopathy (pathway C)?
- Do cerebral structural anomalies cause signs of birth asphyxia during and after delivery (pathway C)?
- Can other antenatally acquired cerebral deficits such as those resulting from ascending bacterial infection or intracranial haemorrhage mimic signs of birth asphyxia (pathway D)?

The answers to these questions will be extremely important in the formulation of preventive policies appropriate to each of these situations.

What causes the signs of birth asphyxia?

Figure 9.3 shows the variety of situations and conditions which may lead to signs of 'birth asphyxia' or 'intrapartum fetal distress' being observed in the term fetus or newborn child. Surprisingly there are few studies of total birth populations that describe the antecedents of signs of fetal distress or birth asphyxia using good epidemiological methods (Adamson *et al.* 1995, Badawi *et al.* 1997). We postulate that only rarely are these signs due solely to intrapartum events occurring in a normal fetus after an uneventful pregnancy and that the majority are associated with problems arising before labour and delivery. Some possible pathways are described below.

Which causes are on a pathway to cerebral palsy?

This section discusses the evidence for the occurrence of each of the pathways shown in Figure 9.3.

MALFORMATIONS AND NEURONAL MIGRATION DISORDERS

Malformations and neuronal migration disorders are discussed in Chapter 6. There is now considerable evidence that signs compatible with birth asphyxia, including neonatal enceph-alopathy, are likely to occur in infants who have these brain anomalies (Nelson and Leviton 1991, Paneth 1993, Evrard *et al.* 1997, Grant and Barkovich 1997).

MULTIPLE BIRTH

There are several antenatal problems specific to multiple births that may result in signs of fetal distress in labour. It has also been believed that multiple births are at greater risk of intrapartum complications, particularly the second or later born children. However, there are factors which may confound these observations, as discussed in Chapter 10.

INTRAUTERINE GROWTH RESTRICTION AND OTHER PREGNANCY COMPLICATIONS

Intrauterine growth restriction, from whatever cause, may increase the vulnerability to intrapartum hypoxia (Fig. 9.2, pathway B). This vulnerability could result from insufficient substrates or reserves in the fetus for it to mount adequate compensatory responses and is discussed further in Chapter 8.

Pathways involving other pregnancy complications, such as maternal thyroid disease, are discussed in Chapter 6.

PLACENTAL PROBLEMS

The placenta is a veritable storehouse of information pertaining to events and conditions in pregnancy, including infection and others described below. However, relatively little work has yet been done to determine to what extent placental examination can elucidate aetiological pathways to cerebral palsy.

Placental infarcts

Beebe *et al.* (1996) studied placental infarcts, as morphological markers of reduced utero-placental blood flow, and found that they were significantly associated with prenatal cerebral ischaemic lesions in a large autopsy study. Placental infarcts were not associated with spas-tic cerebral palsy in the Western Australian case–control study of 183 cases (Blair and Stanley 1993a), but retrospective studies cannot apply the rigorous protocols for placental examination necessary to study the possibility of an association.

Antepartum haemorrhage

Chronic placental abruption with first and second trimester bleeding, extensive marginal damage to the placenta and haemosiderin in the membranes and chorionic plate is a relatively straightforward pathological diagnosis suggesting early pregnancy problems which could have interfered with neuronal migration and resulted in cases of cerebral palsy (H. Chambers, personal communication 1998). However, antepartum haemorrhage does not feature prominently in aetiological studies of cerebral palsy. It is not mentioned in reports from the Swedish Register (Hagberg *et al.* 1996). The NCPP cohort study found an association only with third trimester bleeding, which was present in 22 per cent of cases of cerebral palsy compared with 13.7 per cent of the total population (Nelson and Ellenberg 1986a). In contrast, the Western Australian study of spastic cerebral palsy found that third trimester bleeding was protective against cerebral palsy (odds ratio 0.27, 95% CI 0.1–0.8) but that severe mid-trimester haemorrhage was significantly positively associated. While the association was strong (odds ratio 5.2, 95% CI 0.8–34) it was found in only four of 183 cases (three of whom were born before 30 weeks gestation) and four of 549 controls (Blair and Stanley 1993a). Three of the four cases had placental anomalies and two had more than one severe bleed, while none of the four controls had either factor. Torfs *et al.* (1990) found premature separation of the placenta (without specifying gestation or severity of bleed) in four of 41 cases of cerebral palsy compared with 1.4% of controls, giving a relative risk of 7.6 (95% CI 2.7–21).

The lack of standardized criteria for this factor is obvious and may be responsible for the conflicting reports. However, the risk associated with antepartum haemorrhage may not be confined to early haemorrhage nor to very preterm births. For further discussion of antepartum haemorrhage, preterm birth and cerebral palsy, see Chapter 7.

Chronic hypoxic stress
Chronic hypoxic stress may be suggested by examination of the placenta (Redline 1995). Phelan *et al.* (1995) describe an association between abnormally high numbers of nucleated red blood cells in cord blood and long-term neurological impairment. The highest levels of nucleated red blood cells were found in infants with evidence of the most recent and most severe hypoxic stress. Their rate of disappearance was also faster with more recent injury (Phelan *et al.* 1998). These observations suggest that measurement of nucleated red blood cell concentrations over time may be helpful in timing recent fetal hypoxic damage, though Korst *et al.* (1996) have pointed out problems with this conclusion.

Fetal thrombotic vasculopathy
Thrombi in fetal stem arteries suggest a fetal hypercoagulable state. This may be associated with maternal antiphospholipid antibodies or hereditary deficiencies in coagulation and is likely to predispose to fetal cerebral injury (Redline and Pappin 1995, Kraus 1997, Debus *et al.* 1998). While significant associations between avascular villi (a putative marker of a fetal vascular thrombotic event) and various adverse perinatal outcomes, such as ECG abnormalities and intrauterine growth restriction, have been seen in a very small study (J. Kingdom, personal communication 1998), it needs to be replicated with larger numbers (see also Chapter 6).

Reports of placental pathology may be used to challenge claims of intrapartum mismanagement on the grounds that preexisting pathology makes it less likely that alternative management would have be able to prevent brain damage (Williams and Lucci 1990, Redline 1995). However, while associations between long-term adverse neurodevelopmental sequelae and various chronic placental lesions have been reported (Benirschke 1994, Redline 1995), placental pathology would be more useful in the elucidation of aetiological pathways if placental lesions were more accurately defined using standardized terminology (Beebe *et al.* 1996).

Pathway A in Figure 9.2 is the mechanism that has traditionally been assumed to occur in the aetiology of cerebral palsy. Clinically, intrapartum electronic fetal heart rate monitoring is most often used to diagnose impending asphyxia and to guide interventions. Electronic fetal monitoring has been shown by randomized trial to be ineffective in reducing the occurrence of later cerebral palsy (Lumley 1988; Grant *et al.* 1989; MacDonald 1996a,b; Nelson *et al.* 1996). Nonetheless, a recent review suggested that fetal monitoring had prevented birth asphyxial deaths, disputed the evidence from randomized trials, and ignored the possibility that these monitoring abnormalities may be signs of a previously damaged infant (Spencer 1998).

Inter- and intraobserver variability in interpretation of the traces is a major problem now increasingly being acknowledged (Spencer *et al.* 1997). Not only do different obstetricians interpret the same heart rate patterns differently, but when reassessing a trace *blinded* to their previous assessment, they do not agree with themselves more often than by chance (Spencer *et al.* 1997). Using such an unreliable tool to guide decisions about interventions to avoid brain damage from birth asphyxia has resulted in very expensive litigation and a crisis in obstetric care (Freeman 1990, Stanley and Blair 1991, Stanley *et al.* 1994, Stanley 1994b, Nelson *et al.* 1996).

The catastrophic intrapartum events most likely to cause acute fetal asphyxia are a prolapsed cord, massive intrapartum haemorrhage, prolonged or traumatic delivery due to cephalopelvic disproportion or abnormal presentation, a large baby with shoulder dystocia, or maternal shock from a variety of causes including uterine rupture, infection, cardiac complications or trauma.

Nelson and Grether (1998) reported a study where the obstetric records of cerebral palsy cases without evidence of prenatal damage, and of controls, were searched for potentially asphyxiating events by researchers blinded to the outcome. Such events were 12 times more common in cases of spastic quadriplegia than in controls, a tight nuchal cord being the most common, although placental abruption was also reported. The authors did not rule out the possibility that where babies were in a poor condition at birth the presence of a tight nuchal cord was more likely to have been noted. However, they suggested that if the potentially asphyxiating conditions they found were sufficient causes for the cerebral palsy, they would account for approximately 6 per cent of total cerebral palsy in children with a birthweight ≥2500 g, 13 per cent of otherwise unexplained cerebral palsy and 43 per cent of otherwise unexplained spastic quadriplegia. The incidence, mortality and long-term neurological morbidity associated with umbilical cord prolapse were studied by linking the Oxford obstetric data on 56,283 births to their Register of Early Childhood Impairments (Murphy and MacKenzie 1995). The incidence of cord prolapse was 2.3 per 1000 births, with 9 per cent perinatal mortality, but only one baby died from birth asphyxia. The other deaths were due to lethal malformations, placental abruption and extreme preterm birth. Only one child who was delivered very preterm by caesarean section had cerebral palsy at 3 years of age. Thus, in spite of their high risk, neonates born after cord prolapse do not die from asphyxia or have poor neurological outcomes as often as might be expected, particularly in centres with good obstetric care.

There is some evidence that occurrence of cerebral palsy and perinatal mortality is associated with levels of care assessed by obstetricians as poor. A case–control study from Oxford (Gaffney *et al.* 1994a) showed that there was a relationship between suboptimal care and abnormal fetal outcome, although Blair (1996a) has suggested that the role of obstetric care may have been somewhat overestimated. This relationship was stronger for perinatal death than for cerebral palsy and, in confirmation of previous estimates, probably affected less than 10 per cent of all cases of term cerebral palsy. The problem with any observational study like this is that it is a *post hoc* attempt to evaluate the impact of care, and one can never be sure that the association of poor care and cerebral palsy is not due to some common confounding factor.

SORTING OUT THE DIFFERENT ANTECEDENTS AND PATHWAYS
Unless there is an extraordinary intrapartum event (Fig. 9.2, pathway A), only the unusually vulnerable fetus will be neurologically damaged by intrapartum hypoxia (pathway B). However, evidence suggesting that a fetus is vulnerable is also compatible with preexisting neurological damage. What is difficult to determine in any individual case is whether birth asphyxia is the irreversible brain damaging event (pathway B) or whether preceding factors were important in influencing either the birth asphyxial conditions or the fetal response to them (pathway C).

In a few cases, *in utero* or early neonatal cranial imaging has confirmed a cerebral anomaly such as porencephaly or hydrocephalus prior to delivery. In such cases, whether the origin is genetic (*e.g.* lissencephaly), developmental (*e.g.* abnormal neuronal migration due to CMV) or vascular (*e.g.* twin to twin transfusion syndrome), there can be no doubt of prior cerebral damage (pathways C or D), although it is possible that the stresses of labour may exacerbate the damage. More usually, the relevant imaging was not performed, and the likelihood of prior neuronal damage can only be suggested from the presence of factors which may also increase the vulnerability of the fetus to hypoxic stress (pathway B).

Conclusions
The 'traditional' pathway of fetal heart rate abnormalities, as measured by electronic monitoring in labour, followed by a 'suboptimal' obstetric response (not expediting delivery), birth asphyxia, neonatal encephalopathy and cerebral palsy does not occur for most cases of cerebral palsy. Even where clinical signs are suggestive it is impossible to prove.

In the 1970s obstetricians suggested that if the sequence was altered by making care more 'optimal' (which they defined as emergency caesarean section for abnormalities on the electronic fetal monitor) then the cerebral palsy would be avoided (Quilligan and Paul 1975). The major effects of electronic monitoring of the fetal heart in labour are an increase in caesarean section rates and a reduced rate of neonatal seizures; it has had no impact on the rates of cerebral palsy (Stanley and Watson 1992, Nelson *et al.* 1996). This may be because few cases of cerebral palsy result from this pathway. Even those cases in which brain damage is caused by excessive intrapartum hypoxia, clinical signs sufficient to warrant emergency caesarean section may only be recognizable after the damage is done. And of course caesarean section may not be the 'optimal' response.

Getting this sequence so markedly out of perspective has had adverse effects both on obstetrics and on disabled people and their families. It is thus very important that epidemiology delivers better information to guide perinatal interventions in the future—the major reason for the proper elucidation of causal pathways.

Birth asphyxia is a theoretical concept implying a causal relationship between hypoxia in labour and lasting neurological damage. There are no clinical observations specific to birth asphyxia, and a definitive diagnosis is not possible. The best criteria currently available are outlined in an international consensus statement (MacLennan *et al.* 1999). Ideally these require full antenatal, intrapartum and neonatal histories, of which the antenatal history is the most likely to be incomplete. Examination of the placenta may well provide valuable information about intrauterine pathology which may affect fetal responses to labour (as well as contributing to intrauterine growth restriction—see Chapter 8—and very preterm birth— see Chapter 7). Placental pathologists are now developing standard placental examinations and classifications to facilitate the prediction of normal and abnormal pregnancy outcomes (Benirschke 1994, Redline 1995, Beebe *et al.* 1996). Representative samples of placentae must be made available for study. Randomized controlled trials of interventions to rescue asphyxiated infants (see Chapter 12) await the development of accurate methods of recognizing and timing asphyxial events.

In developed countries, in the late 20th century it has been estimated that intrapartum events are responsible for about 10 per cent of cerebral palsy, but this estimate must be conjectural given the difficulties in accurately recognizing birth asphyxia. Methodological problems make similar estimates in developing countries and in previous epochs even harder, but they are likely to be significantly greater. It is likely that:

(a) Birth asphyxia may not currently be as important in the aetiology of the cerebral palsies as previously thought, quite possibly because it is no longer responsible for as large a proportion as it may previously have been.

(b) Neonatal signs of birth asphyxia, such as difficulty in initiating and maintaining respiration and abnormal neonatal neurological signs such as seizures, may be early manifestations of cerebral palsy from a variety of causes, of which birth asphyxia is only one.

(c) The majority of children with cerebral palsy who have signs compatible with birth asphyxia probably had some antenatal insult or condition that either was the cause of their impairment or made them particularly vulnerable to birth events.

(d) Infants neurologically damaged by intrapartum hypoxia may not have fared better even if they had received alternative obstetric care.

10
THE SPECIAL CASE OF MULTIPLE PREGNANCY

A pregnancy carrying more than one fetus is referred to as a multiple pregnancy. Multiple pregnancy can result from the fertilization of a single ovum which divides (monozygotic) or from the fertilization of more than one ovum (polyzygotic). The proportion of pregnancies that are multiple, and whether they are mono- or polyzygotic, varies with factors such as maternal age, parity, nutritional status, genetic constitution, and whether they were the result of infertility treatment. The rate of monozygotic twinning is relatively constant at around 3–4 per 1000 pregnancies, but the population rate of spontaneous and nonspontaneous dizygotic twinning is more variable, ranging from 3–40 per 1000 pregnancies. This means that when making international comparisons, allowance must be made for geographical variations in the rate of multiple birth and type of zygosity. The highest rates of twin births have been observed in Nigeria where only 5 per cent were monochorionic (necessarily monozygotic) and the lowest in Japan, where more than 60 per cent were monochorionic (Derom *et al.* 1995).

Since the 1980s the proportion of multiple pregnancies has risen within developed countries. This has been attributed in part to a natural increase in multiple rates (James 1997) and to the increase in mean maternal age as more mothers are delaying child bearing. However, the widespread use of fertility enhancing drugs and the rapid development of therapies for infertility is primarily responsible for the increase, particularly of higher order multiple pregnancies (Derom *et al.* 1995, Dunn and Macfarlane 1996, Westergaard *et al.* 1997). Assisted reproduction results principally in higher rates of polyzygotic pregnancy, although the incidence of monozygotic multiples is also increased slightly (Derom *et al.* 1987). In Western Australia during the 1980s, the simultaneous replacement of several zygotes after *in vitro* fertilization (IVF) contributed to rising rates of multiple pregnancy. Figure 10.1 shows that in the early 1990s, the rate of triplet pregnancy dropped, perhaps because growing awareness of the problems associated with multiple pregnancy led to the Reproductive Technology Accreditation Committee recommendation that no more than three embryos be replaced in any one cycle (Watson *et al.* 1996). Subsequently this was legislated for in the Human Rights Act of 1991.

The rate of cerebral palsy is higher among births following multiple pregnancy (Petterson *et al.* 1990, 1998). This association fits all the traditional criteria for a step in a causal path. It rises with the number of fetuses carried, thus showing a 'dose' response, and the association of cerebral palsy with multiple pregnancy is strong and consistent. Multiple pregnancies are associated with poor intrauterine growth, preterm delivery, birth defects and intrapartum

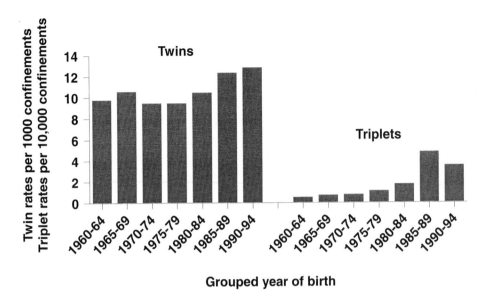

Fig. 10.1. Twinning rates per 1000 confinements and triplet rates per 10.000 confinements in Western Australia, 1960–1994.

complications, all of which are associated with cerebral palsy in singletons. However, these factors do not entirely account for the increased prevalence of cerebral palsy, which is contributed to by other problems specific to multiple pregnancy, including the intrauterine death of a co-fetus.

The increasing survival of preterm and very low birthweight babies (see Chapter 4), together with increasing rates of multiple pregnancy are responsible for an increase in the proportion of children with cerebral palsy attributable to multiple pregnancy (Petterson *et al.* 1993a). Their study is facilitated by the fact that the majority are identifiable in even rudimentary perinatal data sets, but multiple births raise new methodological issues and demonstrate unique causal pathways. These facts and the preventive possibilities secondary to their association with fertility treatments justify their consideration in a separate chapter.

Epidemiology
METHODOLOGICAL CONSIDERATIONS SPECIFIC TO MULTIPLE GESTATION
Units
The most evident problem is that the number of births (individuals) is greater than the number of pregnancies. The research objective will determine the optimal choice of units: *confinements* when considering antenatal care or *individuals* when considering outcome. However, it is always necessary to define clearly the units of both numerator and denominator when reporting multiple pregnancy rates. For example, a twinning rate expressed as per 1000 births will be approximately twice that expressed as per 1000 confinements.

Definition of multiple conception, multiple pregnancy and multiple birth

Defining multiples poses problems (rarely made explicit), which arise because each individual may die at any gestational age. Plurality is based on the number of fetuses in a pregnancy, but not all multiple conceptions become multiple pregnancies, many being lost before the fetal period (defined as commencing 9–10 weeks after the onset of the last menstrual period). A birth is variously defined as a delivery after a gestation of specified duration, or as one of more than a specified weight. The multiplicity of the pregnancy may therefore exceed that reported at birth if some fetuses do not meet the minimal legal limits for registration. For example, some stillborn co-multiples who die early in a pregnancy that results in the birth of a liveborn infant may not be registered. As far as *birth* registration is concerned this is correct, but the fact that the birth was the product of a multiple conception then goes unreported.

Hospital records may be a more reliable source of plurality in pregnancies in which an early antenatal death has occurred. However, hospitals vary in the completeness with which they search for, ascertain and record evidence of early multiplicity in a pregnancy. Earlier ascertainment of multiplicity is becoming possible as a result of the increasing use and sensitivity of ultrasonography. Reliable recognition of multiple pulsatile cardiac activity is now possible after seven weeks of amenorrhoea (Bessis 1995), before the fetal stage has been attained. Early ultrasound studies of multiple conception show that the loss of one or more individuals before 20 weeks is not uncommon (Landy and Nies 1995). In the past, and in many places even now, many surviving co-twins of individuals dying before 20 weeks have been considered to be singletons and registered as such. For the construction of valid trends in multiple birth rates over time, the chance of being counted as a multiple birth should remain constant. This might best be achieved by using a definition of a multiple birth as one in which at least two fetuses survive past 20 weeks, since their recognition by the time of birth is likely in most places. However, the use of such a definition would mean that the effect of co-multiple losses before 20 weeks could not be studied.

Zygosity and chorionicity

Di- or polyzygotic multiples may be no more similar genetically than other siblings. Genetically dissimilar multiples will each have their own amnion, chorion and placental connections even if their individual placentae fuse to appear as one placental mass at delivery. In contrast, the placental architecture and membrane complement of monozygotic multiples depends on the time at which the conceptus splits. If division occurs before implantation, they may be as separate as polyzygotic multiples. If the split occurs a little later there is a single chorion and placenta (monochorionic multiples) and the rare occurrences of still later splits result in a single amnion as well as chorion (monochorionic mono-amniotic multiples) (Derom *et al.* 1995, Wigglesworth 1995).

As pregnancy proceeds, all multiples incur risks associated with restricted maternal supply and uterine crowding. Monozygotic multiples have additional risks. Monozygosity, which can itself be considered a congenital anomaly, is associated with other congenital anomalies. Monochorionic multiples have a high probability of vascular anastomoses (interfetal connecting blood vessels within the shared placenta) and may have grossly unequal sharing of the placenta (Machin and Still 1995). Monochorionic multiples that are also monoamniotic have the additional risk of cord entanglement. Zygosity and the extent of placental and membrane sharing therefore determine the effects of multiplicity. Unfortunately, precise data on placentation and blood supply are seldom available for retrospective study. However, even when they are, comparing outcomes of mono- and polyzygotic multiple births to assess heritability of various outcomes, including cerebral palsy, does not adequately control for the additional noninherited but shared environmental risks associated with multiplicity.

Relative risks
The consequences of multiple pregnancy are usually expressed as the risk relative to that for singletons. The risk per confinement and the risk per individual born must then be clearly differentiated. However, comparisons may also usefully be made between different pluralities (*e.g.* twin vs triplet), between different categories of twins (*e.g.* mono- vs dichorionic, mono- vs dizygotic or term vs preterm) or within sets of multiples (*e.g.* first vs second twin). In making comparisons between categories of a given plurality, only plurality is matched, but within a set of multiplies many potential confounders are matched.

Which factors constitute confounders? How should samples be selected and when should we adjust for what?
The rationale for adjusting for confounders must be carefully considered. When doing so it is important to remember that multiple pregnancy itself can be the initiator of chains of events, including factors associated with cerebral palsy such as poor growth and preterm birth. If the aim is to measure the overall contribution of multiple pregnancy to cerebral palsy, it is inappropriate to control (by stratification or inclusion in a multivariate regression model) for factors associated with multiple pregnancy or to use these as criteria for selection. For example, if the pathological consequences of twinning are sought in a sample selected on birthweight or gestational age, effectively the consequences of different causes of low birthweight or preterm birth are being compared (*e.g.* the effect of multiple pregnancy is compared with that of other causes such as chorioamnionitis or pre-eclampsia), rather than assessing the overall effect of multiple pregnancy. Such comparisons are, of course, important research questions in their own right, but fail to answer questions about multiples.

There are research questions for which controlling for preterm birth and/or appropriateness of intrauterine growth is appropriate—for example, whether the pathological effects of growth restriction or preterm delivery resulting from multiple pregnancy are different from those resulting from other causes.

Control for preterm birth is achieved by matching on gestational age, but controlling for appropriateness of intrauterine growth is more difficult. Logically, multiple gestation should be considered potentially pathological if its negative effects are being sought. In that case the best measure of appropriateness of growth may be the ratio of observed birthweight to the birthweight expected for a singleton of the same gestational age, gender and birth order.

Birthweight is a robust measure that has been used extensively as a surrogate for preterm birth. However, birthweight is the product of duration of gestation and rate of intrauterine

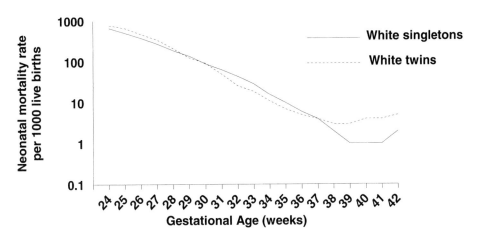

Fig. 10.2. Neonatal mortality by gestational age in White twins and singletons born in the USA 1983–1985. (From data reported by Powers *et al.* 1995.)

growth, so controlling for birthweight makes it impossible to differentiate the individual effects of each (Blair 1996c; see Chapter 8)—for example, the rate of intrauterine growth in multiples is reduced, particularly in the third trimester. Use of birthweight matched comparisons between twins and singletons born in the third trimester will tend to favour twins because they are likely to be compared to earlier born but appropriately grown singletons. Gestational age at delivery is a stronger determinant of mortality and of cerebral palsy than is appropriateness of intrauterine growth. The opposite may be true in the second trimester before the onset of growth restriction induced by multiple gestation. Thus twins delivered in the second trimester may be less likely to be growth restricted than singletons of similar gestational age who tend to be growth restricted as a result of the cause of their preterm delivery. For such reasons the use of birthweight as an explanatory variable, rather than its component variables, may lead to erroneous conclusions (Blair 1996c). A further pitfall of using birthweight to estimate growth, specific to monochorionic twin sets, is the possibility of chronic twin–twin transfusion leading to weight differences. It is this phenomenon, rather than differences in placental supply, that is primarily responsible for the poorer outcomes of twin pairs of widely differing weight and for the tendency for outcome of the larger twin of such sets to be less optimal than that of the smaller twin (Fujikura and Froehlich 1974, Sonntag *et al.* 1996).

Should there be specific norms for gestational age and growth for multiple births?
Should the earlier delivery and lower third trimester growth rates in multiple pregnancies be considered as pathological or as normal? Figure 10.2 compares the neonatal mortality rates in each gestation week for White singletons and twins born in the USA during 1983–1985, plotted from data presented by Powers *et al.* (1995). The gestational age of the nadir of gestation-specific mortality rates suggest that the optimal gestational age at delivery

113

TABLE 10.1
Risk of cerebral palsy for twins (A) and triplets (B) relative to singletons, estimated from population studies

A. Twins

Study	Twins n/N	Singletons n/N	Relative risk[1] (95% CI)[2]	Weight[1] %	Relative risk[1] of CP (95% CI)
Grether et al. (1993)	20/2985	172/152,587		7.8	5.94 (3.75–9.43)
Petterson et al. (1993a)	38/4915	362/224,687		18.2	4.80 (3.44–6.70)
King and Johnson (1995)	46/6237	598/265,716		32.3	3.28 (2.43–4.42)
Nelson and Ellenberg (1995)	10/1079	189/49,737		9.4	2.44 (1.29–4.59)
Pharoah and Cooke (1996)	64/5073	582/253,232		26.9	5.49 (4.25–7.10)
Williams et al. (1996)	17/2289	104/101,271		5.4	7.23 (4.34–12.06)
Total	195/22,578	2007/1,047,230		100.0	4.49 (3.88–5.20)

χ² 15.10 (df=5); Z = 20.12

(scale: 0.1 0.2 1 5 10)

B. Triplets

Study	Triplets n/N	Singletons n/N	Relative risk[1] (95% CI)	Weight[1] %	Relative risk[1] of CP (95% CI)
Petterson et al. (1993a)	6/215	362/224,687		52.6	17.32 (7.82–38.38)
Pharoah and Cooke (1996)	6/136	582/253,232		47.4	19.20 (8.74–42.15)
Total	12/351	944/477,919		100.0	18.21 (10.41–31.87)

χ² 0.03 (df=1); Z = 10.17

(scale: 0.1 0.2 1 5 10)

[1]See Glossary.

[2]For an explanation of the symbols used here, see Glossary, under Meta-analyses.

114

for multiples is lower, at 38–39 weeks, than for singletons, at 40 weeks. However, the neonatal (and infant) mortality of multiples born at their optimal gestational age is higher than that for singletons born at their optimal gestation. Successful adaptation would appear to make the best of the limited availability of maternal resources and intrauterine space imposed by multiple pregnancy, but does not entirely remove its disadvantages. It is therefore not appropriate to use specific standards of gestational duration or growth for multiples when assessing the effect of multiplicity on outcome. However, when making comparisons within a multiplicity—for example, when assessing whether an individual multiple has reached her/his optimal weight and gestational duration, specific standards of growth and gestational duration for multiples are appropriate.

RATES OF CEREBRAL PALSY IN MULTIPLE BIRTHS
Six population-based studies have measured rates of cerebral palsy in multiple births (Table 10.1). However, the denominators and the inclusion criteria for cerebral palsy used to calculate the rates varied between studies: for example, all but one study excluded children with postneonatally acquired brain damage, the risk of which is not enhanced by multiple pregnancy (see Chapter 11). The risk of cerebral palsy in multiple births relative to singleton births within each study, shown in Table 10.1, is therefore likely to be more comparable between studies than are the absolute rates. After weighting for sample size, the average rate of cerebral palsy in twins was 4.5 (95% CI 3.9–5.2) (Table 10.1A), and in triplets 18.2 (95% CI 10.4–31.9), times that in singletons (Table 10.1B).

Type of cerebral palsy
Compared with singletons, cerebral palsy in multiple births is more likely to be either spastic hemiplegia or spastic diplegia. In Western Australian births occurring in 1980–1989, the rate of spastic diplegia in multiples was what might be anticipated given the lower birthweight distribution of twins, but lower birthweights did not account for all the excess of spastic hemiplegia (Petterson *et al.* 1993a). In twins with cerebral palsy, the distribution of cognitive ability and of severity of motor impairment did not differ from that in singletons with cerebral palsy, and their tendency to exhibit less epilepsy did not reach statistical significance.

Time trends
While confidence intervals around the relative rate estimated from each study in Table 10.1A are wide, there is a suggestion that the estimate of relative risk in the Nelson and Ellenberg (1995) study may be the lowest. The births in this study occurred in 1959–1966, whereas all the other studies considered births in the 1980s. Excluding this early study gives a summary rate of cerebral palsy in twins of 4.7 (95% CI 4.1–5.5) times that of singletons, almost twice the 2.44 (1.3–4.6) found in the Nelson and Ellenberg study, though not statistically significantly different at the $p = 0.05$ level. This suggestion of changes in relative rate over time is supported by Figure 10.3 which shows five-year moving averages of cerebral palsy rates in singletons and multiples from the Western Australian Cerebral Palsy Register where consistent methodology has been maintained since its inception.

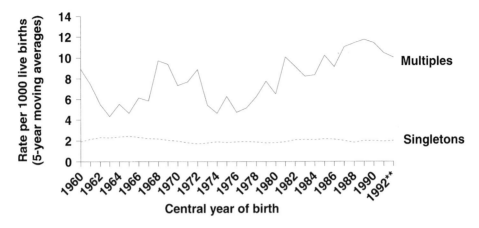

Fig. 10.3. Rates of cerebral palsy (excluding cases due to postneonatal causes) in multiple and singleton births in Western Australia, 1960–1992, by five-year moving averages. (1992 rates are based on preliminary data for 1993–1994.)

Neonatal intensive care was introduced in Western Australia about 1974–75 and could not therefore be responsible for the unexpectedly large number of twins with cerebral palsy (nine cases) born in 1970 which is entirely responsible for the first peak in Figure 10.3. The subsequent increase is more consistent and has continued to 1992.

Higher order multiple pregnancies
Few individual studies have sufficient numbers of higher order multiple pregnancies to allow meaningful estimates of their relative rates of cerebral palsy compared with those of twins. However, the summary estimate for triplets (derived using Revman software—Cochrane Collaboration 1998b) of a relative risk of 18.2 is statistically significantly higher than that for twins of 4.5 (Table 10.1). Further evidence that the relative risk may continue to increase with increasing multiplicity comes from two studies. A Japanese study of multiple births reported cerebral palsy rates of 9, 31 and 111 per 1000 twins, triplets and quadruplets respectively (Yokoyama *et al.* 1995), but this was based on self-selected volunteers. A study of triplets and higher order multiples in England and Wales reported an overall rate of 17.4 per 1000 (Macfarlane *et al.* 1990). Neither was a cohort study and both either excluded (England and Wales) or tended to exclude (Japan) sets with prenatal or early deaths. Since co-multiple death is associated with cerebral palsy and occurs more frequently in higher multiples, the rates of cerebral palsy in the higher orders reported by these studies are likely to be underestimated since the higher order itself, as well as fetal and embryonic deaths, were under-ascertained.

ORIGINS OF THE HIGHER RATES OF CEREBRAL PALSY IN MULTIPLE PREGNANCIES
Malformations
There is a greater potential for cerebral anomaly in multiple than in singleton pregnancies

throughout development. The splitting of the conceptus in monozygotic twinning is an abnormal event associated with an excess of congenital anomalies (Bomsel-Helmreich and Al Mufti 1995), including those of the central nervous system (Myrianthopoulos 1976), and with an enhanced potential for chromosomal abnormalities. Multiple ovulation, which results in polyzygotic pregnancy, is not apparently associated with an increased frequency of congenital anomalies arising early in pregnancy (Burn 1995, Keeling 1995), but the mechanisms which cause it are not well understood (Bomsel-Helmreich and Al Mufti 1995). Few studies have examined the association between congenital anomalies, multiple pregnancy and cerebral palsy because of the large sample sizes necessary. However, among Western Australian twin births 1980–1992, cerebral anomalies were present in four (6.5 per cent) of the twins with cerebral palsy but in only 0.3 per cent of those without cerebral palsy. Nevertheless in three of the four twins with cerebral palsy the cerebral damage observed was of the type most likely to be caused by the haemodynamic shock sustained at the time of death of a co-fetus, and thus more probably part of the effect rather than the cause of the cerebral palsy.

Placental complications
As described above, zygosity and the timing of ovum splitting in monozygotic pregnancies determines placentation and the likelihood of placental vascular anastomoses. Placental anastomoses were seen in 80 per cent of a series of 69 monochorionic sets (Machin and Still 1995), but it is generally considered that the proportion is usually larger. Any anastomosis of significant diameter links the blood pressure of the two fetuses, thus rendering both twins vulnerable to the effects of sudden changes in blood pressure initiated by events such as death or delivery of either twin.

Arteriovenous links uncompensated by other anastomoses, which were seen in 20 per cent of the series of 69 monochorionic sets (Machin and Still 1995), can result in twin–twin transfusion, even in the absence of any sudden haemodynamic changes. In its severe form this results in one small, anaemic oligohydramniotic twin and one large, plethoric, poly-hydramniotic twin. In the past nearly all these twin pairs died. Therapeutic strategies such as amniocentesis or laser ablation of placental vessels have recently been developed and have reduced mortality, but may have increased neurodevelopmental disability (Reisner *et al.* 1993, De Lia *et al.* 1995, Ville *et al.* 1995, Cincotta *et al.* 1996).

With or without shunting or anastomoses, monochorionic twins may have unequal shares of the placenta. A twin with significantly less than half the volume of venous drainage is at very high risk of intrauterine deprivation. Monoamniotic twins and monochorionic twins in whom the dividing amniotic membrane ruptures, share the same amniotic space. They are vulnerable both to cord entanglement, which is associated with intrauterine deprivation and asphyxia, and to twin–twin entanglement (locking) which creates intrapartum difficulties.

Fetal growth and birthweight
Independent of zygosity, limited maternal supply results in relatively low fetal growth rates in the third trimester of multiple pregnancies (MacLennan 1984), and intrauterine crowding results in earlier delivery. Thus the birthweight distribution is shifted to lower values with

TABLE 10.2

Risk of cerebral palsy for twins relative to singletons by birthweight, estimated from population studies

Study	Twins n/N	Singletons n/N	Relative risk[1] (95% CI)[2]	Weight[1] %	Relative risk[1] of CP (95% CI)
A. Birthweight ≥2500g					
Grether et al. (1993)	4/1667	997/145,479		7.3	3.58 (1.32–9.72)
Petterson et al. (1993a)	11/2636	233/214,918		17.9	3.85 (2.11–7.04)
King and Johnson (1995)	4/2920	343/251,334		36.2	1.00 (0.37–2.69)
Pharoah and Cooke (1996)	11/2602	326/236,733		30.9	3.07 (1.69–5.59)
Williams et al. (1996)	3/1095	57/93,832		7.6	4.51 (1.41–14.38)
Total	33/10,920	1056/935,388		100.0	2.70 (1.91–3.82)
χ² 6.37 (df=4); Z = 5.61					
B. Birthweight 1500–2499 g					
Grether et al. (1993)	4/1143	33/6226		7.8	0.66 (0.23–1.86)
Petterson et al. (1993a)	16/2031	66/8688		18.2	1.04 (0.60–1.79)
King and Johnson (1995)	21/2807	138/12,533		32.3	0.68 (0.43–1.07)
Pharoah and Cooke (1996)	24/2096	141/11,608		26.9	0.94 (0.61–1.45)
Williams et al. (1996)	5/983	33/5127		5.4	0.79 (0.31–2.02)
Total	70/9060	411/44,182		100.0	0.83 (0.65–1.07)
χ² 1.91 (df=4); Z = 1.43					
C. Birthweight <1500 g					
Grether et al. (1993)	12/177	42/882		10.9	1.42 (0.77–2.65)
Petterson et al. (1993a)	9/248	59/1147		16.1	0.71 (0.35–1.40)
King and Johnson (1995)	21/510	117/1849		38.9	0.65 (0.41–1.02)
Pharoah and Cooke (1996)	29/260	115/1264		30.2	1.23 (0.83–1.80)
Williams et al. (1996)	9/127	14/577		3.9	2.92 (1.29–6.60)
Total	80/1322	347/5719		100.0	1.08 (0.79–1.27)
χ² 13.30 (df=4); Z = 0.04					

Forest plot axis: 0.1 0.2 1 5 10

[1]See Glossary.

[2]For an explanation of the symbols used here, see Glossary, under Meta-analyses.

118

increasing plurality (Petterson *et al.* 1993a). Cerebral palsy rates of multiple births relative to singleton births are shown stratified by birthweight in Table 10.2. With one exception, register-based studies of births in the 1980s suggest that cerebral palsy rates in multiples of at least 2500 g birthweight are higher than those in singletons of the same birthweight (Table 10.1A). Despite the exceptional result observed in the largest study, the summary estimate obtained by sample size weighted average of all studies suggests that twins of at least 2499 g birthweight have a rate of cerebral palsy 2.7 times that of singletons. Thus irrespective of their distribution of birthweight for gestational age, multiples have increased risks of both death (Fig. 10.2) and cerebral palsy (Table 10.2).

The rates of cerebral palsy in smaller babies are, of course, much higher than in babies of normal birthweight, but the rates in multiples of low birthweight are not higher than those in singletons in the same birthweight stratum (Table 10.2B,C) and may even be lower in infants of 1500–2499 g birthweight. However, it must be remembered that multiple pregnancy is the cause of the low birthweight and thus cannot be considered either benign or protective. A lower relative rate among low birthweight twins implies only that twinning is a lower risk than other causes of low birthweight. A possible explanation is that since twins are more likely than singletons to be growth restricted in the third trimester, twins in the middle birthweight category are likely to be more mature than singletons in the same birthweight category and, at least for singletons, duration of gestation is a stronger risk factor for cerebral palsy than is poor intrauterine growth. A singleton pregnancy is much more likely to produce an appropriately grown fetus at term, for whom the likelihood of cerebral palsy is much lower.

Similar rates of cerebral palsy do not necessarily mean that the causal paths are the same. Analysis by birthweight cannot tell us the relative importance of poor intrauterine growth as opposed to preterm delivery. This requires analysis by duration of gestation and appropriateness of intrauterine growth. Of the five studies in Table 10.2, only Williams *et al.* (1996) reported cerebral palsy rates by gestational age, giving results for four gestational age strata. Table 10.3 combines their data with 1980–1992 data from the Western Australian Cerebral Palsy Register. The weighted average cerebral palsy rate for twins is equal to that for singletons in the 29–32 week stratum and is not lower in any gestational age stratum. When analysed in these gestational age categories, twinning is associated with a doubling of the cerebral palsy rate for deliveries before 28 weeks and between 33 and 36 weeks, rising . to a three-fold increase at term (Table 10.3). However, for this stratification to give an accurate picture, the gestational age distribution within each stratum should be the same for singletons and multiples. Since gestation is systematically shorter in twin births there are no grounds for making this assumption. This is shown by Western Australian population-based data of survivors to 1 year born 1980–1992. A far greater proportion of multiples born after 36 completed weeks of gestation were born in the 37th week of gestation than were singletons (40 per cent compared with 6.5 per cent). Thus, finer divisions of gestational age are necessary to give an accurate picture of relative rates of cerebral palsy by gestational age. In the same Western Australian data there were very few survivors and no cases of cerebral palsy among twins born before 24 weeks or after 40 weeks. Regression analysis limited to births at 24–40 weeks inclusive showed a U-shaped relationship between the rate of cerebral palsy and gestational age in twins relative to singletons. Though numbers are

TABLE 10.3

Risk of cerebral palsy in multiple births relative to singleton births by gestational age at delivery, estimated from population studies

Study	Multiple n/N	Singleton n/N	Relative risk[1] (95% CI)[2]	Weight[1] %	Relative risk[1] of CP (95% CI)
20–28 weeks					
WA CP Register	15/123	50/786		89.0	1.92 (1.11–3.31)
Williams et al. (1996)	2/51	7/376		11.0	2.11 (0.45–9.87)
Total	17/174	57/1162		100.0	1.94 (1.16–3.24)
χ^2 0.01 (df=1); Z = 2.52					
29–32 weeks					
WA CP Register	16/511	80/2241		86.7	0.88 (0.52–1.49)
Williams et al. (1996)	5/101	22/866		13.3	1.95 (0.75–5.03)
Total	21/612	102/3107		100.0	1.02 (0.65–1.62)
χ^2 2.10 (df=1); Z = 0.09					
33–36 weeks					
WA CP Register	16/2299	52/15761		88.8	2.11 (1.21–3.69)
Williams et al. (1996)	3/326	12/4363		11.2	3.35 (0.95–11.80)
Total	19/2625	64/20,124		100.0	2.25 (1.35–3.74)
χ^2 0.43 (df=1); Z = 3.11					
37–44 weeks					
WA CP Register	15/3745	404/277,325		92.2	2.75 (1.64–4.60)
Williams et al. (1996)	3/704	63/94,077		7.8	6.36 (2.00–20.22)
Total	18/4449	467/371,402		100.0	3.04 (1.90–4.86)
χ^2 1.72 (df=1); Z = 4.64					

Forest plot axis: 0.1 0.2 1 5 10

[1]See Glossary.
[2]For an explanation of the symbols used here, see Glossary, under Meta-analyses.

small, these data suggest that birth at <29 weeks of gestation is a greater risk factor for cerebral palsy in twins than in singletons. This is not explained by mortality since mortality is also greater in twins than in singletons within each gestational week below 29 weeks (see Fig. 10.2). By 29–32 weeks the rates of cerebral palsy are similar in twins and singletons.

A Western Australian study of the association between intrauterine growth in twins and their risk of cerebral palsy shows that affected twins tend to be better grown than normally surviving twins. This is primarily a result of the earlier delivery of twins with cerebral palsy compared with all twins because, in contrast to singletons, adequacy of growth in twins is inversely proportional to gestational age of delivery. Statistical analysis controlling for gestation at delivery suggested that very preterm twins subsequently diagnosed as having cerebral palsy were better grown than equally preterm twins who showed normal development. Moderately preterm twins with cerebral palsy tended to be somewhat more growth restricted than normally developing twins, as found with singletons, but there was no difference in the distributions of the proportion of expected birthweight for twins with and without cerebral palsy who were born at term. In summary, gestational age at delivery appears to be a stronger determinant of risk of cerebral palsy in twins than in singletons, and the growth restriction resulting from multiple pregnancy is not as strongly associated with cerebral palsy as (some) other causes of growth restriction.

Zygosity/gender combination
Given the larger number of pathological mechanisms specific to monozygotic twins, the increased risk of cerebral palsy observed in twins might be anticipated to arise predominantly in monozygotic twins or, in the absence of zygosity data, in like-sex twins, but this is not the case (Grether *et al.* 1993, Petterson *et al.* 1993a). The observed rate of cerebral palsy represents the balance between death and normal survival, and it may be that the higher rate of poor outcome anticipated in monozygotic twins is primarily mortality.

Intrapartum factors and birth order
The intrapartum difficulties that can be associated with multiple delivery are another potential source of their increased risk of cerebral palsy. In the past, higher rates of disability have been reported in second born twins (Russell 1961, Ellis *et al.* 1979) and were assumed to be the result of intrapartum difficulties. More recent studies have shown no difference between rates of cerebral palsy in first and second born twins. Furthermore, combining the studies of Grether *et al.* (1993) and Petterson *et al.* (1993a), of 11 cases with stillborn co-twins, nine of the surviving twins were first-born. Hence birth order may be determined by factors which are themselves determinants of survival and cerebral palsy and should not be viewed as a simple marker for intrapartum difficulties. Studies failing to take this into account may underestimate the importance of intrapartum difficulties in the aetiology of cerebral palsy in multiple pregnancy.

Co-fetal death
The antenatal death of the co-twin is associated with cerebral damage in several case histories (Fusi *et al.* 1991, Liu *et al.* 1992, van Bogaert *et al.* 1996) as well as in four of the

121

TABLE 10.4

Risk of cerebral palsy for twins whose co-twin died antenatally relative to twins whose co-twin survived to birth, estimated from population studies

Study	Co-twin death n/N	Co-twin survival n/N	Relative risk[1] (95% CI)[2]	Weight[1] %	Relative risk[1] of CP (95% CI)
Rates per confinement					
Grether et al. (1993)	4/33	14/1504		12.2	13.02 (4.53–37.45)
Petterson et al. (1993a)	5/52	30/2530		24.5	8.11 (3.28–20.07)
Pharoah and Cooke (1996)	6/63	52/2572		50.4	4.71 (2.10–10.56)
Williams et al. (1996)	1/16	25/1242		12.9	3.10 (0.45–21.54)
Total	16/164	121/7848		100.0	6.35 (3.85–10.47)
χ^2 3.11 (df=3); Z = 7.24					
Rates per child					
Grether et al. (1993)	4/33	16/3008		12.5	22.79 (8.05–64.51)
Petterson et al. (1993a)	5/52	31/4844		23.8	15.02 (6.08–37.11)
Pharoah and Cooke (1996)	6/63	58/5144		50.7	8.45 (3.78–18.85)
Williams et al. (1996)	1/16	28/2484		12.9	5.54 (0.80–38.32)
Total	16/164	133/15,480		100.0	11.44 (6.95–18.81)
χ^2 3.12 (df=3); Z = 9.60					

Forest plot axis: 0.01   0.1   1   10   100

[1]See Glossary.
[2]For an explanation of the symbols used here, see Glossary, under Meta-analyses.

studies referred to in Table 10.2. Meta-analysis of these four studies (Table 10.4) shows that co-fetal death is associated with a six-fold increase in rate of cerebral palsy per twin confinement, or an 11-fold increase in rate per child. Further analysis by gestational age at delivery using Western Australian data for twins born 1980–1992 showed a history of antenatal death of a co-twin in three of 15 children with cerebral palsy born before 29 weeks gestation, 0/16 born 29–32 weeks, 3/16 born 33–36 weeks and 1/15 born after 36 weeks. Although these numbers are small, this risk does not appear to be confined to delivery at particular gestations. What is perhaps of greater interest is whether it is confined, as anticipated, to monochorionic twins and whether the damage was initiated at the gestational age at which the co-fetus died (Scheller and Nelson 1992, Pharoah and Cooke 1997).

Grether *et al.* (1993) (Table 10.4) reported that three of the four cases of cerebral palsy following co-fetal death in their study were known to be monozygotic, while the fourth followed fertility enhancement treatment and was therefore likely to be dizygotic. Petterson *et al.* (1993a) included additional retrospectively ascertained twins in an appendix to their report, and indicated that only one of six twin pairs with co-fetal death in which the gender of both twins was known were of unlike gender. Unlike gender is found in about 30 per cent of the twin populations in these studies, so while twins with cerebral palsy and co-fetal death may be less likely to be of unlike gender they are not exclusively of like gender. However, since all twins are at higher risk of cerebral palsy, it is possible that the co-fetal death in this case was coincidental. Individual cases of co-fetal neurological damage have been documented for twin deaths before 20 weeks of gestational age, the earliest reported as at about 13–14 weeks (Anderson *et al.* 1990). Since twin pregnancies with early co-fetal losses are seldom registered and may not even be recognized as twin conceptions, the risk of cerebral palsy associated with first and early second trimester co-fetal loss cannot be estimated.

Perinatal outcome of 100 cases of selective termination of an abnormal co-fetus in dichorionic multiple pregnancy have been reported (Berkowitz *et al.* 1997). Gestational age at termination varied between 12 weeks and 23 weeks. In 5.4 per cent of those terminated before 16 weeks, the remaining fetuses were aborted spontaneously, compared with 14.4 per cent of those terminated later in gestation. Termination of the presenting fetus was an additional risk factor for spontaneous abortion. Longer term follow up was only reported for the infant born at 23 weeks who was developing normally at 3.5 years. No neonatal problems were noted in infants born at later gestations.

Postnatal death of the co-twin is also associated with cerebral palsy, but this is largely attributable to the excess of preterm birth in multiple births which result in postnatal death.

Conclusion

Multiple pregnancy is associated with cerebral palsy through a number of different mechanisms. The risk of cerebral palsy attributable to this complication may increase as medical care improves and the mortality of multiples continues to be reduced. This underlines the need to avoid births of high plurality secondary to fertility treatment. In view of our uncertainties about the effects of co-fetal death and the potentially adverse effects of multifetal reduction (see Chapter 12), primary prevention, through carefully regulated infertility management, is preferable.

11
POSTNEONATALLY ACQUIRED CEREBRAL PALSY: INCIDENCE AND ANTECEDENTS

"There can be no keener revelation of a society's soul than the way in which it treats its children."

Nelson Mandela (in Williams 1997)

A significant proportion of all cerebral palsy is acquired after the neonatal period as the result of a recognized brain damaging event. By definition these aetiologies are well understood. Postnatal onset of cerebral palsy without recognized cause is usually included with congenital cases because it is far more likely that an antenatal cause would be undetected (Blair and Stanley 1993b). However, children labelled as acquiring cerebral palsy postneonatally have been reported to have an excess of ante- and perinatal risk factors such as low birthweight, neonatal respiratory problems or CNS abnormalities (Blair and Stanley 1982, Pharoah *et al.* 1989). The pathway to a postneonatally acquired lesion may therefore commence before the postneonatal period, although this may not be recognized. Morton *et al.* (1991), for example, described a series of cases of cerebral palsy labelled as postneonatally acquired because impairment was first observed following early childhood infection. They were subsequently recognized as having glutaric aciduria type I, a metabolic defect that rendered them peculiarly susceptible to cerebral damage under conditions of stress (see p. 7). Other metabolic abnormalities, such as pyruvate dehydrogenase deficiency, may give rise to motor disorders as may clotting disorders which are a risk factor for cerebral thrombosis (Thorarensen *et al.* 1997, Debus *et al.* 1998). Such disorders are also more likely to be associated with antenatal and/or repeated damage which then appears to be a progressive condition.

Despite a growing awareness of such uncertainties (Badawi *et al.* 1998c), the aetiologies of postneonatally acquired cases are considerably better understood than those of congenitally acquired cases. This should render it easier to devise preventive strategies. However, *because* their aetiologies are considered to be well understood, postneonatally acquired cerebral palsies have often been ignored or largely excluded from aetiological research. Since these represent a significant proportion of all cerebral palsy cases and often show severe impairments, it is important not to forget them, especially as may be the easiest to prevent.

Three reports (Blair and Stanley 1982, Arens and Molteno 1989, Pharoah *et al.* 1989) deal exclusively with postneonatally acquired cerebral palsy. Some studies of all cases of cerebral palsy also identify them as a separate group and provided additional details.

Definition of postneonatally acquired cerebral palsy

The problems of defining cerebral palsy are discussed in Chapter 2. There is no standard method of categorizing cases acquired after birth. Earlier studies described a *postnatally* acquired group, often without well defined criteria. Some workers have included cases acquired from neonatal causes, most of which have their origins during pregnancy, labour and delivery. For example, neonatal kernicterus has been included among the postnatal causes (Haque 1986, Laisram *et al.* 1992). Others have sought to identify a group without perinatal problems, usually termed post*neo*natally as distinct from postnatally acquired. To be classified as postneonatally acquired there must be a history of a potentially brain damaging event after the neonatal period in a child thought to be neurologically normal. There is considerable variation in the age limits in publications describing postneonatally acquired cerebral palsy. The earlier limit ranges from birth to 2 months. However, as suggested above, postnatal age at the time of the damaging insult may not in itself be sufficient evidence that its effect was independent of ante- and perinatal events. With improved resuscitation at birth and neonatal intensive care, increasingly compromised infants are now surviving. They may be particularly vulnerable to postnatal insults and for a longer period than healthy babies of the same age.

On the other hand, it is not reasonable to classify a cerebral injury sustained by an apparently normal term infant in a motor vehicle accident at 14 days as congenitally acquired, even if it is still within the neonatal period (commonly defined as 0–28 days after birth). Neither is it postneonatally acquired. Conversely, an infant delivered very preterm who sustains an intracerebral haemorrhage more than 28 days after birth as a result of immaturity does not meet the criteria for postneonatal acquisition. To circumvent these difficulties a third category of aetiological timing is used in Western Australia. This comprises cases with a history of a potentially brain damaging postnatal event that is either within the neonatal period but not obviously related to ante- or perinatal events, or past the neonatal period but very likely to be related to ante- or perinatal events. Although very few cases were placed in this category between the years 1975–1992, by creating a separate category these cases can be identified and then grouped appropriately for whatever reason the data are being sought (see Chapter 3).

The upper age limits vary from 2 to 10 years (see Appendix) and are chosen for pragmatic rather than methodological reasons. From a therapeutic point of view, the management of children damaged after the acquisition of motor skills differs from that of those who have never acquired them. From the point of view of prevention, the profile of aetiologies changes with increasing age, from more infectious to more accidental aetiologies with increasing immunological competence and motor independence, merging into that of adolescent and then adult brain damage.

What proportion of cerebral palsy is acquired postneonatally?

The frequency of postneonatally acquired cerebral palsy is generally reported as a proportion of all cerebral palsy, because it is most often measured as a subset of all cerebral palsy. The proportions reported in the literature vary between 1.4 and 60 per cent (Table 11.1). Little of this variation is accounted for by differences in age limits. Many estimates were based

TABLE 11.1

Postneonatally acquired cerebral palsy as a proportion of all cerebral palsy in several studies

Reference	Place	Years	All CP N	Age limits*	Postneonatally acquired CP N	%
A. Population based estimates						
Pharoah et al. (1989)	Mersey, UK	1966–77	833	28d–5y	147	17.6
King and Johnson (1995)	4 UK counties	1984–90	617	28d–5y	46[1]	7.5
Murphy et al. (1993)	Atlanta, USA	1985-87	204	1m–10y	33	16.2
Haerer et al. (1984)	One county, Mississippi, USA	1978[2]	50	pnn–2y	7	14.0
Riikonen et al. (1989)	Türkü, Finland	1968–72	42	8d–3y	6	14.3
		1978–82	70	8d–3y	1	1.4
Uvebrant (1988)	Göteborg, Sweden		117[3]	birth–2y	18	15.3
Hagberg and Hagberg (1989)	Göteborg, Sweden	1979–82	162	birth–2y	11	6.8
Hagberg et al. (1993)	Göteborg, Sweden	1983–86	192	birth–2y	15	7.8
Hagberg et al. (1996)	Göteborg, Sweden	1987–90	216	birth–2y	10	4.6
Dite (1995)	Victoria, Australia	1970–92	1846	birth–6y	213	11.5
Blair and Stanley (1982)	Western Australia	1956–75	802	birth–5y	89	11.1
Unpublished	Western Australia	1980–92	801	28d–5y	121	15.1
Arens and Molteno (1989)	Cape Town, S. Africa	1986[2]	588	birth–13y	146	24.8
White			91		12	13.2
Coloured			375		90	24.0
Black			122		44	36.1

126

B. Clinic or hospital based estimates

Reference	Location	Years	N	Age*	n	%
Haque (1986)	Riyadh, Saudi Arabia	1978–82	208	7d–2y	67[4]	32.2
Taha and Mahdi (1984)	Riyadh, Saudi Arabia	1980–83	102[5]	birth–5y	29	28.4
Özmen et al. (1993)	Istanbul, Turkey	1982–89	308	14d–2y	49	15.9
Duggan and Ogala (1982)	Zaria, Nigeria	1974–77	44	pnn	20	45.0
Sathiakumar and Yakubu (1987)	Zaria, Nigeria	1981–83	141	pnn	8	5.7
Makwabe and Mgone (1984)	Dar es Salaam, Tanzania	1983	50	postnatal–4y	30[3]	60.0
Dyer (1997)	Zambia				>50	>50
Laisram et al. (1992)	New Delhi, India	1981–89	544	postnatal	134[4]	24.6
O'Reilly et al. (1981)	Missouri, USA	1947–	1503	postnatal		14.8[1]

*Ages when postneonatally acquired cerebral palsy is thought to have occurred.
[1]Excludes tumours.
[2]Prevalence from cross-sectional population survey.
[3]Hemiplegic cerebral palsy only.
[4]Excludes those attributed to neonatal jaundice or kernicterus.
[5]Excludes hereditary syndromes.

on clinic populations whose representativeness is questionable. For example, a single clinic in Zaria, Nigeria reported 45 per cent of their cerebral palsy as being postneonatally acquired between 1974 and 1977 (Duggan and Ogala 1982), but only 6 per cent between 1981 and 1983 (Sathiakumar and Yakubu 1987). While this may be an extreme case where small numbers in the earlier period add statistical uncertainty to selection bias, it highlights the problem of studying causation in data that are not population based. For this reason, Table 11.1A presents estimates based on populations separately from those from clinics (Table 11.1B).

Population based data are seldom available from developing countries. The exception is the study from Cape Town municipal area (Arens and Molteno 1989) which used multiple sources of ascertainment. Even so, the authors had little confidence in the accuracy of their estimates for non-White populations. It is, however, striking that the estimated proportions of postneonatally acquired cerebral palsy tend to be substantially higher in developing than in developed countries. Little, in his classic paper presented in London in 1862, observed that postneonatally acquisition of cerebral palsy was 20 times more common than intrapartum acquisition. Thus recent rates in developing countries may be similar to rates of 19th century London and reflect potentially preventable causes that have been largely addressed in developed countries.

Absolute rates of postneonatally acquired cerebral palsy

Table 11.2 gives estimates of absolute rates of postneonatally acquired cerebral palsy. Not all the studies represented in Table 11.1 reported rates, and the small numbers involved make for unstable estimates as shown by the confidence intervals in Table 11.2. The two estimates using neonatal survivor denominators are higher than those using live birth denominators. The only traditionally estimated prevalence (at age 10 years) is higher still. Confidence intervals of the estimates obtained using births as the denominator do not overlap those of the other estimates. Since neonatal and childhood mortalities are unlikely to be sufficient to account for the difference, the apparent trend with choice of denominator may be due to chance, researchers in those studies with the lowest rates of postneonatal acquisition choosing to use live births as the denominator. The narrowest confidence intervals come from the largest samples obtained by collecting over long time periods. If postneonatally acquired cerebral palsy is dependent primarily on social conditions, there is little point in obtaining more stable estimates of rate by summing over time or geographical location if the social conditions are changing over time and between locations.

TRENDS BY YEAR OF BIRTH

Three groups have reported cerebral palsy rates by birth cohorts over more than a decade of births, to which may be added more recent unpublished data from the Western Australian register. The Swedish Register estimated rates per 10,000 live births of 1.5 (95% CI 0.6–2.3) in 1979–1982 (Hagberg and Hagberg 1989), 1.95 (1.0–2.9) in 1983–1986 (Hagberg et al. 1993) and 1.09 (0.4–1.8) in 1987–1990 (Hagberg et al. 1996), showing neither a consistent trend nor significant differences. It is difficult to compare rates prior to these cohorts without the raw data (Hagberg et al. 1984), but they do not appear to have varied greatly since 1959.

TABLE 11.2
Rate of postneonatally acquired cerebral palsy

Denominator	Reference	Place	Birth cohorts	Postneonatally acquired cerebral palsy		
				N	Rate per 10,000 births	(95% CI)
Live births	King and Johnson (1995)	Oxford	1984–90	46	1.9	(1.4–2.5)
	Riikonen et al. (1989)	Turku, Finland	1968–82	7	1.3	(0.3–2.2)
	Hagberg (1989), Hagberg et al. (1993, 1996)	Göteborg, Sweden	1979–90	36	1.5	(1.0–2.0)
Neonatal survivors	Pharoah et al. (1989)	Mersey, UK	1966–77	147	3.3	(2.8–3.9)
		W. Australia	1956–92	210	3.1	(2.7–3.5)
Prevalence at 10 years	Murphy et al. (1993)	Atlanta	1975–77	33	3.7	(2.4–4.9)

129

Similarly, the Merseyside Register reported annual rates varying between 1.6/10,000 and 5.7/10,000 neonatal survivors between 1966 and 1977, but again there was no trend over time. In contrast, the Western Australian Register has shown a significant increase. Between 1956 and 1975 the average rate per 10,000 neonatal survivors was 2.4 (1.9–2.9) with a small rise over time that did not reach statistical significance (Blair and Stanley 1982). Between 1976 and 1990 the average rate per 10,000 neonatal survivors was significantly higher at 4.1 (3.4–4.8), composed of 4.3 (3.0–5.6), 3.5 (2.4–4.6) and 4.5 (3.3–5.7) over the three five-year periods. The Western Australian collection was started in 1977, thus cases born before the mid-1970s were ascertained retrospectively. It is therefore possible that the apparent jump in rates around 1975 is an artefact arising from incomplete retrospective ascertainment. Evidence against this being due to underascertainment is the consistency of the rate of congenitally acquired cerebral palsy over the entire collection period, which results in an increase in proportion of cerebral palsy classified as postneonatally acquired, shown in Table 11.1.

Causes of postneonatally acquired cerebral palsy
The classification of causes of postneonatally acquired cerebral palsy should lead to the development of preventive strategies. Broad classifications, *e.g.* traumatic, infectious and hypoxic, are not very helpful because they each cover such a variety of causes. However, there is no universally accepted (or obvious) more detailed classification system, and it is not always self-evident how a given cause should be classified. For example, severe gastroenteritis leading to dehydration and cerebrovascular accident has been classified as a cerebrovascular accident (Arens and Molteno 1989), an infectious cause (Taha and Mahdi 1984) and in a category on its own (Blair and Stanley 1982, Pharoah *et al.* 1989). In many case series it is not mentioned as an individual cause, even in developing countries where it might be expected to be more common. This complicates the comparison of aetiological profiles between different reports and does not help to suggest preventive strategies. It is therefore more useful to report causes in greater detail, even though numbers due to any one cause may be very small and principally of parochial interest.

DEVELOPING COUNTRIES
Data from hospitals and clinics suggest that cerebral infections and febrile convulsions are the most common causes in African countries. Duggan and Ogala (1982), citing four African studies, mentioned only meningitis and febrile convulsions, though not all cases were accounted for. Makwabe and Mgone (1984) in Tanzania, and Dyer (1997) in Zambia highlighted cerebral malaria as the principle cause of the febrile convulsions. Sathiakumar and Yakubu (1987), on the other hand, reported that five of their northern Nigerian series of seven postneonatally acquired cases had had septicaemia. In India, Laisram *et al.* (1992) reported a similar pattern with 74 per cent due to cerebral infection and 16 per cent due to convulsions (cause not specified), but the remaining 10 per cent were attributed to head injury. In Turkey, Özmen *et al.* (1993) reported that more than half of 300 postneonatally acquired cases had had either meningitis or septicaemia. Two reports from Saudi Arabia indicate more varied causes: Taha and Mahdi (1984) reported that of 26 postneonatally

acquired cases, two were due to home accidents, one to near-drowning, six to gastroenteritis and dehydration, seven to meningitis, four to pertussis, three to measles and three to respiratory tract infections, while Haque (1986) reported that of 55 cases with a specified cause, four were due to trauma, 10 to dehydration, 26 to CNS infection and 15 to sepsis (otherwise unspecified). This resembles the aetiological profiles seen in developed countries.

DEVELOPED COUNTRIES

The Swedish Register indicates an evolution in postneonatal causes. Almost two-thirds, 14 of the 22 postneonatally acquired cases born 1954–1970, resulted from infection, five from hypoxia and two from trauma, while one was acquired perioperatively (Hagberg and Olow 1975). Of the 15 cases born 1983–1986 only four resulted from CNS infection, two from hypoxia and one from cerebral haemorrhage (cause not specified), one was associated with convulsions, but nearly half (seven of the 15) followed operations for congenital malformations (Hagberg et al. 1993). In the latest report of 1987–1990 births, none of the postneonatally acquired cases resulted from CNS infection: one was due to pertussis, one to cerebrovascular accident, one to QT syndrome (see Glossary), two to skull trauma (cause not specified) and three to near-miss sudden infant death syndrome (now called apparently life-threatening events or ALTE—see Chapter 12), while two were acquired postoperatively (Hagberg et al. 1996). Numbers are very small, not because the denominators are so small, but because the 1987–1990 rate of postneonatally acquired cerebral palsy (1.09/10,000 live births) is the lowest reported in the world, largely because of the absence of CNS infection as a cause.

The Western Australian Register has larger numbers of postneonatally acquired cases with consistent methods of classification of the aetiological profile. One reason for the higher rate in Western Australia is that about 5 per cent of their births are to Aboriginal mothers whose infants are at increased risk of postneonatally acquired cerebral palsy (see p. 133). Table 11.3 shows the distribution of causes in two cohorts of Western Australian births and indicates that it is changing in a manner similar to that in Sweden. Cerebral infections are decreasing in importance, as are gastroenteritis and malnutrition, but all other causes are increasing, with cerebrovascular accidents associated with surgery and ALTE representing new causes. Some of the emerging causes are likely to represent the use of medical technology to salvage young children from causes that would previously have been fatal (e.g. ALTE, major congenital malformations and accidents). What is of particular concern in Western Australia is the statistically significant increase in the rate of nonaccidental injury. It is conceivable that in the later period, caregivers had a higher index of suspicion and/or were more willing to report nonaccidental injury than in the earlier period. However, numbers in the other categories in which nonaccidental injury is most likely to been placed (unknown cause or head injury due to falls or without specified cause) are all either higher or unchanged in the second period.

Infections still dominate the aetiological profile in other reports from the developed world. From the Mersey Register, 43 per cent (63/147) of postneonatally acquired cases born 1966–1977 (Pharoah et al. 1989), 32 per cent born 1970–1990 in the State of Victoria, Australia (Dite et al. 1995) and 39 per cent born 1984–1990 in the Oxford region, England

TABLE 11.3
Distribution of causes of postneonatally acquired cerebral palsy in
two cohorts of Western Australian births

Causes	1956–1975[1] (N = 89)		1980–1992[2] (N = 121)	
	n	%	n	%
Infections				
Cerebral infection	45	50.6	32	26.4
Pertussis	3	3.4	0	—
Post-DTP[3]	2	2.2	1	0.8
Gastroenteritis + dehydration	6	6.7	2	1.7
Head injury				
Motor vehicle accident	11	12.4	20	16.5
Nonaccidental	3	3.4	18	14.9
Falls	2	2.3	4	3.3
Unspecified head injury	3	3.4	5	4.1
Unspecified cause	0	—	5	4.1
Cerebrovascular accident				
Spontaneous	4	4.5	13	10.7
Postoperative	0	—	7	5.8
Other				
ALTE[4]	0	—	6	5.0
Status epilepticus	4	4.5	2	1.7
Suffocation	2	2.3	1	0.8
Near-drowning	1	1.1	4	3.3
Malnutrition	2	2.3	0	—
Unknown	0	—	5	4.1

[1]Blair and Stanley (1982).
[2]Unpublished data from the Western Australian Cerebral Palsy Register.
[3]Diphtheria–tetanus–pertussis immunization.
[4]ALTE = Apparently life-threatening event (formerly called near-miss sudden infant death syndrome or SIDS).

(King and Johnson 1995) were associated with infection. Head injury was the next most important cause, accounting for between 17 and 24 per cent of cases in these three studies. The reported proportions of nonaccidental injury were between 6 and 9 per cent; however, it is possible that this is underreported or included with unknown or miscellaneous causes or with the means by which the nonaccidental injury was inflicted. Cerebrovascular accidents accounted for five of the 147 Mersey cases (3 per cent), four of 46 Oxford cases (9 per cent) and 34 of 213 Victorian cases (16 per cent), and a postoperative cause was found in three (2 per cent), seven (15 per cent) and 15 cases (7 per cent) in the respective studies. Convulsions and dehydration following gastroenteritis were only important in the Mersey study, accounting for 9 per cent and 15 per cent respectively. Other causes that were mentioned were near-drowning, accidental suffocation, electrocution, shock following a burn (which may represent household accidents), ALTE and Reye syndrome.

A similar aetiological profile, primarily of infection followed by trauma, cerebrovascular accident and surgical complications, was reported by Uvebrant (1988) for postneonatally acquired hemiplegic cerebral palsy. This study also drew attention to the importance of *Haemophilus influenzae* meningitis as the principal type of cerebral infection in developed countries.

A small number of cases are attributed to pertussis or to the adverse effects of immunization against pertussis. However, many more children are immunized than are not, and whilst there is rarely uncertainty about an attribution to pertussis, attribution to triple antigen vaccine usually relies on a temporal sequence *only* and is far less certain. These two facts suggest that even if pertussis immunization could be on a causal path to cerebral palsy, not to be immunized is a far greater risk factor for cerebral palsy, and this danger will increase if levels of vaccination fall (see Chapter 12).

A Western Australian survey (Hanna and Wild 1991) found that the most common bacterial organisms involved in children with meningitis between 4 weeks and 60 months of age were *H. influenzae* type b, *Streptococcus pneumoniae* and *Neisseria meningitidis*. The population surveyed for the study comprised 114,018 children aged 0–5 years, of whom 186 were known to have developed haemophilus meningitis. Of these, 10 children died and six developed cerebral palsy, accounting for 13.9 per cent of all cases of postneonatal cerebral palsy in Caucasians and 33 per cent in the Aboriginal children in those birth cohorts. This gave some indication of the size of the preventive effect which was to be achieved by the implementation of effective immunization (see Chapter 12).

COUNTRIES WITH RACIALLY MIXED POPULATIONS

The existence of studies from countries with racially mixed populations in which the social conditions vary systematically by race gives the opportunity to measure the effect of social conditions independent of the methods of data collection. In these studies, rates of postneonatal acquisition vary by race. In Atlanta, Georgia, the rate in the Black population was 1.6 times that in the White population (Murphy *et al.* 1993). In Cape Town, the rate in Coloureds was 2.3 times and the rate in Blacks was 2.6 times that in Whites (Arens and Molteno 1989). In Western Australia the rate in Aboriginal Australians was about six times that in Caucasians (Blair and Stanley 1982) in 1956–1975, rising to almost eight times the caucasian rate by 1980–1992 (unpublished data).

In Cape Town, while cerebral infection was the most important cause in all racial groups it accounted for only five of 12 White cases compared with 49 of 90 Coloured cases and 28 of 44 Black cases (Arens and Molteno 1989). The remainder was largely accounted for by cerebral trauma which accounted for one-third of White cases, one-quarter of Coloured cases but only two out of the 44 Black cases. Pedestrian–motor vehicle collisions were the most common cause of head trauma, though nonaccidental injury was reported for one of 12 White children, one of 90 Coloured children and no Black children. Further comparisons are difficult on account of the broad aetiological categories used.

In Western Australian births 1956–1975, 17 of the 20 Aboriginal cases were attributed to infection, including dehydration following gastroenteritis, two to malnutrition and only one to an accident. In contrast, 37 of 69 non-Aboriginal cases were attributed to infection, one-quarter to head injury, principally motor vehicle accidents but including three that may have been nonaccidental. The aetiological pattern has changed for both groups in the

133

1980–1992 birth cohorts. Infections still accounted for the majority of Aboriginal cases (19/35), but only 13 of 82 non-Aboriginal cases. Head injury accounted for one-quarter (9/35) of Aboriginal cases, only one of which was nonaccidental. In comparison, head injury caused 36 of 82 non-Aboriginal cases, 15 of which were nonaccidental (race was not recorded in two of the cases of nonaccidental cause in Table 11.3). Cerebrovascular accident accounted for two of 35 Aboriginal cases, compared with 18 of 82 non-Aboriginal cases.

Epidemiology

The epidemiology of postneonatally acquired cerebral palsy naturally varies with the cause. Since this is changing both within and between different societies, the distribution of impairments and causal pathways also varies with place and time.

AGE OF ACQUISITION

Age of acquisition varies with cause, but both Arens and Molteno (1989) and Blair and Stanley (1982) report an exponential fall in number of cases with increasing age, with more than half the cases occurring before 5 years of age being acquired in the first 12 months after birth. The number may increase again in later childhood. Murphy *et al.* (1993) reported that in 27 per cent of their postneonatally acquired sample, acquisition was between the ages of 5 and 10 years, and Pharoah *et al.* (1989) point out that head injury often occurs after the age of 2 years, while infections and nonaccidental injury occur principally before the age of 2 years.

TYPE OF MOVEMENT IMPAIRMENT

The distribution of type of impairment in postneonatally acquired cerebral palsy is compared with that in congenitally acquired cases in two cohorts of Western Australian births in Table 11.4. Compared with congenitally acquired cerebral palsy, a higher proportion of postneonatally acquired cases are spastic in type, though the difference may be diminishing. In the past very few postneonatally acquired cases (1.4 per cent—Pharoah *et al.* 1989; 1.1 per cent—Blair and Stanley 1982) have been dyskinetic. In the more recent Western Australian cohort, seven of 121 cases were dyskinetic (Table 11.4) as were 15 of 90 Coloured cases in Cape Town (Arens and Molteno 1989). Of 10 postneonatally acquired dyskinetic cases in Western Australia, three were caused by cerebrovascular accident following surgery (compared with 6.6 per cent of the entire postneonatally acquired cohort), three by cerebral infection, one each by near-drowning, ALTE and nonaccidental injury, and one was of unknown cause. The newly emerging causes of cerebrovascular accident, ALTE and nonaccidental injury, may therefore be associated with dyskinetic cerebral palsy.

As anticipated, there is a significant excess of hemiplegic spastic cerebral palsy which is most often associated with head injuries, a less significant excess of quadriplegic cases, and very few diplegic cases compared with congenitally acquired cases. Similar differences are seen in data from the Merseyside Register birth cohorts 1966–1977 (Pharoah *et al.* 1987, 1989), except that the dearth of spastic diplegia is even more marked. In that study hemiplegia accounted for 42 per cent of postneonatally acquired cases, quadriplegia for 53 per cent, and diplegia for only one of the 147 cases (Pharoah *et al.* 1989).

TABLE 11.4
Distribution of type of cerebral palsy in postneonatally and congenitally acquired cases of cerebral palsy in two cohorts of Western Australian births

| | 1956–1975 cohort[1] | | | | 1980–1992 cohort[2] | | | |
| | Postneonatal (N = 89) | | Congenital (N = 810) | | Postneonatal (N = 121) | | Congenital (N = 669) | |
	n	%	n	%	n	%	n	%)
Spastic								
Hemiplegia	39	43.5	173	21.4	67	55.4	225	33.6
Diplegia	12	13.5	209	25.8	8	6.6	199	29.7
Quadriplegia	26	29.2	193	23.8	33	27.3	121	18.1
Total	80[3]	90.0	612[3]	75.6	108	89.3	545	81.5
Nonspastic								
Ataxia	4	4.5	55	6.8	6	5.0	51	7.6
Dyskinesia	1	1.1	85	10.5	7	5.8	67	10.0
Hypotonia	3	3.4	57	7.0	0	—	6	0.9
Total	9[3]	10.0	198[3]	24.4	13	10.7	124	18.5

[1]Blair and Stanley (1982).
[2]Unpublished data from the Western Australian Cerebral Palsy Register.
[3]Balance of cases did not meet the criteria for inclusion in any of the three subcategories.

SEVERITY OF MOVEMENT IMPAIRMENT

There was no difference in distribution of severity of movement impairment between congenitally and postneonatally acquired cerebral palsy in either the 1956–1975 or the 1980–1992 birth cohorts. The proportion with severe impairment is increasing in both congenital and postneonatally acquired cases. In the 1980–1992 cohort, 29 per cent of cases were described as severe and a further 26 per cent as moderate.

ASSOCIATED IMPAIRMENTS AND SURVIVAL

In common with congenital cerebral palsy, many postneonatally acquired cases have very significant additional impairments. In the 1980–1992 Western Australian cohort, 22.3 per cent of postneonatally acquired cases have severe or profound learning disability compared with 19.5 per cent of congenitally acquired cases; 13.6 per cent are nonverbal compared with 24.6 per cent; 17.9 per cent are blind compared with 8.8 per cent; 45 per cent have epilepsy compared with 32 per cent; but only 1 of 121 is deaf compared with 2.3 per cent. By the age of 5 years 8.3 per cent were known to have died, compared with 8.1 per cent of congenitally acquired cases.

GENDER

As with congenital cerebral palsy, males tend to be at greater risk of postneonatally acquired cerebral palsy. In Western Australia the gender ratio was 1.37:1 in 1980–1992, not statistically significantly different from the ratio of 1.61:1 in the period 1956–1975. Gender ratios of 1.3:1 (Pharoah *et al.* 1989), 2.5:1 (Murphy *et al.* 1993) and 1.0:1 (Arens and Molteno 1989) have been reported elsewhere. Examining the distribution of cause of postneonatal acquisition by gender in the 1975–1992 Western Australian birth cohort shows that boys were slightly but not statistically significantly more likely to have an infectious cause (of 161 cases with recorded cause, 27 of 95 boys vs 15 of 66 girls), not more likely to have accidental head injury (26 of 95 boys vs 22 of 66 girls) and significantly more likely to be the target of nonaccidental injury (16 of 95 boys vs four of 66 girls: odds ratio = 3.1, 95% CI 1.0–9.9). Cause was coded as missing for an additional four girls and one boy. If it is assumed that all these unknown causes were in fact unreported nonaccidental injury, the odds ratio for a nonaccidental cause reduces to 1.7 (95% CI 0.7–4.1).

This suggests that males of less than 5 years are not at greater risk of postneonatally acquired cerebral palsy on account of their adventurousness, in contrast to the origin of injury in adolescents and young adults. In the same Western Australian 1975–1992 birth cohort there were no significant differences in distribution of age of acquisition: males were slightly more likely to acquire their cerebral palsy under 12 months of age, the age at which nonaccidental injury and cerebral infections are most likely.

PERINATAL RISK FACTORS
Birthweight and gestational age at delivery
Both Merseyside and Western Australian Registers have noted an association between birthweight and postneonatal acquisition. Pharoah *et al.* (1989) note a doubling of risk of postneonatal acquisition for infants with <2500g birthweight. In the 1956–1975 West Australian cohort an association was found only with birthweights between 2500 and 3500g. This may be an artefact as postneonatal acquisition was less likely to be assigned in cases with low birthweight (Blair and Stanley 1982). In the 1975–1992 cohort, analysis by race (Aboriginal or otherwise) and birthweight shows that much of the association with low birthweight is confounded by Aboriginal race, since Aboriginal babies tend to be of lower birthweights (Blair 1996d). There is, however, a small excess of birthweights below 2500g in both Caucasian and Aboriginal children with postneonatally acquired cerebral palsy, though not nearly as pronounced as that observed with congenitally acquired cerebral palsy. No postneonatally acquired case had a birthweight <1500g nor were any delivered before 33 weeks of gestation, though a higher proportion (14/121) were born preterm (before 36 completed weeks) than in the total population of neonatal survivors (odds ratio 1.7, 95% CI 1.0–2.9).

Maternal age and parity
The 1956–1975 Western Australian cohort analysis reported a weak association with increasing maternal age (Blair and Stanley 1982). In the more recent cohort an association was seen with maternal age below 20 years, but this disappears on stratification by race, since Aboriginal women tend to commence child-bearing at younger ages. There was a significant trend in rate of postneonatal acquisition with increasing maternal parity in the 1956–1975 cohort, and this has persisted in the 1980–1992 cohort. Aboriginal race also confounds this association because Aboriginal women tend to have a larger number of children than Caucasians. On stratification by race the association with parity does not reach statistical significance and is seen only among Aboriginal children, for whom there is a 60 per cent increase in rate for the fourth and subsequent births. While maternal age

and parity are confounded with Aboriginal race, it is possible that adolescent child-bearing and large numbers of children to care for may be on causal pathways to postneonatal acquisition of cerebral palsy in Aboriginal infants.

Plurality

Multiple births are not at higher risk of postneonatally acquired cerebral palsy. Of 121 postneonatally acquired Western Australian cases there was only one multiple birth, a twin. This is not only lower than among congenitally acquired cases (see Chapter 10), but is lower than the 2.2 per cent of multiples in the total population of Western Australian survivors to 1 year (Stanley and Petterson 1995).

Conclusions

Postneonatally acquired cerebral palsy accounts for a significant proportion of all cerebral palsy. It is no less severe and is equally disabling as congenitally acquired cerebral palsy, with a similar mortality rate to 5 years.

Most postneonatally acquired cerebral palsy is acquired in the first 12 months following birth. Males are at greater risk but not apparently as a result of their greater adventurousness. While postneonatally acquired cases tend to be more likely to have a birthweight <2500 g than the total population of live births, they are not born very preterm or of very low birthweight, and there is no strong evidence for predisposing medical or biological factors increasing their vulnerability to injury.

In less developed societies, postneonatally acquired cerebral palsy is principally due to cerebral infection and febrile convulsions in infancy. As societies develop, causes change and diversify rather than disappear entirely. Infectious causes become less important, and head injury becomes more important. Small numbers also result from causes that might previously have been fatal. The strong association with social disadvantage makes it likely that postneonatally acquired cerebral palsy is primarily a social disease of poverty and ignorance combining to create barriers to effective parenting.

12
POSSIBILITIES FOR THE PREVENTION OF THE CEREBRAL PALSIES: SOCIAL AND MEDICAL FACTORS

"The basic incongruity in American perinatal care lies in our superb ability to care for the individual patient and our dismal failure to address the problems of the larger society."

(Rosenblatt 1989)

"In recent years it has been suggested that it is unethical for new treatments to be introduced without proper evaluation using randomised controlled trials. Perhaps it is equally unethical if inappropriate endpoints for such trials are used: long term follow up of the baby should be regarded as an integral and essential part of well designed trials of interventions in the perinatal field."

(Johnson 1997)

It has been suggested in earlier chapters that the causal pathway model increases our potential to devise preventive strategies. The earlier a causal pathway can be interrupted the more effective the prevention is likely to be, as there is less chance the fetus will be compromised. Earlier interventions tend to be of a social or public health nature applied to a population, whereas later interventions tend to be medical care applied to a sick or compromised individual mother or neonate. Moving away from a single cause (*e.g.* birth asphyxia) or epoch (*e.g.* intrapartum) allows more effective but often less directly measurable preventive strategies.

For example, better diet (vitamin D) and housing (more sunlight) in England in the 19th century reduced the numbers of girls with rickets. When these children became mothers, they were less likely to have small rachitic pelves and had fewer obstructed and traumatic labours with reduced risk of intrapartum damage to the brains of their infants.

Table 12.1 lists the social conditions and social and medical risk factors that may initiate and interact on the considerable number of causal pathways to cerebral palsies, and outlines various preventive strategies. Links may plausibly be drawn between many factors in the table. Many may interact. Not all the social conditions shown are unequivocally bad. Unemployment *per se* is not always bad as it may allow time for optimal parenting and health care in pregnancy, whereas strenuous and tiring employment for women obliged to work in pregnancy can be damaging. However, involuntary unemployment coupled with poverty can be devastating and is often associated with poor education and limited access

TABLE 12.1
The importance of social conditions in pathways to cerebral palsy and possible preventive strategies

Social conditions	Unemployment	Poverty
	Poor education	Social disintegration
	Group isolation	Individual greed
	Environmental degradation	Social isolation
	Delayed childbearing	Declining communities
	Overpopulation	
Social risk factors	Domestic violence	Early motherhood
	Poor nutrition	Poor hygiene
	Substance abuse	Promiscuity
	Close child spacing	Toxic exposures
	Consanguinity	
Medical risk factors	Stress	Maternal abdominal trauma
	Nutritional deficiencies	Infection
	Sexually transmitted diseases	Infertility
	Reproductive technology	Recessive genetic defects
	Preterm birth	Intrauterine growth restriction
	Child abuse	Multiple births
	Individual morbidity	
Preventive strategies	Marriage/relationship counselling	Social security
	Universal literacy (particularly girls)	Sex/parenthood education
	Vaccines	Parenting programmes
	High quality, inexpensive child care	Genetic counselling
	Part time employment	Parental leave support
	Iodized salt	Dietary education
	Widely available family planning	Infant health programmes
	Alternative infertility treatment/	(infections, trauma, sudden infant
	counselling	death syndrome)

to information important for health. Many of these factors will cycle through families and generations.

Perinatology in the developed world has made a huge investment in research and care to treat high risk mothers and infants with resulting increases in individual survival. This overemphasis on expensive 'late' interventions to save life and the virtual neglect of the problems in the broader society which give rise to the causal pathways, and the resulting poor quality of life of the survivors, has been called the 'perinatal paradox' (Murphy 1993, Williams 1994, Kliegman 1995, Leviton 1995).

This paradox is reflected in the increasing numbers of very preterm infants with disabilities, and the static levels of preterm births and of indicators of poor maternal and child health in our populations (Kliegman 1995, Guyer *et al.* 1997). The level of cerebral palsy in the community is a balance between many contributing pathways. Social conditions which improve general maternal health may be counterbalanced by those which increase cerebral palsy; *e.g.* medical care which reduces both deaths and cerebral palsy also results in the increased survival of small sick neonates ever more vulnerable to cerebral damage.

Considering causal pathways encourages new and broader ways of thinking about cause, increasing the number of options for prevention. Currently, funding and commitment still favours later medical interventions rather than earlier social and public health programmes. While those working to provide perinatal care may feel that the population-based interventions are beyond their jurisdictions, they should be encouraged to think about causal sequences, and collectively we may be powerful enough to influence government and non-government agencies to develop policies to address some of the important social conditions in Table 12.1. In the meantime, it is important for those providing care to ensure that what they do is based on firm evidence. This chapter aims to summarize what is known of the effectiveness of specific current public health, obstetric, neonatal and postneonatal interventions in reducing cerebral palsy risk. An important aspect of this is the quality of the evidence available upon which we can base our recommendations for prevention.

Levels of evidence
SOME STUDIES ARE MORE RELIABLE THAN OTHERS
Many types of epidemiological studies have been used to assess causality—where either an intervention causes a reduction in cerebral palsy, or an exposure causes cerebral palsy. These range from interpretations of the results of ecological studies (*e.g.* trends in rates of cerebral palsy under different circumstances as assessed by aggregated data) to comparing how frequently cerebral palsy occurs in the different arms of randomized controlled trials of specific interventions. Table 12.2 lists the different types of epidemiological studies in order of increasing levels of confidence in causal inference. Causal inference from descriptive studies is the least secure while that from randomized controlled trials is the most secure.

Descriptive studies (Table 12.2A)
In studies that compare rates of cerebral palsy in different populations (ecological studies), such as in time periods before and after the availability of neonatal intensive care, we may not be aware of other factors which may influence the rates and thus incorrect assumptions are made about the effects of the exposure of interest. In studies of a series of individuals with cerebral palsy, the frequency of various interventions can be described. However, if these frequencies cannot be compared with those found in individuals without cerebral palsy, we cannot evaluate effectiveness.

Controlled studies (Table 12.2B)
Case–control studies allow the comparison of frequencies between cases and controls of a variety of risk factors including whether they had been exposed to a preventive strategy or not. The major problem with these studies is bias: (i) in either case or control selection; (ii) in who gets the intervention; (iii) in data collection since it is almost always retrospective; and (iv) in control of confounding factors. There is also the frustrating problem of crucial data being unrecorded and therefore unavailable for study. Cohort studies can overcome bias both in subject selection (provided losses to follow-up are minimal) and in data collection, particularly in prospective cohort studies, as data are collected closer to the time of exposure. However, even prospective cohort studies suffer from bias because the intervention being investigated is not randomly allocated.

TABLE 12.2

TABLE 12.2
Levels of evidence in epidemiological studies to evaluate effectiveness of preventive strategies

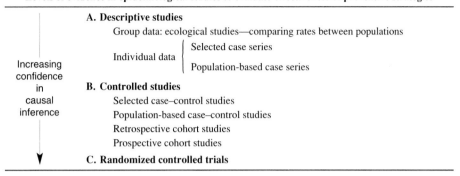

	A. Descriptive studies
	Group data: ecological studies—comparing rates between populations
	Individual data — Selected case series
	Individual data — Population-based case series
Increasing confidence in causal inference	**B. Controlled studies**
	Selected case–control studies
	Population-based case–control studies
	Retrospective cohort studies
	Prospective cohort studies
	C. Randomized controlled trials

Randomized controlled trials (Table 12.2C)

The easiest studies to interpret are those with random allocation of interventions in a way that avoids bias and confounding—the randomized trials.

The difficulties in drawing causal inferences from observational studies of obstetric or neonatal care practices should discourage their use in the evaluation of care. There has been a significant movement in many areas of medical care evaluation toward randomized trials, which are, when properly performed, the most trusted method of assessing interventions, and provide the most reliable and thus highly persuasive evidence on which to base practice (Tarnow-Mordi and Brocklehurst 1997). A recent paper by Jordens *et al.* (1998) reported a survey of all neonatologists (with a 95% response rate) and a sample of obstetricians (87% response rate) in Australia and ascertained that the majority felt that their practice had been influenced considerably by the results of randomized trials and systematic reviews of randomized trials. However, a national survey of obstetric practice in Canada suggested that considerable use of procedures and technologies known to be unnecessary or potentially harmful still continues (Kaczorowski *et al.* 1998).

SYSTEMATIC REVIEWS AND THE COCHRANE COLLABORATION

Paralleling the increase in randomized trials, the International Cochrane Collaboration has initiated the systematic review of their results in many areas and encouraged researchers to fill the gaps in knowledge about the effects of medical care. This worldwide expansion of scientifically conducted and disseminated systematic reviews had its origins in the peri-natal arena (National Perinatal Epidemiology Unit 1996). The Oxford Data Base of perinatal trials (Sinclair and Bracken 1992) has now grown into the Cochrane Pregnancy and Childbirth Data Base. This data base is continually updated, available electronically and aims to provide unbiased, accurate and up to date information of the effects of obstetric, midwifery and neonatal practice (Henderson-Smart and Crowther 1997, Neilson and Levene 1997). It includes public health as well as clinical interventions. It is part of a major and mostly voluntary international collaborative activity, conducting systematic reviews in many areas of health care. We have used this data base as a source of systematic reviews throughout this chapter. For information on reading and interpreting systematic reviews, see Klassen *et al.* (1998).

WHY ARE CEREBRAL PALSY AND OTHER LONG TERM OUTCOMES NOT EXAMINED IN RANDOMIZED TRIALS OF PERINATAL INTERVENTIONS?

Few trials or meta-analyses of perinatal interventions are large enough or last long enough to allow the proper assessment of their effects on cerebral palsy or other long term outcomes (Villar *et al.* 1995, Johnson 1997, Mongelli *et al.* 1997, Tarnow-Mordi and Brocklehurst 1997). Trials and meta-analyses which provide conclusive evidence about perinatal mortality or surrogate measures of long term outcomes but which are inconclusive about major long term outcomes such as cerebral palsy may stop further research, with the result that effects on cerebral palsy are not measured (Tarnow-Mordi and Brocklehurst 1997). The inferences from many small trials pooled together in meta-analyses are not as secure as those from large, well conducted, multicentre trials with good follow-up. For example, we still need trials with long term follow-up of antibiotic therapies for preterm pre-labour rupture of membranes which reduce infections and prolong pregnancy: their effects on mortality and brain pathology are unknown and could be adverse. Many neonatal interventions could improve the chances of survival but at the expense of an increased risk of disability among the surviving children. As Johnson (1997) states, parents are most concerned about the risk of later disability in their child.

Practical difficulties are the main barrier to long term follow-up being incorporated into perinatal trials. These difficulties include the diversity of long term outcomes, their low prevalence (2 per 1000 for cerebral palsy), decisions about the best time to trace and examine the children, losses to follow-up and their impact on the accuracy of estimates of disability, as well as the time and costs inherent in any follow-up study (Wariyar and Richmond 1989, Fooks *et al.* 1997, Johnson 1997). Cerebral palsy registers such as the ones in Western Australia, Sweden and Oxford enable cerebral palsy among study participants to be recognized very easily provided out-migration by the age of registration is low. Networks of Neonatal Intensive Care Units have been established in the USA, Europe and Australia to encourage large, randomized trials of new therapies and to monitor the impact of their introduction (Donoghue 1997, Wright and Papile 1997). These should be encouraged and where possible linked into data bases that allow cerebral palsy and other outcomes to be studied (see Chapter 14).

The extent to which improvements in obstetric and neonatal care over the past three decades have resulted in improved population measures of fetal outcome such as perinatal mortality or cerebral palsy is of great interest to obstetricians, paediatricians and those organizing and funding perinatal services. We feel it is now self-evident that, particularly in obstetrics and neonatology, no new treatment should be introduced without good evidence of its effectiveness and, above all, its safety. However, there are many situations, including the offer of prenatal diagnosis, use of operative delivery, and invasive investigations, where it has been difficult to randomize patients to treatment or no treatment groups (Lumley *et al.* 1985b); hence much of the available evidence is not based on randomized controlled trials but on observational studies with their inherent problems of interpretation.

Evidence for prevention

For this review we have sought the most reliable evidence available for systematic reviews—*Effective Care in Pregnancy and Childbirth* (Chalmers *et al.* 1989), *Effective Care of the Newborn Infant* (Sinclair and Bracken 1992), *Cochrane Pregnancy and Childbirth Data Base* (Cochrane Collaboration 1998a)—before interpreting other published sources more cautiously. Recommendations for further research are made. The sequence of this chapter follows the order of the chapters relating to causal pathways.

Prevention of causal pathways commencing before conception or early in pregnancy (Chapter 6)

As discussed in Chapter 6, these pathways included those with inherited genetic factors, infertility and endocrine problems, and the range of factors (teratogens, toxic compounds, infections, vascular accidents) which result in cerebral and other organ malformations and in defects such as porencephaly and neuronal migration disorders. Some specific maternal exposures such as methylmercury, alcohol and carbon monoxide poisoning and severe iodine deficiency are also implicated in causing early brain pathology and cerebral palsy.

Effective interventions to reduce cerebral palsy arising early in pregnancy are listed in Table 12.3. The other factors mentioned in Chapter 6 require more research either to prove they are on causal pathways to cerebral palsy or to determine how the pathways can be interrupted.

Routine Ultrasound in Early Pregnancy

The assumed benefits of one routine ultrasound in early pregnancy have been better assessment of gestational age, earlier detection of multiple pregnancy, and detection of fetal malformations at a time when offering termination of pregnancy is still an option (Neilson 1998).

The detection of clinically unsuspected fetal anomalies early enough in pregnancy to offer termination to the parents of an affected fetus has been addressed in detail in two trials. One showed improved detection, increased terminations and reduced perinatal mortality (Saari-Kemppainen *et al.* 1990). This, if implemented as a public health strategy in large populations of pregnant women, would presumably translate into fewer surviving children with cerebral palsy due to malformations if ultrasound detected those with nonlethal defects. The other trial had much lower detection rates, reflecting poor diagnostic acumen, and had minimal impact on mortality (Ewigman *et al.* 1993).

The meta-analysis overall showed an increase in terminations for abnormalities, a decrease in undiagnosed twins at early gestational ages, fewer inductions for post-term pregnancies (reflecting better gestational age assessments), a nonsignificant reduction in perinatal death rates, and no differences in long term adverse outcomes. One study noted an increase in left handedness, which could have been a chance finding but may have some worrying aspects (Paneth 1998). In practice, prenatal ultrasound may alter the management of labour but not neonatal outcome (Skari *et al.* 1998); more research is needed.

The rapid increases in antenatal screening and diagnosis bring certain problems. Certain chromosomal anomalies, such as those of the sex chromosomes, are relatively common and

TABLE 12.3
Interventions to reduce cerebral palsy arising from early pregnancy pathways

A. *Effective*—good levels of evidence
 1. Rubella vaccination
 2. Iodine supplementation in areas of severe iodine deficiency
 3. Cleaning environments contaminated with methylmercury
 4. Anti-D vaccination to prevent kernicterus

B. *Probably effective*—less evidence and needs more data with regard to recommendations
 1. One routine early ultrasound
 2. Reducing excessive fetal alcohol exposure
 3. Avoiding toxoplasmosis
 4. Screening for toxoplasmosis in endemic areas

compatible with a reasonable quality of life, and yet may be associated with some motor impairment. Even when there is certainty about the presence of a structural anomaly of the brain, such as a cyst, or partial or complete agenesis of the corpus callosum, not enough is known about the natural history of such anomalies to predict which are compatible with normal motor development and which are associated with severe disability. Where such anomalies are found it is not easy to judge whether offering termination of pregnancy is justified.

When screening with fetal imaging, additional problems of specificity and sensitivity of diagnosis arise because interobserver error is likely to be greater than in karyotyping or biochemical estimations. Before a screening programme is introduced into practice it is therefore important to be sure that it will do more good than harm. For each abnormality the screening detection sensitivity, specificity, false negative and false positive rates need to be estimated, together with the medical and financial costs of screening which must be balanced against the benefits. This is particularly important for findings of uncertain or little medical consequence that may lead to worry and further unnecessary obstetric intervention (Wald and Kennard 1998). Screening should be organized in the context of a well run genetic counselling service (D'Ercole *et al.* 1998).

RUBELLA VACCINATION TO PREVENT CONGENITAL RUBELLA SYNDROME
Following the development of the rubella vaccine most countries developed a policy of vaccinating young teenage girls with the aim of immunizing them before they became pregnant. Whilst this was successful in reducing the incidence of congenital rubella syndrome quite dramatically in the years following the programmes (Stanley *et al.* 1985), cases continued to be born to women who had not seroconverted following vaccination or who, for a variety of reasons, were not vaccinated.

Although preventive programmes vary from place to place, now all young children are usually immunized with a combined measles–mumps–rubella vaccine, with the aim of reducing the infection in the community generally and thus the chances of any pregnant woman being exposed (Centers for Disease Control 1998). This is usually backed up by screening for maternal antibody status, ideally preconceptionally but more usually in pregnancy. Mothers shown to be nonimmune in pregnancy will be counselled to avoid exposure to rubella if possible and offered postpartum vaccination. Offering gammaglobulin as passive protection has not been shown to prevent rubella after exposure, and the US Centers for Disease Control (1998) do not recommend it in pregnancy or at any other time. Infants with congenital rubella have been born to women who received gammaglobulin after exposure. In the UK, maternal rubella infection in early pregnancy is a ground for legal termination if the parents wish it. So far all women inadvertently vaccinated in pregnancy have had normal babies and thus this group can be reassured (Preblud and Williams 1985).

The costs of congenital rubella syndrome outweigh those of vaccination several fold (Wang and Smaill 1989). There is evidence of an increase in congenital rubella in the USA with recent falls in vaccinations levels (Lee *et al.* 1992, Centers for Disease Control 1997).

IODINE SUPPLEMENTATION IN AREAS OF SEVERE DEFICIENCY TO PREVENT MATERNAL IODINE DEFICIENCY AND ENDEMIC CRETINISM
A randomized controlled trial from Papua New Guinea comparing iodized oil with saline given to alternate households in an area with high rates of endemic cretinism demonstrated that the condition could be prevented if iodine was given before pregnancy (Pharoah *et al.* 1971, Pharoah and Connolly 1987). An epidemic of endemic cretinism had been described in New Guinea in the 1950s after the local population obtained iodine free salt, having previously used naturally occurring iodine rich salt. Subsequent use of iodized salt resulted in a virtual abolition of the condition (Pharoah *et al.* 1971, Hetzel 1994b). In spite of this knowledge, the condition remains endemic in many areas of the world in spite of efforts by WHO and UNICEF, and we believe that it is the most important preventable cause of cerebral palsy worldwide. This is an excellent example of the need for political action for an effective public health intervention to prevent a major cause of cerebral palsy.

ELIMINATION OF METHYLMERCURY FROM THE FOOD CHAIN TO PREVENT FETAL NEUROTOXICITY
Environmental disasters such as the methylmercury poisoning in Minamata, Japan (Kurland *et al.* 1960) caution us that the fetus is vulnerable to chemical teratogens and neurotoxins. Our commitment should be to clean environments and to public health policies to ensure that pregnant women are not in hazardous situations either at work or where they live (see Table 12.1).

ANTI-D VACCINATION FOR THE PREVENTION OF KERNICTERUS IN PREGNANCIES AFFECTED BY RH BLOOD GROUP INCOMPATIBILITY
Vaccination with anti-D has been one of the most important prevention strategies in obstetrics, to which the major part of the reduction in Rhesus isoimmunization, kernicterus, death and cerebral palsy has been attributed (Gravenhorst 1989). Considerable contribution also resulted from the significant reduction in large families in which the disease is more likely.

A series of controlled trials were carried out in the late 1960s following the discovery of anti-D (Clarke *et al.* 1963, Freda *et al.* 1964). Women receiving anti-D had no antibodies months after their immunizing pregnancy, and deaths and cerebral palsy due to this disease have been eliminated in those places where anti-D programmes are in place (Stanley and Alberman 1984).

Prevention strategies applied later in the causal pathway include exchange transfusion to reduce the damaging effects of isoimmunization on the fetus or neonate (Gravenhorst 1989). Exchange transfusions, either intrauterine or neonatal, whilst effective, have considerable complication rates, and a proportion of those transfused are still neurologically damaged (Ellis 1980).

MATERNAL CLOTTING DEFECTS

Genetic clotting defects are increasingly being implicated in fetal cerebrovascular accidents with resulting porencephalic cysts and even hydranencephaly (Thorarensen *et al.* 1997, Debus *et al.* 1998). Further research into detecting these defects (such as factor V Leiden and maternal antiphospholipid antibodies) may eventually elucidate preventable pathways. A controlled trial comparing aspirin with aspirin plus heparin for women with previously affected pregnancies has already commenced (Perinatal Trials Group 1998).

PREVENTING EXCESSIVE FETAL ALCOHOL EXPOSURE IN PREGNANCY

Programmes specifically aimed at preventing fetal alcohol syndrome can be population-based health education or specific pre-pregnancy counselling sessions targeting individual women (Newman 1986, Lumley and Astbury 1989). The aims of such programmes should be to avoid heavy exposures rather than to avoid all alcohol. Women who drink heavily also tend to abuse other substances which may also adversely affect pregnancy outcomes and their health generally.

Campaigns to increase public awareness of the dangers of alcohol in pregnancy make pregnant women anxious, particularly if they drank significantly before they realized that they were pregnant. There has been considerable debate about safe limits of alcohol recommended in public health programmes. In a large cohort study in Australia no untoward fetal effects were noted in women drinking up to two standard drinks every day (Lumley *et al.* 1985a). A meta-analysis showed a lower prevalence of preterm delivery and fetal growth restriction in those drinking one or two alcoholic drinks per day than in those drinking either more or none (Holman *et al.* 1996a,b). Drinking some as opposed to no alcohol in pregnancy reduced the risk of neonatal encephalopathy (Badawi *et al.* 1998a).

SCREENING FOR, OR AVOIDING CONTACT WITH, TOXOPLASMOSIS AND CYTOMEGALOVIRUS (CMV)

As there is no vaccine to prevent toxoplasmosis, debate has centred around two other possible preventive strategies. The first is to screen for toxoplasmosis in pregnancy with treatment of those women found to be seropositive. However, major uncertainties exist regarding risk of infection, efficacy of treatment regimes and the costs of implementing such programmes, particularly in low prevalence areas. The population incidence in Western Australia (Walpole *et al.* 1991a) is too low to suggest that screening would be cost-effective. Alternatively, health education campaigns could be introduced advising pregnant women against preparing or eating undercooked meat and to avoid handling cats (Henderson *et al.*

1984). In the case of CMV, which may be the most common congenital infection associated with cerebral palsy, methods of prevention have not yet been established. Work is proceeding on possible vaccines, but as yet no safe vaccine has been developed. If available it might prevent somewhere between 1 and 10 per cent of all cerebral palsy, depending on the risk status of the population concerned. The risk of contracting this infection varies with maternal age, parity and opportunities for exposure such as in day care centres or workplaces (Murph *et al.* 1998). No effective public health message is available.

Evidence for prevention of causal pathways to cerebral palsy involving very preterm birth (Chapter 7)

An immense amount of research has focused on very preterm birth since it is the most important cause of both infant death and childhood morbidity. In spite of the close correlation between cerebral palsy risk and decreasing gestational age, very preterm birth alone is not a 'sufficient' cause of cerebral palsy. The majority of very preterm survivors do not develop cerebral palsy, and a proportion of those who do are damaged antenatally. This is known from imaging studies as discussed in Chapter 7. Delaying preterm delivery can prevent brain damage resulting only from specific neonatal complications of very preterm delivery, not that incurred antenatally. There has been little emphasis on global social interventions to reduce the rate of preterm births, which seem to be more successful at targeting moderately rather than extremely preterm births (Leviton 1995).

INTERVENTIONS TO PREVENT PRETERM BIRTH

Only France appears to have successfully reduced its preterm birth rate, halving the proportions born before 33 weeks gestation nationally between 1972 and 1981 (Papiernik 1993). Over the same period the total cerebral palsy rate fell slightly from 1.07/1000 to 0.98/1000 births (Rumeau-Rouquette *et al.* 1994). However, a causal link cannot be assumed, particularly since the largest decreases in rates of cerebral palsy were for spastic hemiplegia and quadriplegia rather than diplegia, the type most commonly associated with very preterm birth.

The evidence concerning strategies aimed at the primary prevention of preterm birth is now reviewed, followed by those which may reduce the neonatal morbidity associated with very preterm delivery and which may impact on cerebral palsy rates. This concentrates on aspects of obstetric and neonatal care as this is where most of the research has been done.

Table 12.4 summarizes the recent systematic reviews of main interventions for preventing very preterm birth, together with their effects on other outcomes and cerebral palsy rates. Few have been successful in delaying or avoiding very preterm delivery, and *none* has been shown to have any impact on cerebral palsy.

Social support in pregnancy

The meta-analyses of social support in pregnancy of trials with large numbers of women showed no benefit in terms of preterm birth, neonatal mortality, need for intensive neonatal care admission or other factors which might indicate an improved neurological outcome for the baby (Blondel and Bréart 1995, Hodnett 1998). However, social and emotional

TABLE 12.4
Prevention of preterm birth (PTB): evidence of effectiveness from meta-analyses

Intervention (Reference)	Effect on preterm birth	Other effects	Effect on cerebral palsy
1. Antenatal social support (Hodnett 1998a)	None	Positive psychosocial	Not known; ? ↓ postneonatally acquired cerebral palsy
2. Bed rest in hospital for multiple births (Crowther 1997)	None overall; may ↑ PTB (<34 w)	?Better growth; may ↓ maternal hypertension	Not known
3. Antibiotics			
• Asymptomatic bacteriuria (Smaill 1998)	↓ PTB	None	Not known
• PPROM (Kenyon and Boulvain 1998)	Prolongs pregnancy	↓ Chorioamnionitis ↓ Neonatal infection	Not known[1]
• Preterm labour, intact membranes (King and Flenady 1998)	None	↓ Chorioamnionitis ↓ Neonatal encephalopathy ↑ Perinatal deaths	Not known (no IVH effects)
4. Tocolysis in active preterm labour (Keirse et al. 1989)			
• Betaminetics	↓ Delivery <48 h ↓ Delivery <37 w	None on respiratory distress syndrome (RDS) or perinatal death	Unknown[2]
• Indomethacin	↓ Delivery <48 h ↓ Delivery <37 w	None on RDS or perinatal death	
• Magnesium sulphate for previous preterm birth	Weak effects	Not known; ? ↑ PVH	Unknown
5. Low dose aspirin for prevention of pre-eclampsia (Darling 1998)	None	None on IUGR	None

[1]Nonsignificant reduction in neonatal cranial ultrasound abnormality.
[2]Major benefits on cerebral palsy may be to delay delivery long enough to allow maternal transfer to a tertiary centre and to give steroids to reduce the risk of respiratory distress syndrome.

outcomes were improved for the mothers who had less postnatal depression and more confidence with parenting and caring for the child. Such effects could translate into better postnatal care for children and prevention of postneonatally acquired cerebral palsy (see Table 12.1).

Hospitalization with bed rest for multiple pregnancy
Bedrest in hospital for multiple pregnancy with no additional pathology showed no evidence

of reducing rates of preterm delivery; in fact there was a significant increase in births before 34 weeks. There was no long term follow-up so the effects on cerebral palsy are not known.

Antibiotics in pregnancy

The effect of antibiotics for asymptomatic bacteriuria, premature prolonged rupture of membranes (PPROM) or in preterm labour with intact membranes is of considerable interest given the observational studies reviewed in Chapter 7. No clear evidence of a significant effect of antibiotics on cerebral palsy rates was reported in any of these various situations, although as both chorioamnionitis and neonatal infection tended to be reduced (non-significantly) one would have anticipated a beneficial effect on mortality and cerebral palsy. There was some concern about the increase in perinatal mortality in one review which was unexpected and significant (King and Johnson 1995). An international, multicentre, random-ized controlled trial of antibiotics in preterm labour with ruptured membranes (the ORACLE trial) is currently underway which will be large enough to investigate infections and deaths and is seeking additional funding for long term follow-up to an age at which cerebral palsy can be recognized (W. Tarnow-Mordi, personal communication 1998). Thus it is premature to introduce large scale programmes aimed at eradicating maternal reproductive tract infections in pregnancy. Bacterial vaginosis is a common condition, being found in at least 10 per cent of pregnant women. Its treatment involves the use of powerful and expensive antibiotics and the effect on risk of cerebral palsy is not known. One recent editorial has recommended that more trials of treatment be undertaken (Goldenberg and Andrews 1996), and another has counselled caution before a "rush to obliterate genital tract colonisation" (Pearlman and Faix 1997). Even if the putative damaging effects of inflammatory cytokines and chemokines in preterm births is confirmed, there is as yet no effective treatment. Nevertheless this is a promising field of research which demands a collaborative approach.

Tocolysis

Trials of several therapies such as betamimetics and indomethacin prolong pregnancy (Table 12.4), but they have not been shown to have any beneficial effect on perinatal outcomes. Their benefit appears to be only to prolong delivery long enough to intervene with other useful activities such as giving the mother corticosteroids or transferring her to deliver in a tertiary centre to improve neonatal outcome. Both of these may reduce the risk of cerebral palsy but definite evidence is lacking.

A recent trial of magnesium sulphate for maintenance treatment after threatened preterm labour (Crowther and Moore 1998) showed no effect on periventricular haemorrhage when compared with other tocolytics but a significant increase when compared with placebo. This suggests that any tocolysis may increase haemorrhage; however, these trials were felt to be of poor quality (Crowther and Moore 1998). There was no effect on preterm birth. Mag-nesium sulphate cannot therefore be recommended for tocolysis on the currently available randomized trial evidence, although it is widely used in the USA for both tocolysis and for preventing fits in pre-eclampsia (for which there is good evidence) (Keirse *et al.* 1989).

Adverse short term side-effects and inadequate data on any long term outcomes of tocolysis should encourage both caution in its use and further research in this area.

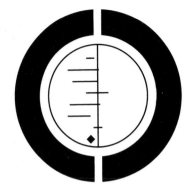

Fig. 12.1. The Cochrane Collaboration logo: the summary meta-analysis demonstrating the significant reduction in respiratory distress syndrome in infants born preterm to mothers who had received antenatal corticosteroids.

Reducing the incidence or severity of pre-eclampsia

Reducing the incidence or severity of pre-eclampsia (and hypertensive disease of pregnancy) would have an important effect on the incidence of preterm birth, as it is responsible for a significant percentage of elective preterm deliveries, but few studies of the prevention of pre-eclampsia are available. Several trials of low dose aspirin have been done, based on the underlying plausible hypothesis of preventing thrombi in placental vessels. An overview of these trials (Darling 1998) showed no reduction in pre-eclampsia, poor fetal growth or preterm delivery either in all or in high risk groups. There are currently no clinically accurate tests for detecting either pre-eclampsia or growth restriction resulting from it, nor any effective means of prevention. The complex pathogenesis associated with pre-eclampsia and its consequences demands multidisciplinary investigation. Several trials and a meta-analysis (Chien *et al.* 1996, Coetzee *et al.* 1998, Duley *et al.* 1998) now strongly support the use of magnesium for preventing maternal eclamptic seizures, but no data are yet available for the effects on cerebral palsy (see p. 153).

No studies could be identified to provide any information on the reduction of preterm birth due to antepartum haemorrhage or idiopathic causes; multiple births are discussed later.

INTERVENTIONS IN LATE PREGNANCY TO REDUCE THE INCIDENCE OF THE NEONATAL COMPLICATIONS OF VERY PRETERM BIRTH

Interventions to improve the neonatal condition of the very preterm baby can be implemented provided there is sufficient time from signs indicative of threatened preterm labour to the birth. Such an interval can be created by tocolysis as mentioned earlier.

Antenatal corticosteroids in preterm labour

The Cochrane Collaboration logo (Fig. 12.1) depicts the summary meta-analysis demonstrating the significant reduction in respiratory distress syndrome in infants born preterm to mothers who had received antenatal corticosteroids.

The most recently updated review of this meta-analysis (Crowley 1999) also shows a significant reduction in ultrasound diagnosed periventricular haemorrhage and, not surprisingly, reductions in mortality, and in duration and cost of hospital stay. This review includes data

TABLE 12.5

Studies of corticosteroids for preterm delivery: numbers with long-term neurological abnormality in subject vs control (placebo or no treatment) populations*

Study	Subjects n/N	Controls n/N	Peto odds ratio[1] (95% CI)[2]	Weight[1] %	Peto odds ratio[1] (95% CI)
Auckland 1972	12/139	15/111		47.4	0.60 (0.27–1.35)
Amsterdam 1980	2/64	2/58		7.7	0.90 (0.12–6.59)
US Steroid Trial 1981–1989	9/200	15/206		44.9	0.61 (0.27–1.38)
Total	23/403	32/375		100.0	0.62 (0.36–1.08)
χ^2 0.14 (df=2); Z = 1.67					

0.1   0.2   1   5   10

*Adapted from Crowley (1999)—see source for relevant study references.

This is an abstract of a regularly updated systematic review prepared and maintained by the Cochrane Collaboration.

[1]See Glossary.

[2]For an explanation of the symbols used here, see Glossary, under Meta-analyses.

TABLE 12.6

Impact of prenatal dexamethasone on the odds of intraventricular haemorrhage or periventricular leukomalacia—multiple logistic regression analysis[1]

Hours prior to delivery of dexamethasone treatment	IVH or PVL Odds ratio (95% CI)	
<24 hours	0.07 (0.01–0.65)	p=0.02
1–14 days	0.05 (0.01–0.32)	p=0.001
>14 days	4.8 (0.29–79.0)	p=0.3

[1]Adjusted for gestational age, birthweight, sex and maternal hypertension. Reproduced by permission from Kari et al. (1994).

on effect on long-term neurological abnormality for survivors followed for one to two years. Compared with placebo and no treatment groups, the group of babies whose mothers were treated were found to have a clinically important, though not statistically significant, reduction of 38 per cent in such abnormalities (Table 12.5). Given that those in the cortico-steroid group had many more survivors at lower gestations than those whose mothers had received placebo, this finding is encouraging as more with poor neurological function would have been expected in the corticosteroid group due to their greater degree of immaturity. This is a biologically plausible finding given what is known about fetal and neonatal physiology and consistent with observational studies associating antenatal steroids with lower levels of intraventricular haemorrhage (Leviton et al. 1993) and cerebral palsy (O. Dammann, personal communication 1998).

A recent trial (Kari et al. 1994) of antenatal corticosteroid (dexamethasone) treatment in 77 pregnancies for threatened labour between 24 and 32 weeks, together with rescue neonatal surfactant, reported a marked reduction of intraventricular haemorrhage and periventricular leukomalacia compared with 80 pregnancies in a placebo group, although there was no significant difference in mortality (Table 12.6). The infants in the dexamethasone group had lower requirements for surfactant, shorter duration of ventilatory support and oxygen therapy, and higher neonatal survival without ventilation than those in the placebo group. They also had a higher mean blood pressure in the first three days of life. The reduction in incidence of IVH/PVL was only significant in those with treatment close to delivery and more marked in those infants who also had surfactant (odds ratio 0.11, 95% CI 0.02–0.58) than in those who did not (odds ratio 0.55, 95% CI 0.14–2.18). Only one trial (Salokorpi et al. 1997) has data on neurological outcomes (at 2 years): the incidence of cerebral palsy was 10 per cent (5/50) in the dexamethasone group and 22 per cent (7/32) in the placebo group (odds ratio 0.15, 95% CI 0.03–0.84).

O. Dammann (personal communication 1998) has reviewed the current evidence for the short and long term protective effect of this treatment and makes a strong recommendation for its use. However, meta-analyses have suggested that increased risk of maternal or neonatal infection is a possible adverse effect (Crowley 1989), and the effects of multiple courses of treatment in women threatening to go into preterm labour over an extended period are unknown (Quinlivan *et al.* 1998). The risk associated with multiple courses is currently being evaluated in a new multicentre randomized controlled trial (A. Johnson, personal communication 1998). Concomitant glucocorticoids appear to diminish the beneficial effects of antibiotics given to prevent sepsis in infants with preterm premature rupture of membranes (Leitich *et al.* 1998).

The reduction of both mortality and cerebral palsy in children of mothers treated antenatally with steroids compared with children of those randomized to no treatment suggests either that in some preterm births respiratory distress and IVH are on the causal chain leading to cerebral palsy, or that the corticosteroids provide a neuroprotective effect independent of the effect on respiratory function. The latter possibility, if confirmed, would represent a very important advance in our understanding of the preventive process. Either way, these findings provide evidence against the assumption that a reduction of mortality in very preterm infants is inevitably associated with a rise in the rate of cerebral palsy.

Thyrotropin releasing hormone
There is no evidence that the addition of thyrotropin releasing hormone (TRH) to the antenatal steroids provides any additional benefit, in spite of basic research suggesting a possible rationale (Crowther *et al.* 1998a). No effect on cerebral haemorrhage was observed in these infants. In fact there were significantly more maternal side-effects with TRH; and in babies born more than 10 days after trial entry (the majority), more died, needed oxygen and had respiratory problems than those whose mothers had received only corticosteroids. The Australian Collaborative Trial of Antenatal TRH (ACTOBAT) (Crowther *et al.* 1997) has reported an increase in motor delay (odds ratio 1.51, 95% CI 1.11–2.05) and in other minor neurological impairments at 1 year of age. They recommend longer follow-up to ascertain more accurately any permanent adverse effects on the nervous system.

Antenatal indomethacin
Randomized controlled trials of antenatal indomethacin for tocolysis demonstrate no benefit in terms of reducing intraventricular haemorrhaege in very preterm birth, although inadequate follow-up and small sample size precludes proper analysis (Keirse *et al.* 1989). In addition, several observational studies have suggested adverse effects neonatally, including an increased incidence of periventricular haemorrhage and bronchopulmonary dysplasia (Eronen *et al.* 1994, Chang *et al.* 1997, Souter *et al.* 1998).

Magnesium sulphate
In spite of the weakness of the evidence that magnesium sulphate is a tocolytic, its wide use in the USA has enabled the results of some controlled studies to lead to the hypothesis that it reduces the rate of cerebral palsy in preterm infants (Nelson and Grether 1995, 1996, 1997; Nelson 1997; Grether *et al.* 1998). Other reports have not been able to confirm this effect (for review, see Paneth *et al.* 1997). It has been suggested that the reduced odds ratios may reflect confounding (Blair *et al.* 1996). Whilst magnesium does not seem to reduce white matter damage in low birthweight infants (Leviton *et al.* 1997), there are biologically plausible mechanisms whereby magnesium could be protective, and there is general

agreement that this is an important hypothesis which needs to be tested. Thus several large randomized trials of antenatal magnesium sulphate in preterm deliveries have been set up, including the Australian ACTOMgSO$_4$ (Crowther *et al.* 1998b) and the French Premag (Bénichou *et al.* 1998). However, MAGnet (the US Magnesium and Neurologic Endpoint Trial) was stopped early after reporting nine paediatric deaths among preterm infants born to 75 mothers exposed to magnesium compared to only one death in 75 whose mothers were not exposed. Five were due to sudden infant death syndrome, two to twin-to-twin transfusion syndrome, one to congenital malformation and three to perinatal causes (Mittendorf *et al.* 1997). There were criticisms of the MAGnet investigators' interpretation of their data (Bénichou *et al.* 1998, Crowther *et al.* 1998b), and its design differed considerably from the other continuing trials. Answers will eventually emerge from these as to whether or not antenatal magnesium is a safe and effective preventive strategy for cerebral palsy in preterm infants.

TERTIARY CARE

There has long been suggestive evidence that delivery in a tertiary care unit results in reduced mortality and morbidity in babies of very low birthweight. Preterm neonates born outside and transported in to tertiary centres have higher mortality and cerebral palsy rates than those 'inborn' (Ozminkowski *et al.* 1988, French *et al.* 1996, Truffert *et al.* 1998). Grether *et al.* (1996) have shown that very low birthweight singletons in a Level 1 unit had a six-fold risk of cerebral palsy compared with those born in better resourced units; this risk was magnified if delivery occurred rapidly from the time of admission, suggesting confounding in terms of both gestational age and precipitous delivery. In addition, both selection and referral bias would influence the results of these observational studies. Good tertiary centres include good perinatal (obstetric and immediate newborn) care as well as good neonatal intensive care aimed at maintaining homeostasis (warmth, fluids, nutrition, etc.).

Mode of delivery

Whilst there has been a tendency for caesarean section to be used more for women in preterm labour, no good evidence exists to support this practice (Grant 1998). Only five trials were available for Grant's 1995 review, with a total of only 104 women recruited.

There appear to be few benefits in terms of immediate neonatal morbidity; the reduction in intracranial pathology was not significant either statistically or clinically; and more postpartum complications and less breast-feeding occurred amongst those women randomized to the caesarean section group than those delivering vaginally. However, observational data (Murphy *et al.* 1995) suggest that elective caesarean section reduces cerebral palsy risk in very preterm infants (odds ratio 0.3; 95% CI 0.2–0.7). Few studies of any type have examined the effects of elective or emergency caesarean sections on outcome, in either preterm or term infants with fetal distress (see p. 167).

Thus while there may be benefits from caesarean section in terms of cerebral palsy risk, it is unlikely that this will be proven. Lumley *et al.* (1985b) describe the difficulties of conducting such a trial when obstetric practice has already moved towards caesarean sections for very preterm deliveries.

TABLE 12.7

Interventions in late pregnancy to reduce cerebral palsy in very preterm infants

A. **Good levels of evidence : effective**
   Antenatal dexamethasone*
   Delivery in a tertiary centre

B. **Only fair levels of evidence: needs more research**
   Magnesium sulphate in preterm labour

C. **No evidence: not effective**
   Antenatal thyrotropin releasing hormone
   Antenatal indomethracin
   Operative delivery

*Needs more long term outcome research.

TABLE 12.8

Neonatal intensive care for very preterm infants: evidence for activities which may reduce cerebral palsy rates

A. **Good levels of evidence[1]**
   Indomethacin for patent ductus arteriosus
   Treatment of neonatal infections, *e.g.* meningitis, group B streptococcus, encephalopathy
   Phototherapy to reduce bilirubin
   Breast-feeding/preterm formulae

B. **Only fair levels of evidence[2]**
   Surfactant
   Management of thermal environment
   Maintaining glucose homeostatis

C. **No evidence[3]**
   Intensive neonatal resuscitation
   Mechanical ventilation
   Oxygen or nitric oxide (inhaled)
   Drug therapy to prevent IVH/PVH
   D-penicillanine to prevent retinopathy of prematurity
   Maintaining homeostasis

[1]From randomized trials.
[2]Observational studies suggestive, but no adequate data on cerebral palsy.
[3]Based on physiological research and mortality data.

Table 12.7 summarizes these late pregnancy interventions in terms of whether the available evidence supports their use, whether more research is needed, or whether there is no evidence of effectiveness.

NEONATAL INTENSIVE CARE FOR VERY PRETERM BABIES: A REVIEW OF THE EVIDENCE FOR ACTIVITIES WHICH MAY REDUCE CEREBRAL PALSY RATES

Table 12.8 summarizes the aspects of neonatal care for which there is good, fair or no evidence of effectiveness in reducing the risks of cerebral palsy in very preterm infants. We would know much more if the numerous randomized trials of specific treatments had followed survivors for long enough to ascertain cerebral palsy incidence. It is not possible

TABLE 12.9

Studies of synthetic surfactant for respiratory distress syndrome in preterm infants: (A) mortality at 1 year, and (B) cerebral palsy in survivors examined in subject vs control populations*

Study	Subjects n/N	Controls n/N	Peto odds ratio (95% CI)[2]	Weight[1] %	Peto odds ratio[1] (95% CI)
A. Mortality at 1 year					
Long (1991)	44/615	59/622		32.4	0.74 (0.49–1.10)
US Exosurf Study (1991)	34/206	62/213		25.4	0.49 (0.31–0.77)
McMillan (1995)	47/174	47/170		23.5	0.97 (0.60–1.56)
Smyth (1995)	64/113	67/111		18.7	0.86 (0.51–1.46)
Total	189/1108	235/1116		100.0	0.73 (0.58–0.92)
χ^2 4.65 (df=3); Z = 2.70					
B. Cerebral palsy in survivors examined					
Wilkinson (1985)	4/9	2/10		3.6	2.92 (0.44–19.25)
Long (1991)	28/482	36/475		50.3	0.75 (0.45–1.25)
US Exosurf Study (1991)	6/138	14/122		15.5	0.37 (0.15–0.92)
McMillan (1995)	12/144	13/118		18.9	0.95 (0.42–2.18)
Smyth (1995)	8/47	9/42		11.7	0.75 (0.26–2.16)
Total	58/790	74/767		100.0	0.74 (0.52–1.06)
χ^2 4.65 (df=4); Z = 1.64					

Forest plot axis: 0.1 0.2 1 5 10

*Adapted from Soll (1999a,b)—see source for relevant study references.
This is an abstract of a regularly updated systematic review prepared and maintained by the Cochrane Collaboration.
[1] See Glossary.
[2] For an explanation of the symbols used here, see Glossary, under Meta-analyses.

to assess the role of neonatal intensive care from changes in the frequency of cerebral palsy in very preterm infants, as has been attempted in the many published follow-up studies (see Chapters 4 and 7).

Intensive neonatal resuscitation
This is covered in the section on birth asphyxia (pp. 168–169).

Surfactant
Several controlled trials of prophylactic and 'rescue' surfactant, both natural and synthetic, in very preterm infants have demonstrated marked improvements in many, but not all, immediate neonatal outcomes (Soll 1999a,b). Those with established respiratory distress syndrome treated with synthetic surfactant have been shown to have a decreased risk of pneumothorax, pulmonary interstitial emphysema, intraventricular haemorrhage, broncho-pulmonary dysplasia, neonatal mortality, and mortality prior to hospital discharge and at 1 year of age. It may, however, lead to an increase in apnoea of prematurity. It has also been shown that natural surfactant may be preferred to the synthetic form in respect of a decreased risk of pneumothorax. Few data are available on long term follow-up of infants. One observational analysis suggested surfactant therapy may be a risk factor for cerebral palsy (Allan *et al.* 1997). However, a small number of the randomized controlled studies of the effects of synthetic surfactant for respiratory distress syndrome in preterm infants included some follow-up of survivors using cerebral palsy as an outcome, as well as looking at mortality at 1 year: meta-analyses of their findings (Soll 1999a) are reproduced in Table 12.9. Although neither of these meta-analyses shows a significant difference between the surfactant-treated cases and controls, risks of both mortality and cerebral palsy in the treated group were about 75 per cent of those in the controls.

Comparisons suggest that prophylaxis with surfactant is more effective than 'rescue' therapy in terms of immediate respiratory and other morbidity (Morley 1998; Soll 1999a,b). Thus surfactant appears to reduce mortality from respiratory distress syndrome in very preterm infants without increasing the risk of impaired survival; however, more data are needed. Extending the duration of follow-up of existing (and future) surfactant trial popu-lations to ascertain cerebral palsy incidence would be the quickest and most cost-effective way of obtaining this important information.

Indomethacin for patent ductus arteriosus (PDA)
Nehgme *et al.* (1992) reviewed the use of indomethacin to both prevent and treat PDA in very preterm infants and included IVH among the outcomes studied. Indomethacin given prophylactically early in life significantly reduced both PDA and IVH (odds ratio 0.74; 95% CI 0.62–0.88) but not mortality (see comments on prevention of PVH/IVH, p. 160–161).

Treating neonatal infections
Preterm births are at considerable risk of bacterial infections such as septicaemia, enterocolitis, encephalitis and meningitis. A number of different organisms may be involved, including group B streptococcus, meningococcus, listeria, *Haemophilus influenzae*, herpes simplex

virus, *Escherichia coli* and *Klebsiella* spp., some of which have high rates of mortality and neurological sequelae. Randomized controlled trials show that antibiotic therapy, particularly the third generation cephalosporins, reduce both mortality and longer term sequelae (Baley and Fanaroff 1992b). There is growing concern over the rapid growth of resistance to antibiotics of many serious bacterial infections, and it has been suggested that some of these powerful antibiotics should be reserved for the most severe infections, with careful typing of the organisms and their antibiotic sensitivities before therapy is contemplated (see also iatrogenesis and cerebral palsy, p. 00).

There are three systematic reviews of the effects of intrapartum antibiotics in reducing the incidence of early onset group B streptococcal disease in neonates (Allen *et al.* 1993, Ohlsson and Myhr 1994, Smaill 1998). All three concluded that the incidence of neonatal colonization from a group B streptoccus carrying mother was reduced with antibiotic treatment. A descriptive paper from a Sydney population showed that over eight years, universal screening and intrapartum antibiotics for maternal infection was associated with a reduced rate of neonatal infection as measured by blood or urine testing (Jeffery and Lahra 1998). Evidence from both randomized controlled trials and observational study suggests that screening and treatment has the potential to reduce the incidence of this disease from 2 to about 0.2 per 1000 live births, which should also reduce rates of death and brain damage. Questions remain about when to screen, rescreen and treat, and these need further trials.

Necrotizing enterocolitis, which may be on a causal pathway to cerebral palsy, is the most important gastrointestinal complication in very preterm births. Its aetiology appears complex, involving ischaemia, infection and feeding. There is some evidence that both the incidence and severity of necrotizing enterocolitis is reduced by antenatal steroids (Bauer *et al.* 1984, Halac *et al.* 1990), by feeding breast milk and by IgA supplements (Baley and Fanaroff 1992b). There are few relevant randomized controlled trials or meta-analyses, and more research is needed to know what are the best treatments and whether they improve neonatal neurological outcomes.

Neonatal herpes simplex virus infections are rare but have very high mortality and rate of neurological sequelae. Acyclovir is the only available treatment, and the few small trials that have been conducted suggest that it is effective (see Baley and Fanaroff 1992b).

Unless treated promptly and effectively, neonatal infections involving the central nervous system may lead to irreparable brain damage. The decreased mortality and morbidity of very preterm infants treated in well staffed and resourced neonatal intensive care units (see below) may be due in part to earlier diagnosis and more effective treatment of such infections. The whole package of neonatal intensive care provides a host of co-interventions such as warmth, fluids, nutrition, surgery and homeostatic support, all of which may influence the outcome of very preterm infants (see pp. 154 and 159).

Phototherapy to reduce hyperbilirubinaemia in preterm infants
There is good randomized trial evidence that phototherapy is very effective in reducing jaundice and improving morbidity and mortality from hyperbilirubinaemia from any cause in preterm neonates (Maisels 1992), decreasing the need for exchange transfusions.

Management of the thermal environment
This is well reviewed by Sinclair (1992). Paying attention to the thermal environments of very preterm infants has been shown by randomized trials to reduce mortality and respiratory distress. It may therefore be effective in reducing brain damage, but these trials did not have long term follow-up.

Maintaining glucose homeostasis
Lucas *et al.* (1988) have reported the increased risk of cerebral palsy in preterm infants with hypoglycaemia in modern neonatal intensive care units in the UK, with the risk increasing with decreasing blood sugar. However, there appears to be significant debate as to appropriate therapy as few trials are available (DiGiacomo and Hay 1992). Research is needed to better define 'normal' and 'abnormal' blood glucose levels in newborns at various gestational ages, to identify more rapid and accurate methods of measurement, and to obtain randomized trial evidence of prevention as well as treatment.

Special feeding for very preterm infants
There is a large literature on infant feeding which has been well reviewed (Steer *et al.* 1992). The aim of promoting postnatal growth at the same rate as would have occurred had the preterm infant remained *in utero* seems to have been justified in terms of better outcomes as demonstrated by randomized trials. Important beneficial effects on neurological sequelae in very preterm infants have been reported following early feeding with exclusive breast milk or with preterm formula.

Mechanical ventilation
There is good randomized trial evidence of reduced mortality and respiratory morbidity with ventilation of the preterm infant in a neonatal intensive care setting (Bancalari and Sinclair 1992). Cerebral palsy was not included in this meta-analysis.

Bhuta and Henderson-Smart (1998) have reviewed new methods of ventilating preterm infants for respiratory distress syndrome and other neonatal lung problems. While some trials showed beneficial effects on immediate and longer term respiratory morbidity, the longer term neurological outcomes (PVL, developmental abnormality at follow-up) were variable depending on the techniques and other co-interventions used. For example, elective high frequency jet ventilation and high frequency oscillatory ventilation both differed in terms of neurological outcome depending on volume strategies used or whether surfactant was also given.

It is thus vital in recommending these therapies to be aware that while they may benefit immediate outcome, whether their long term effects on the brain are positive or negative may depend on how each is applied and whether other therapies are also given. The whole package of neonatal care against which new interventions are evaluated needs to be clearly defined (see also Chapter 13).

Oxygen
It is important for those seeking new treatments to remember the 'parable' of oxygen use

in neonatal intensive care (Silverman 1980). It illustrates well the balance between enhancing survival and increasing impairments, and is a constant reminder of the importance of properly investigating *all* therapies, however harmless they may appear (Silverman 1980, 1998). Duc and Sinclair (1992) reviewed the evidence illustrating this dilemma for neonatologists. Oxygen decreases mortality, but at certain levels increases retinopathy of prematurity and possibly may have other adverse consequences in survivors. The authors suggest that a comprehensive evaluation of oxygen is required in the context of its neonatal intensive care co-interventions such as the treatment of acidosis. Research is required to elucidate the antioxidative defences of the very preterm neonate and to find interventions to enhance them. Randomized trials are needed of oxygen monitoring, of how to wean infants from oxygen therapy, and of the effects of ambient oxygen on survival, on retinopathy and on the brain.

Inhaled nitric oxide
Inhaled nitric oxide improves oxygenation in very preterm newborns with severe hypoxaemic respiratory distress syndrome, sepsis/pneumonia and pulmonary hypoplasia (Kinsella and Abman 1998). However, the potential risks warrant a cautious approach; clinical use should currently be limited to randomized trials investigating both safety and efficacy. Inhaled nitric oxide also appears to benefit oxygenation in term infants with persistent pulmonary hypertension and reduces the need for extraporporeal membrane oxygenation: inhaled nitric oxide in term infants also needs randomized trial evaluation as there are concerns about harmful effects. Such a trial (INNOVO) is being conducted with disability at 1 year as an outcome (Perinatal Trials Group 1998).

D-penicillamine to prevent retinopathy of prematurity
D-penicillamine (Phelps *et al.* 1998) has been shown to dramatically reduce the risk of retinopathy of prematurity in <2000 g and <1500 g infants. The effect on abnormal neurological outcome was also measured and showed no difference from placebo.

Therapy for periventricular and intraventricular haemorrhage (PVH/IVH)
In evaluating the impact on permanent neurological sequelae, it is important to differentiate between preventive strategies that reduce the incidence in high risk infants and rescue therapy of existing IVH/PVH. Horbar (1992) carefully reviewed the randomized controlled trial evidence of a variety of therapies in obstetric and neonatal intensive care in very preterm neonates to reduce IVH.

There are no data for very preterm births on the effects of management of labour and delivery such as electronic fetal monitoring, duration of labour, mode of delivery or episiotomy on the occurrence of IVH/PVH or cerebral palsy. There is a similar paucity of data on the effects of any early neonatal practices on IVH/PVH or cerebral palsy. The list of such practices is shown in Table 12.10. A plea for more trials which are larger and with longer follow-up is made again and again by the dedicated Cochrane reviewers. In addition Horbar calls for more basic research to identify better treatments and noninvasive methods for measuring cerebral blood flow in the human neonate. As mentioned earlier (p. 157) and in another systematic review (Horbar 1992), indomethacin reduced all IVH/PVH (odds ratio

TABLE 12.10
Early neonatal practices in very preterm infants
which may impact on cerebral haemorrhage and
hence cerebral palsy*

Early intubation
Handling
Suction of airways
Sodium bicarbonate
Continuous monitoring of blood pressure and gases
Blood volume expansion
Pressors to reduce blood pressure
Sedatives
Umbilical artery catheter placement
Heparinization of catheters
Ductal ligation
Super oxide dismutase

*Adapted from Horbar (1992).

0.71, 95% CI 0.6–0.85) and severe IVH/PVH (odds ratio 0.64, 95% CI 0.43–0.94) but not death, if given within 24 hours after birth. However, there is concern about its effects on cerebral blood flow and metabolism, and long term studies are needed. These drugs often have other indications, and decisions about their use are complex and require consideration of other morbidities. There is no good evidence that phenobarbitone, ethamsylate, vitamin E , fresh frozen plasma or antenatal vitamin K reduce mortality or haemorrhage, although there is enough suggestive evidence to warrant more research. The effects of antenatal steroids and surfactant have been mentioned already. Horbar (1992) suggests that general prevention of preterm birth such as has occurred in France has not yet been shown to reduce haemorrhage (see p. 147). The data evaluating the impact of transporting mothers to deliver in tertiary centres, thus reducing the proportions of very preterm births in level 1 centres, have shown enormous variability in levels of IVH, suggesting that many factors are involved.

IATROGENESIS AND CEREBRAL PALSY IN PRETERM INFANTS
The contribution of the iatrogenic effects of neonatal intensive care to cerebral palsy have not been adequately researched. Aggressive resuscitation and treatment of babies with an obviously very high risk of cerebral damage such as those with multiple congenital malformations, severe neonatal encephalopathy or extremely preterm birth is not necessarily good neonatal care. Baley and Fanaroff (1992a) provide an excellent review of the history of the iatrogenic risks of infection in neonatal nurseries, but otherwise the published literature is sparse.

Some pharmacological products have been investigated with respect to their potential for increasing infections or IVH, which may translate into increased rates of cerebral palsy. There is no evidence that surfactant for respiratory distress, postnatal steroids for broncho-pulmonary dysplasia, or indomethacin for patent ductus arteriosus have increased the rates of infection. As mentioned earlier there is concern about the effects of antenatal steroids on rates of infection in the newborn and any untoward effects in women who require repeated doses.

Causes of intrauterine growth restriction and cerebral palsy: possible preventive strategies (Chapter 8)

Figure 8.5 (p. 89) shows the various causes of intrauterine growth restriction. Strategies for prevention of fetal causes such as chromosomal and birth defects and congenital infections have been discussed earlier in this chapter (pp. 143–147), and those associated with multiple births are discussed on pages 169–170. A meta-analysis of 126 trials evaluated 36 antenatal interventions aimed at preventing or treating impaired fetal growth (Gülmezoglu et al. 1997). Most antenatal interventions do not show any effect on short term perinatal outcomes such as birthweight for gestational age. Factors associated with reductions in very low birthweight rates and therefore possibly having an effect on growth were cessation of smoking (odds ratio for reducing low birthweight = 0.8; 95% CI 0.65–0.98) and antimalarials in primigravid women in endemic malarious zones (odds ratio 0.34; 95% CI 0.15–0.74), while a possible effect (odds ratio 0.76; 95% CI 0.58–1.01) was seen with protein/energy supplement, particularly in malnourished women in rural Africa during the 'hungry' season (Ceesay et al. 1997) (see below). Given the importance assigned to poor fetal growth in the literature, the small number and poor methodological quality of trials of prevention are surprising. A few trials did follow up children to ascertain neurodevelopmental status (see below).

Several authors have reviewed the possibilities suggested from animal and some human data of new therapies for the treatment of intrauterine growth restriction (Gluckman 1997, Harding et al. 1997, Robinson et al. 1997). Currently there is no evidence that nutritional supplementation will reverse intrauterine growth restriction once it is established. Fetal growth hormone and insulin-like growth factor 1 show promise in animal models, and fetal and maternal hormone supplementation increase placental function and may help by increasing the availability of fetal substrates. Quoting early Australian data, Robinson et al. (1997) raised the issue of the possible impact of severe eating disorders in pregnant women on fetal growth restriction. No current recommendations are possible.

Several meta-analyses relevant to the management of the growth restricted pregnancy may impact on cerebral palsy risk. They are summarized in Table 12.11.

NUTRITIONAL SUPPLEMENTS IN PREGNANCY TO REDUCE GROWTH RESTRICTION AND IMPROVE NEUROCOGNITIVE OUTCOMES

A meta-analysis of several trials in both developed and developing countries showed no effect of nutritional supplements in pregnancy on neurocognitive outcomes (Kramer 1998). Such supplements had modest effects on small for gestational age (odds ratio 0.75, 95% CI 0.6–1.0) and preterm babies (odds ratio 0.8, 95% CI 0.6–1.05), the effects appearing to be greater in well than in undernourished women. de Onis et al. (1998) in a broadened and updated overview supported Kramer's conclusions. They and Gülmezoglu et al. (1997) suggest that some dietary micronutrients such as zinc, folate and magnesium merit further research as several trials showed beneficial effects on growth (p=0.05). Observational data suggested

TABLE 12.11
Interventions to prevent cerebral palsy
associated with poor fetal growth

Good evidence
None

Fair: need more research
Micronutrients—zinc, folate, magnesium
Fish oil
Dopper ultrasound in high risk pregnancies

No evidence
Nutritional supplements in pregnancy
Bed rest in hospital
Operative delivery in compromised fetus
Timing of delivery

a significantly lower risk of cerebral palsy in babies born to mothers reporting a high consumption of fish oil in pregnancy (Petridou *et al.* 1998). However, trials have not provided any evidence that fish oil given either prophylactically or therapeutically increased birthweight for gestational age. If fish oil does reduce the risk of cerebral palsy it may act directly on the brain rather than by increasing fetal growth rate. These individual dietary components should be investigated further.

HOSPITALIZATION FOR BED REST IN SUSPECTED IMPAIRED FETAL GROWTH
A review on hospital admission for bed rest (Gülmezoglu and Hofmeyr 1998) suggested a reduced operative delivery rate for fetal distress and improved 1 and 5 minute Apgar scores, but no information on childhood outcomes was available. Further research is needed before supporting this expensive and socially disruptive intervention.

DOPPLER ULTRASOUND IN HIGH RISK PREGNANCIES
This meta-analysis was conducted by Neilson and Alfirevic (1998). Using Doppler ultrasound in high risk pregnancies (variously defined in each of the trials) to diagnose a compromised fetus and instigate some clinical response, reduced perinatal mortality by 30 per cent (not quite statistically significant). Suggestions of decreases in both intraventricular haemorrhage and clinical signs suggestive of hypoxic–ischaemic encephalopathy make this an important diagnostic tool to evaluate in further large randomized trials with long term follow-up.

AVOIDING PERINATAL RISKS TO FETUSES WITH ANTENATAL NEUROLOGICAL DAMAGE
Where pregnancies with fetal neurological damage are continued, particularly in the presence of a chromosomal anomaly, fetal growth is likely to be restricted, and gestation may be shorter than normal. In such fetuses there may be increased risks of intrapartum hypoxia and asphyxia, and postnatally of delay before regular respiration. It was suggested in Chapter 8 that, although difficult to prove, such babies may be further damaged by intrapartum hypoxia.

In such cases birth events are factors acting late in the causal chain, but their prevention or effective treatment may avoid further and more disabling damage. The challenges are to identify such infants and to obtain evidence as to whether mode of delivery or other aspects of intrapartum management may improve outcome.

GROWTH RESTRICTION INTERVENTION TRIAL (GRIT)—TIMING OF DELIVERY IN
GROWTH RESTRICTED AND COMPROMISED FETUSES
Surveillance for fetal growth restriction is not reliable, and the status of the growth restricted fetus cannot be measured with accuracy. Labour may be induced unnecessarily when signs of fetal distress occur in the absence of potentially damaging hypoxia (Patel and Owen 1995). Moreover, hard decisions have to be made when there are choices between the risk of leaving a compromised baby *in utero* or delivering it at a very early gestational age.

A survey was done of 49 obstetricians in three European countries as to when they would deliver a preterm growth restricted fetus with certain adverse signs; there was considerable disagreement and also reluctance to randomize such patients in trials (GRIT Study Group 1996). There was a tendency to support elective delivery as gestational age increased from 24 to 32 weeks. No randomized trials have been done to determine the optimal timing and mode of delivery of severely growth restricted fetuses, and no policies exist. The GRIT trial aims to answer this question.

Hypoxia, hypoglycaemia, hypothermia, polycythaemia, hypocalcaemia, pulmonary haemorrhage and meconium aspiration are the other possible intrapartum or neonatal complications of intrauterine growth restriction. Effectiveness of treatments for the first three are discussed in the previous section (p. 159) and below. There are no treatments for the last four that have been adequately evaluated to assess their impact on cerebral palsy.

Evidence for prevention of birth asphyxia and cerebral palsy (Chapter 9)
Figures 9.2 (p. 102) and 9.3 (p. 103) illustrate a number of important antenatal and intrapartum risk factors in causal pathways to neurological impairment in the term infant, which include signs of birth asphyxia (or fetal distress). As with very preterm birth and intrauterine growth restriction there are two approaches to the prevention of cerebral palsy associated with birth asphyxia: the first attempts to identify and interrupt the pathways resulting in birth asphyxia, and the second attempts to prevent permanent neurological sequelae once signs of asphyxia have been observed.

PRIMARY PREVENTION OF BIRTH ASPHYXIA
Primary prevention of birth asphyxia awaits our capacity to understand the causal pathways to catastrophic intrapartum events such as severe intrapartum haemorrhage, prolapsed cord, abnormal presentations, or maternal shock from either cardiovascular causes or infections. Many infants exhibit signs of fetal distress arising in labour without obvious antecedents and which would be difficult to prevent. Other infants exhibiting fetal distress are most likely to have been affected by causal pathways that started early in pregnancy (such as malformations or migration disorders), multiple birth or pregnancy problems, all which have all been dealt with in other sections of this chapter.

Prevention in the perinatal period can only be successful in those cases where the neurological system of the fetus is still intact, though good delivery care may avoid compounding existing damage. This is the assumption behind several accepted obstetric practices aimed at reducing the long term effects of birth asphyxia. These include electronic fetal monitoring, prophylactic tocolysis with betamimetics in the second stage of labour and caesarean section for fetal distress, which are now reviewed.

Efficacy and effectiveness of intrapartum fetal monitoring to detect fetal distress and influence management

The sensitivity, specificity, positive predictive value, and interpretation of methods of surveillance for signs of fetal distress during labour, reviewed in Chapter 8, do not meet the criteria for a good screening test. To have used them for diagnosing birth asphyxia and to act upon their results (by expediting delivery) was a scientific and clinical error of some magnitude. A number of studies have endeavoured to evaluate the success of such measures in terms of infant survival or long term neurological morbidity. No study has proven that any specific intervention is effective in reducing cerebral palsy. A systematic review of nine randomized controlled trials (58,855 pregnant women) found that with the consistent exception of reducing neonatal seizures (odds ratio 0.5; 95% CI 0.3–0.82), the routine use of electronic fetal monitoring had no measurable effect on mortality or short term morbidity (Thacker *et al.* 1995, Thacker and Stroup 1998). However, an increase in rates of caesarean section and instrumental vaginal delivery was found in every trial (odds ratio 1.23, 95% CI 1.15–1.31). Only two studies (Grant *et al.* 1989, Shy *et al.* 1990) followed up the children, reporting that no benefits were seen in terms of neurological abnormalities. There is no evidence that the addition of fetal scalp blood sampling improved outcomes following electronic fetal monitoring (Thacker *et al.* 1995). These randomized trial data are supported by good observational studies (Nelson *et al.* 1996). The evidence concerning electronic fetal heart rate monitoring in labour strongly suggests that it is an ineffective tool for guiding responses aimed at reducing neurological damage ostensibly due to birth asphyxia.

Intrapartum fetal electrocardiograph plus heart rate recording

The impact of adding qualitative assessment of the ST segment on the fetal electrocardiograph to the assessment of electronic fetal heart rate monitoring was reviewed by Mistry and Neilson (1998). Operative delivery for fetal distress was reduced but operative delivery for failure to progress was not. Significant hypoxia as suggested by pH with base deficit >12 mmol/L in cord blood was reduced but in common with all other outcomes did not reach the p = 0.05 level of statistical significance. Thus adding qualitative information about the ST segment decreased obstetric interventions without jeopardizing immediate outcome.

Fetal biophysical profile scoring

An observational study compared two large cohorts of neonates born in the province of Manitoba in Canada between 1987 and 1991 inclusive. One cohort had been assessed antenatally using a fetal biophysical scoring system and the other had not (Manning *et al.*

1998). The fetal biophysical profile score included five assessments—fetal breathing, gross body movements, tone and heart rate reactivity (all reflecting immediate well-being), and semi-quantitative amniotic fluid volume which reflects fetal condition over the previous 7–10 days. The prevalence of cerebral palsy in those tested (N = 26,290) was 1.33 per 1000 compared with 4.74 in the untested group (N = 58,659). This was not a randomized trial, and there are likely to be reasons for testing which may explain some of these differences. However, the group who were tested were at higher risk than those not tested and would therefore have been expected to have a higher, rather than a lower, rate of cerebral palsy. This suggests that antenatal testing of these parameters should be further investigated using more rigorous methods.

Prophylactic tocolysis with intravenous betamimetics in second stage of labour
This treatment is aimed at improving fetal outcome; the outcomes assessed in the systematic review by Hofmeyr (1998d) were method of delivery and neonatal outcome. There were more forceps deliveries in the tocolytic than in the placebo group; there were no differences in neonatal outcome or Apgar scores at 2 minutes. The mean umbilical arterial pH values were similar overall but significantly higher in the treatment group when only those delivered according to protocol (second stage no longer than 30 minutes) were considered. There was no effect on neonatal irritability or feeding difficulties between the two groups, so this treatment is unlikely to affect neurological outcome.

Tocolytics for suspected intrapartum fetal distress
The rationale for use of acute tocolysis in suspected intrapartum fetal distress is that the induced uterine relaxation will improve uteroplacental blood flow and hence fetal oxygenation. Thus, it can be expected to be successful only if excessive uterine activity is the cause of the fetal distress. Kulier and Hofmeyr (1998) have reviewed the few small trials that have addressed this issue. While the odds ratios often indicated clinically significant changes in the immediate outcomes examined, the only significant difference observed was a reduction in persisting fetal heart rate abnormalities (odds ratio 0.26, 95% CI 0.14–0.53) with tocolysis compared with no treatment. There were no data on effect on gestational age at delivery nor on long term outcomes.

Amnioinfusion for umbilical cord compression
Amnioinfusion is the infusion of fluids transabdominally either into the amniotic cavity or into the cord itself. Hofmeyr (1998a,b) reviewed the effects of both interventions applied either prophylactically or when cord compression was suggested by the electronic fetal heart rate monitor. No significant differences in any outcomes were observed with amniotic cavity infusion. With infusion into the cord, there were significantly fewer persistent variable decelerations on electronic fetal monitoring and less meconium stained amniotic fluid, fewer caesarean sections both overall and for fetal distress, and fewer vaginal instrumental deliveries for suspected fetal distress. Fewer infants had Apgar scores below 7 at 1 minute but the Apgar scores were not significantly different at 5 minutes. Significantly fewer infants were born with cord arterial pH <7.2, and fewer stayed in hospital longer than three

days neonatally. There were also some significant maternal benefits. However, further studies are needed to evaluate the effects of amnioinfusion when the diagnosis of fetal distress is not based on fetal heart rate monitoring alone. A multicentre trial of amnioinfusion for the indication of thick meconium is planned (Perinatal Trials Group 1998).

Mode of delivery in fetal distress

A review of the literature concerning the effectiveness of caesarean section (Scheller and Nelson 1994) concluded that although it could be shown to be of benefit in the delivery of babies with particular malformations and infections, it was not associated with any reduction in cerebral palsy.

The most recent systematic review of operative versus conservative delivery management for fetal distress was conducted by Hofmeyr (1998c). Actual operative delivery rates were 61 per cent with 28 per cent by caesarean section in the planned operative group, compared with 20 and 7 per cent respectively in the conservatively managed group. There were no differences in perinatal mortality (14/174 operative vs 12/176 conservative: odds ratio 1.18, 95% CI 0.56–2.48). No details are available for maternal or neonatal morbidity or brain damage.

Hofmeyr (1998c) writes: "The management of 'fetal distress' during labour by expedited delivery of the baby, usually operatively, has become entrenched in obstetric practice without evidence from randomised trials of its effectiveness. Many would regard such evidence as unnecessary, because the need for expedited delivery of fetuses in 'distress' is seen as a self-evident imperative." One reason why no benefits are demonstrated may be that the majority of fetuses with signs compatible with fetal distress do not have impending asphyxia. It is conceivable that in these 'false positive' cases, more harm than good is done by unnecessary interventions, particularly caesarean sections. An alternative reason may be that those fetuses which can benefit from operative delivery may have exhibited more compelling signs of fetal distress and were all delivered operatively in the trials reviewed by Hofmeyr, *i.e.* all those in the conservative arms who could benefit were included in the 20 per cent of operatively delivered infants. It is likely, as has been argued by Blair (1996b), that cerebral palsy due to birth asphyxia may have been more common years ago and that the advent of safe caesarean sections may have prevented many cases. It is reasonable that obstetric mismanagement could be responsible for some cases of cerebral palsy (Gaffney *et al.* 1994b, Richmond *et al.* 1994), but the role of obstetric care may have been overestimated even in these recent case–control studies (Blair 1994). The challenge is to discover which fetuses are likely to benefit from operative delivery given the difficulties of accurately recognizing birth asphyxia.

Johanson and Menon (1998) reviewed trials comparing the use of vacuum extraction with the use of forceps. With vacuum extractors there was significantly less use of regional or general anaesthesia, recourse to caesarian section and severe maternal injury. However, vacuum extractors more often failed to achieve delivery, recourse to forceps being the next step, and was more often followed by maternal concerns for the baby, low Apgar score at 5 minutes, cephalhaematoma and retinal haemorrhages. These results should raise some concerns about the use of vacuum extraction; should we now recommend that it be performed only in the context of large randomized trials to assess its effects on rare but serious adverse outcomes such as neonatal death, intracranial haemorrhage and cerebral palsy?

There is no evidence that epidural versus nonepidural anaesthesia (Howell 1998) or varying episiotomy policies in vaginal births (Carroli *et al.* 1998) have any effect on outcomes relevant to cerebral palsy.

A large multicentre randomized trial is being conducted of planned caesarean section versus planned vaginal birth for the breech fetus at term, with infant follow-up to 2 years (Perinatal Trials Group 1998).

RESUSCITATION AND RESCUE OF ASPHYXIATED BABIES—PREVENTION OF SECONDARY NEURONAL DAMAGE

Immediate neonatal resuscitation
One aspect of care that has changed dramatically over the last 20 years has been the active resuscitation of asphyxiated newborns and all very preterm babies, immediately after postnatal assessments such as Apgar scores. The rationale for the range of interventions used in neonatal cardiopulmonary resuscitation is based on sound neonatal physiology (Ginsberg and Goldsmith 1998, Saugstad 1998). The aim of resuscitation is to 'rescue' the baby from birth asphyxia or to optimize the chances of survival of the very low birthweight preterm infant, with a *secondary* aim of preventing perinatal brain damage. While there is a general consensus as to what constitutes good practice in resuscitation of the newborn, there are few randomized trials either of the package of neonatal resuscitation or of the individual components such as drugs or ventilation regimens (Tyson 1992, Bloom and Cropley 1994, Ginsberg and Goldsmith 1998). A trial comparing oxygen with room air in neonatal resuscitation of asphyxiated neonates found no difference in mortality or in immediate morbidity (Saugstad *et al.* 1998), indicating that room air is as efficient as pure oxygen. Time to first breath or cry was significantly shorter in room air infants; larger trials to evaluate morbidity and mortality outcomes are now required (Tarnow-Mordi 1998). Again few trials follow the infants to an age at which cerebral palsy can be reliably recognized.

Prevention of secondary neuronal damage following birth asphyxia
An important new set of possible strategies has emerged from basic research elucidating the mechanisms underlying secondary neuronal death (see Chapter 9). Suggested methods of preventing long term brain damage in cases of neonatal encephalopathy include specific pharmacological treatments and hypothermia, a trial of which is planned (Williams *et al.* 1993, Vannucci and Perlman 1997, Wyatt and Thoresen 1997, Edwards *et al.* 1998). Peliowski and Finer (1992) reviewed the evidence that hypothermia, hyperbaric oxygen, prophylactic phenobarbitol, steroids and mannitol could benefit infants with hypoxic–ischaemic encephalopathy. None appear beneficial in the short or long term, but there are few randomized trials, and all studies have methodological problems such as insufficient numbers, poor definition of encephalopathy, inadequate randomization and/or observations not being blinded.

Calcium channel blockers, prostaglandin inhibitors (indomethacin), thromboxane synthesis inhibitors, excitatory amino acid transmitter blockade and gangliosides have also been suggested as agents which may block apoptotic neuronal death on the basis of physiological research. A major challenge in taking such research into randomized trials is how to accurately identify the small number of babies in the process of being damaged by intrapartum hypoxia and who would benefit from such rescue therapy. In the experimental situation the use of magnetic resonance spectroscopy and near infrared spectroscopy may prove to be crucial if they can identify the stages of neuronal death in infants with a history of fetal distress who develop neonatal encephalopathy (A.D. Edwards, personal communication 1998).

Extracorporeal membrane oxygenation (ECMO)
Neonates with severe but potentially reversible cardiorespiratory failure have shown high mortality and cerebral palsy rates. The conditions leading to the need for ECMO include congenital diaphragmatic hernia, idiopathic fetal circulation and persistent pulmonary hypertension attributable to meconium aspiration, sepsis, and idiopathic respiratory distress syndrome (Glass *et al.* 1997, Graziani *et al.* 1997). Results for death and disability from a UK trial, which followed up survivors to the age of 1 year, have now been published (Johnson *et al.* 1998a). The trial was stopped early because sufficient data were available to be sure that differences in severe disability would not be large enough to counterbalance the differences in death rates between the two groups. Around one-third (32 per cent) of the ECMO infants and 59 per cent of the conventionally managed infants died before the age of 1 year. Sixteen per cent of the ECMO survivors and 13.5 per cent of the others had tone changes in the limbs, but only two infants, one in each group, were severely disabled. It was concluded that a policy of ECMO support reduces the risk of death in these severely ill term babies without a concomitant rise in severe disability. These results are in accord with the results of a similar trial reported in abstract form only (Gross *et al.* 1994).

Evidence for prevention of cerebral palsy in multiple births (Chapter 10)
Multiple births are more likely to be preterm, small for gestational age and have fetal distress, all important risk factors for cerebral palsy. As outlined in Chapter 10, multiple births increasingly result from infertility drug treatments, such as ovarian stimulation and implanting multiple embryos in IVF and GIFT procedures.

REGULATION OF INFERTILITY TREATMENTS
In Western Australia, reducing the number of embryos implanted has resulted in a decrease in the triplet birth rate (Watson *et al.* 1996), from which one would anticipate a reduction in the rate of cerebral palsy. Others have suggested that, as the costs of multiple births following infertility treatments are so high, more research should be done on alternative methods to treat infertility that are not associated with multiple pregnancies (Callahan *et al.* 1994). It is acknowledged that infertility treatment is a risk factor for preterm birth and neonatal morbidity via twinning and other factors and that it is important that this should now be monitored (Addor *et al.* 1998). Thus population perinatal data sets should routinely collect information on fertility treatments.

The practice of multifetal pregnancy reduction has been introduced as a method for reducing the complications and problems with higher order multiples following infertility treatments (Berkowitz *et al.* 1997). An Israeli study (Geva *et al.* 1998) has quantified the risk of PVL with multifetal reduction in a case–control analysis of preterm infants. The 14 cases of PVL and 1361 controls were selected from the same cohort of <36 week newborns admitted to an intensive care unit. The risk of PVL was 20-fold higher (odds ratio 20.9, 95% CI 5.5–79.4) in those who had had multifetal reduction at 12 weeks following infertility treatment to conceive. Being a twin and infertility treatments were also independently associated with PVL risk, but the significant effect of pregnancy reduction remained when these were controlled. Controlling for such powerful confounders is difficult, particularly in very small studies where inaccuracies in only a few cases can markedly affect results and it may be that they are on a causal pathway. Further evidence, preferably from trials, should be sought before rejecting multifetal reduction. However, a better solution (earlier in the causal path) would be to avoid high plurality births by replacing no more than three embryos in infertility procedures.

Our knowledge about prevention of the cerebral palsy associated with multiple births is limited; much of what is known has been covered in the sections on very preterm births, intrauterine growth restriction and birth asphyxia.

Postneonatally acquired cerebral palsy (Chapter 11)

It is in postneonatally acquired cerebral palsy that the possibilities of prevention are the most obvious. It is considerably more common amongst economically and socially deprived communities, and preventive strategies are more likely to be social than medical (see Table 12.1, p. 139). While postneonatally acquired cerebral palsy is now less likely to follow infections and more likely to follow accidental and nonaccidental head injuries and apparently life-threatening events (formerly called near-miss SIDS) (see Table 11.3, p. 132), a significant proportion still occur as a result of cerebral infections, some of which are now preventable.

The development and use of an effective vaccine against *Haemophilus influenzae* type B (Hib) has virtually eradicated invasive Hib including meningitis and its sequelae when given as part of the infant vaccine programme. The first available vaccines for Hib were for toddlers. As most children under 5 with meningitis get it before the age of 12 months, this vaccine could not be as effective as one given as early in life as possible. Once the switch to infant vaccines occurred, invasive Hib rates fell dramatically. Thus the recommended intervention is primary vaccination with Hib at the same time as the diphtheria–tetanus–pertussis vaccine (in Australia at 2, 4 and 6 months), followed by a booster at 18 months. Figure 12.2 shows how the number of reported cases of Hib meningitis in England and Wales has fallen since immunization was introduced (Salisbury and Begg 1996). A similar picture has been observed in Western Australia (Bower *et al.* 1998). As Hib vaccination was only introduced in Western Australia in October 1992, its impact on postneonatally acquired cerebral palsy rates will not be seen until the cerebral palsy cases from cohorts born after 1992 have

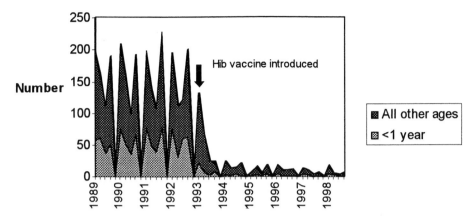

Fig. 12.2. Laboratory reports of *Haemophilus influenzae* type b by age (England and Wales 1989–1998, provisional). (Data from Public Health Laboratory Service, Communicable Disease Centre.)

been ascertained. However, it can be anticipated that it will reduce the rate of postneonatally acquired cerebral palsy particularly among Aboriginal children.

As yet there are no similar programmes of routine immunization against other organisms causing bacterial meningitis, although vaccines for meningococcal disease types A and C and for the many pneumococcal subtypes are available. Vaccination for meningococcus is not generally recommended because the incidence of meningococcal-associated conditions is low, and the majority of cases in any area differ quite markedly by type and occur in children too young to be protected by presently available vaccines (Salisbury and Begg 1996). Conjugated pneumococcal vaccines are currently being developed for use in childhood.

Since immunization, pertussis has been a rare cause of brain damage, but it may well reemerge, ironically due to parents being misinformed about the risks of brain damage *from the vaccine*. There were eight infant deaths in the 1997 Australian pertussis outbreak and an unconfirmed 20 cases of brain damage—all of which could have been avoided if vaccination rates had not fallen to such low levels. Many infants under the age of 2 months were infected in this epidemic, demonstrating how important it is to have high levels of immunization in the community to prevent the passage of the disease to populations too young to be immunized.

Viral encephalitides, including measles, are also a cause of permanent neurological damage. Vaccination has now made it possible for measles to be eliminated in those countries with high levels of vaccination. Recent outbreaks in Australia (and some other developed countries) are again due to falling childhood vaccination levels. More sophisticated public health education campaigns are required to combat apathy combined with ignorance, and to convince parents of the dangers of not vaccinating their children. Data from methodologically very weak epidemiological studies implicating measles vaccination with bowel disorders and autism are damaging to the cause of preventing measles and hence the brain damage associated with it (Nicoll *et al.* 1998).

171

Children who are particularly vulnerable to postnatal CNS infections include those with specific nutritional deficiencies such as vitamin A or zinc; those with anomalies of the immune system; very preterm infants; and those requiring operative intervention for hydrocephalus. Vaccination of these children is essential.

PREVENTION OF HEAD INJURY

The increasing importance of injuries as a cause of postneonatally acquired cerebral palsy is a major public health challenge. Legislation to restrain children in cars needs to be introduced where it is not already mandatory and better methods of restraint devised. In Western Australia, where such legislation was introduced several years ago, 91 per cent of parents regularly use appropriate restraints (J. Kurinczuk, personal communication 1998). Those areas which have introduced legislation for swimming pool fencing have shown that this is effective in reducing brain damage from near-drowning in young children (Nixon 1994).

The most worrying rise in the Western Australian data has been the proportion of children damaged as a result of nonaccidental injury, often associated with alcohol, social difficulties, domestic violence and family breakdown. As such a range of complex and sensitive issues is involved in these cases, there is little research on whether preventive strategies, such as the "Don't Shake the Baby" campaign, are having any effect. Many of the risk factors listed in Table 12.1 (p. 139) create barriers to effective and caring parenting and put children at risk of postneonatal brain damage from child abuse and neglect. Solutions may lie with improving living conditions in society, such as increasing employment, widely available parenthood classes, better pregnancy spacing, avoiding teenage or unwanted pregnancies, and counselling and support for people in relationships.

Support during childbirth from husbands, partners or a trained caregiver has been shown by randomized trial to improve outcomes such as prolonging breast-feeding, finding mothering easier and decreasing postpartum depression (Hodnett 1998b). These may translate into better parenting with beneficial effects for the child.

Support from caregivers for socially disadvantaged (e.g. young, inner city and/or unmarried) mothers comprised home visits from birth and throughout the first year of life. The visits supported parenting by encouraging reading, playing and singing with their child, encouraging healthy behaviours and the use of health services for illnesses (Hodnett and Roberts 1998). Effects of the programmes varied but included better immunization and breastfeeding rates, and lower rates of hospitalization and severe nappy rash in the first year of life and of child abuse. Mothers in supported groups were less tired, unhappy or likely to report negative feelings, fewer were housebound and fewer became pregnant again within 18 months. Olds et al. (1997) reported data on the 15-year follow-up of a randomized trial of infant home visits showing reduced use of welfare and less child abuse and neglect in socially disadvantaged mothers.

PREVENTION OF CEREBROVASCULAR ACCIDENTS

About 17 per cent of postneonatally acquired cerebral palsy is due to cerebrovascular accidents: about 11 per cent occurs spontaneously and 6 per cent postoperatively. Vitamin K administered intramuscularly at birth has long been accepted as a means of preventing haemorrhagic disease of the newborn. A case–control study by Golding *et al.* (1990) suggested a relationship with childhood cancer, which was confirmed in a subsequent study (Golding *et al.* 1992). This conclusion now appears ill-founded but has resulted in a shift toward the use of oral vitamin K which has not (yet) been shown to be as effective (Greer 1995). The evidence would suggest that intramuscular vitamin K is effective at birth and should be continued to prevent cerebral haemorrhage due to vitamin K deficiency in infancy. Other spontaneous cases may be due to various thrombotic or other clotting disorders, or occur without explanation, and are currently unavoidable. Postoperative cases should be investigated to identify any preventable situations.

PREVENTION OF APPARENT LIFE THREATENING EVENTS (ALTE)
Another public health success story of the 1990s has been the dramatic fall in sudden infant death syndrome (SIDS) rates in communities which have introduced a policy of encouraging new parents to lay their babies on their back or side, to stop smoking, to breast-feed and to avoid wrapping the baby up too warmly. This policy resulted from several case–control studies and one influential Australian cohort study (Dwyer *et al.* 1991) and concurrent case–control study (Ponsonby *et al.* 1995) which identified a prone sleeping position as a particularly important factor. Whilst randomized trials were suggested, these have not been conducted and the evaluation to clarify which of the postnatal risk factors contributed to the decline in rates largely consisted of comparing infant care practices before and after the decline in SIDS rates (Mitchell *et al.* 1994, Wigfield *et al.* 1994, Dwyer *et al.* 1995). Thus, a recommendation to reduce ALTE in infants (assuming it has the same pathophysiology as SIDS) would be to continue to follow the SIDS prevention strategy outlined above.

Despite the availability of effective preventive strategies we fear that the frequency of post-neonatally acquired cerebral palsy may not fall as dramatically as might be anticipated. Cases avoided by prevention of infections may be counterbalanced by increases associated with child abuse and accidents and parents deciding against, or becoming apathetic about, infant vaccination. Infant home visiting programmes for high risk families appear to be effective in enhancing parenting and decreasing some of these risks. They are part of a good maternal and child health service and should commence antenatally.

Table 12.12 summarizes the strength of the evidence that various interventions may reduce rates of cerebral palsy. There is sufficient evidence relating to interventions of Group 1 to consider that they are proven to reduce rates of cerebral palsy. There is less evidence pertaining to interventions in Group 2, but what evidence as does exist suggests that they are likely to reduce rates of cerebral palsy. There is very little empirical evidence in humans pertaining to the interventions in Group 3 but biologically they are plausible preventive strategies. The evidence does not suggest that the interventions listed under Group 4 prevent cerebral palsy and they may even have detrimental effects. Groups 2 and 3 comprise the areas where research is most needed. We also hope that those involved in the development of maternal and child health policy and of guidelines for clinical care in obstetrics and neonatology will find the table thought-provoking. Are the interventions of Group 1 implemented as frequently as possible? Are health resources continuing to be used inappropriately

TABLE 12.12
TABLE 12.12
Interventions for the prevention of cerebral palsy: evidence for effectiveness

Group 1. Proven to reduce cerebral palsy
Rubella vaccination
Iodine supplementation in areas of severe iodine deficiency
Cleaning environments contaminated with methylmercury exposure
Anti-D to prevent Rh– women making Rh antibodies
Tocolysis to delay very preterm delivery to enable further preventive treatments
Delivery of very preterm infant in a tertiary centre
Treatment of neonatal infections
Maternal screening for group B streptococcus[1]
Limit number of embryos transferred in infertility treatments to three or less
Infant immunization
Fencing of swimming pools
Home visiting programmes for socially disadvantaged new parents

Group 2. Probably effective in reducing cerebral palsy but more evidence needed
Early routine ultrasound[1,2]
Reduce excessive maternal alcohol ingestion in pregnancy
Screening for toxoplasmosis in endemic areas[1]
Antenatal steroids in very preterm labour[2]
Prophylactic surfactant in very preterm infants[2]
Treating necrotizing enterocolitis
Phototherapy for neonatal jaundice
NICU care in very preterm infants including managing thermal environment, use of oxygen, special feeding,
    mechanical ventilation strategies, assessing and treating hypoglycaemia, and intensive resuscitation at birth[2]
ECMO[2]
Vitamin K at birth to prevent haemorrhage
Special programmes to prevent child abuse
SIDS prevention strategies to reduce apparently life-threatening events (ALTE)
Infant restraints in cars

Group 3. More research needed now: includes some exciting possibilities
Antibiotics/other interruption of causal pathways to PPROM, chorioamnionitis, very preterm birth
Magnesium sulphate
Mode of delivery for very preterm birth including breech
Inhaled nitric oxide for very preterm and term asphyxiated infants
D-penicillamine
Zinc, folate, fish oil to prevent IUGR and/or brain damage
Doppler ultrasound in high risk pregnancies[1]
Timing and mode of delivery of growth retarded fetus
Operative delivery for fetal distress
Methods of detecting/measuring poor fetal growth[1]
Fetal biophysical score[1]
Amnioinfusion for umbilical cord compression
Measures to assess birth asphyxia/encephalopathy (NIRS, MRS)[1]
Rescue therapy for birth asphyxia/hypoxic ischaemic encephalopathy (hypothermia, drug therapy)

Group 4. Doubtful or no evidence of effectiveness
Electronic fetal monitoring for fetal distress—addition of fetal scalp blood sampling or ECG[1]
Antenatal indomethacin
Antenatal thyrotropin-releasing hormone
Bed rest in hospital for multiple pregnancy
Bed rest for growth restriction
Tocolysis in 2nd stage for fetal distress
Multifetal pregnancy reduction for high order multiples

[1]If followed by effective interventions.
[2]Needs further evaluation in terms of brain damage (see text).

on the interventions of Group 4 which do not prevent cerebral palsy and may even have undesirable effects?

Summary and conclusions

Although there are many interventions which either reduce (Group 1) or are very likely (Group 2) to reduce rates of cerebral palsy, the rate of cerebral palsy remains steady. This could mean that it takes more than identifying the appropriate interventions to implement change; that we still fail to understand the complex causal pathways in their entirety, including the social milieux in which people live and make, or fail to make, decisions; or that the balance between death and cerebral palsy is irreducible.

On account of the complexity of causation and the dynamic nature of the application of preventive strategies it is not possible to assess the proportion of those cases arising before the postneonatal period which, given the best possible currently available care, could be prevented. For example, anti-D administration is now standard medical practice: is it still reasonable to project how many cases of kernicterus might have occurred without it and count them as being prevented? Courts of law may now consider failure to administer anti-D appropriately as unwarranted causation, rather than its appropriate administration as prevention.

If it were possible to prevent *de novo* the occurrence of cerebral palsy in those infants who show intrapartum signs compatible with asphyxia (assuming that they had been developing normally *in utero* before the onset of labour), and one quarter of the approximately 24 per cent of cases born very preterm, and the approximately 2 per cent due to congenital infections, then the total reduction would not exceed 20 per cent. Furthermore, this prevented portion, or some part of it, may not be apparent if aspects of the perinatal care preventing these cases allowed the survival of others who would previously have died before recognition of their cerebral palsy.

13
EPIDEMIOLOGICAL ISSUES IN EVALUATING THE MANAGEMENT OF CEREBRAL PALSY

"It is easy to be critical but hard to study the effects of various intervention procedures in CP."

(Forssberg and Tedroff 1997)

In common with many other medical practices, interventions for the management of cerebral palsy have historically been introduced without the objective evaluations currently demanded of new drugs. The Cochrane Collaboration aims to synthesize all available scientifically sound evidence and to encourage research in areas where insufficient evidence is available, as discussed for perinatal management strategies in Chapter 12. However, sound evidence concerning the management of cerebral palsy is not easily obtainable because of the nature and diversity of people with cerebral palsy.

Therapeutic intervention consumes considerable resources and often places considerable demands on the individual. It is only worth doing if it is effective. A sound empirical basis for treatment decreases the guesswork, facilitating the choice of timely interventions that seize opportunities which may be available only once in an individual's lifetime. For example, electromyography (EMG) and video assessment can result in a better appreciation of how and which muscles are working abnormally; three-dimensional computerized gait analysis with force plates can detect where abnormal forces exist. Appropriately applied, this knowledge can decrease the possibility of performing inappropriate and usually irreversible surgery. Reducing spasticity in a muscle during periods of accelerated bone growth may enable the muscle to grow at the same rate, thereby avoiding contracture. Initial choice of optimal management strategies and successful intervention enhances quality of life for patients and their families, increases patient compliance and is more cost-effective. It also increases therapist morale (important since the high staff turnover often seen in cerebral palsy treatment centres has detrimental effects on patient care), and decreases the possibility of complaints and litigation. Evidence-based interventions should benefit all concerned, but few are available (Stine 1990, Forssberg and Tedroff 1997). This chapter discusses the barriers to objective evaluation specific to cerebral palsy management and suggests how they might be overcome.

Requirements of scientific evaluation
Management strategies have been justified by observations of improvements following

their application to case series without comparison (or control) groups. Positive results can be reported following many interventions for children with cerebral palsy because the motor cortex develops and children learn new skills throughout childhood, even when they have disabilities. It is more difficult to find evidence that the intervention makes a difference to this development. Confidence in causality increases with increasingly rigorous research design (Ernst 1995), as shown in Table 12.2 (p. 141), which suggests that, ideally, every management strategy should be tested with a randomized, blinded, controlled clinical trial.

In *controlled* research, the effects of performing an intervention under a given set of conditions are compared with the effects of not performing the intervention under otherwise *identical conditions*. In *randomized* controlled trials the identical conditions are created by the random allocation of subjects to the intervention that they will receive, a process called randomization (see Glossary, and under Subjects below). Uncontrolled research in which the outcome is observed after the intervention is applied equally to all subjects cannot determine whether the intervention was *responsible* for the outcome. Even rare dramatic therapeutic successes, *e.g.* penicillin, the effects of which are so obvious that no formal experimentation is necessary, require for comparison knowledge of what the outcome of the target entity (*e.g.* bacterial infection) would be without that treatment. In order to draw causal inferences and avoid mistaking association for causation, research must be controlled.

Blinding avoids systematic bias resulting from human manipulation. It can be applied at three points.

(i) Blinding the *researchers* as to allocation to treatment avoids them influencing which subjects receive which intervention. *Randomization* is equivalent to blinded treatment allocation because adequate methods of randomization involve blinding the allocator to the identity either of the intervention or of the subject—for example, unlabelled capsules may be provided by an independent agent (unaware of subject identity) for allocation by the researcher (unaware of the identity of the intervention).

(ii) Blinding the *subject* as to which intervention they receive avoids *placebo* effects. These may affect outcome if the subject has preconceived ideas about the relative efficacies of the interventions—for example, if there has been media coverage about a new treatment prior to systematic evaluation.

(iii) Blinding the *assessor* of the outcome as to which intervention each subject has received avoids assessment bias.

While deliberate scientific fraud has been known to occur, subconscious effects are likely to be far more prevalent and harder to control. Blinding removes the necessity for researchers to attempt self-imposed impartiality, which, even with the best of intentions, may not be humanly possible. Effective blinding of intervention allocation and outcome assessment is a statement of a researcher's integrity and should never be misconstrued as a test of an assessor's ability or an admission of dishonest tendencies.

The other source of artefact in experimental research is *random error*. The possibility of false conclusions resulting from random error is measured by estimating confidence intervals around results. A confidence interval is the range of values in which there is a specified probability (usually 95 per cent) that the true value will lie. For a 95 per cent confidence interval there is a 5 per cent chance that the true value lies outside this range.

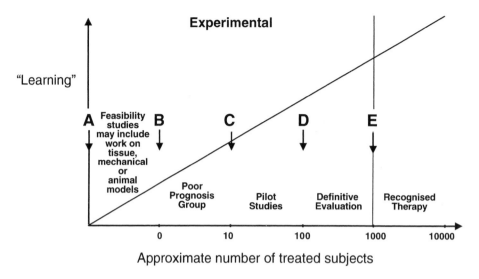

Fig. 13.1. Communal learning curve in a new management for cerebral palsy—or any other condition—becoming a recognized therapy.

The range decreases, and the precision of the estimate increases, as the number of subjects increases. Clinical trials often include large numbers of subjects to minimize the possibility of random error leading to false conclusions. The number of subjects required for a given level of confidence in a specific result can be estimated by guessing the magnitude of the effect (see Sample size estimates, Glossary).

The randomized, blinded, controlled clinical trial research design was conceived for testing drugs to treat common and relatively homogeneous diseases such as infections, heart attacks and strokes, to answer the question, 'Does drug A result in lower mortality than drug B?'. Not only are such trials seldom feasible in the context of cerebral palsy management research, but often we are not yet in a position even to ask such definitive questions.

Therapeutic interventions may be considered to be subject to a communal learning curve, as shown in Figure 13.1. A is the point of the initial idea that an intervention might be useful, but where no data on its effectiveness are available. If feasibility studies suggest a positive cost–benefit ratio, point B is reached at which the therapy is tried on human subjects with a poor prognosis for whom appropriate interventions either do not currently exist or have failed. If this intervention shows an advantageous cost–benefit ratio, point C is reached. At this point it is appropriate to commence pilot studies on small groups of patients in order to define the most appropriate target subjects, optimize therapeutic techniques and devise ways of accurately measuring outcomes in the target population. It is only after reaching D that definitive evaluation (such as controlled trials) is appropriate to compare it with existing therapies. Should it prove superior to existing therapies, point E, the new intervention should cease to be considered experimental and become the recognized therapy. For many interventions in cerebral palsy the communal learning curve has stalled around point C and the therapy has become recognized, at least by some, without a sound empirical basis. Cerebral palsy management is being criticized for the absence of definitive evaluation, but frequently it is too early to attempt definitive evaluation because pilot studies have not yet adequately defined the components of the intervention.

Defining the components of a therapeutic intervention

A therapeutic intervention is designed to achieve a specific outcome in order to ameliorate a particular health problem. Its effectiveness depends on the *intervention* itself as well as at least two other components, namely the *subject* and the *outcome* considered. Another component may be the *provider* of the intervention, whose personal characteristics may influence the character and acceptability of the intervention. Since the aim of a trial is to answer a clinically relevant question, it must be reproducible elsewhere if results are to be generalized beyond the original research setting. All components must therefore be specified carefully and as completely as possible.

The subjects and interventions of perinatal management (described in Chapter 12) tend to be well defined, and the benefits of many outcomes (such as intact survival in contrast to death or neurodevelopmental deficit) are not disputable. In contrast, many interventions used in cerebral palsy management still need answers to questions such as: What exactly is the intervention supposed to accomplish—what are the putative outcomes? How can we ensure that the outcome has been achieved—how can the outcome be measured? What are the optimal intervention techniques? Whom, if anyone, does it benefit—what are the characteristics of appropriate subjects?

Exploratory research to answer these sorts of questions is a necessary precursor of definitive evaluation. It is not substandard evaluation nor should it be mistaken for definitive evaluation. Pilot studies of evaluations, published in order to further research, have sometimes been prematurely interpreted as definitive (Sommerfeld *et al.* 1981, Tirosh and Rabino 1989).

While it is too early to contemplate a randomized trial for some interventions, it is already too late for others. Even without the benefits of recent epidemiological thinking concerning best practice and objective evaluation, decades of sound clinical observation have produced management strategies that are undoubtedly of considerable benefit. They should not be discarded simply because the benefit has not been demonstrated in a randomized controlled clinical trial (Stine 1990). For example, there is compelling evidence that the passive muscle stretching routinely administered to children with spastic and hypertonic muscles is of considerable benefit. Historical accounts of deformities, more contempory anecdotal accounts of isolated cases who have escaped therapeutic attention through childhood, and current observations in developing countries testify that the natural evolution of even mild spasticity or hypertonicity in childhood includes life-limiting and contorting contractures that may result in skeletal deformities and loss of function. Severe acquired deformities in children with mild or moderate impairments are seldom seen in developed countries today, most likely on account of the almost universal practice of passive stretching prescribed and/or provided by physiotherapists. It is no longer ethically possible to subject passive muscle stretching to an evaluation procedure that involves withholding it from a proportion of children with cerebral palsy (Piper *et al.* 1986), since, if contractures are allowed to progress unchecked, the results eventually become irreversible. Research should now be focused on defining the optimum means of providing the stretching by the most rigorous research designs available (Tardieu *et al.* 1982, 1988).

The learning curve in cerebral palsy management shown in Figure 13.1 has stalled because the number of subjects required to fuel it increases rapidly as the existing knowledge about an intervention increases. It is difficult to amass sufficient numbers of suitable cerebral palsy subjects for this research. This is one of many difficulties of defining an intervention's components inherent to the cerebral palsy population. The problems associated with each component are discussed below.

Subjects

For comparable conditions, two groups of patients are required with similar distributions of all factors determining outcome. Some of these factors will be known. For example, walking ability depends on age and the type and severity of impairments. However, it may also depend on other less obvious factors, particularly psychological factors such as intrinsic motivation, parental encouragement or sibling rivalry. While it is possible to match groups on known determinants, it can never be certain that *all* factors determining outcome have been considered. The randomized controlled trial *randomly* allocates subjects to receive or not to receive the intervention, so that *provided enough subjects are randomized*, by chance alone all the factors determining outcome (recognized and unrecognized) will be equally distributed in the two groups of subjects. However, randomization can never *ensure* comparability because, even with sufficient numbers, there remains a small chance of significant inequality. Chance does not work in a dichotomous fashion, and while comparability with respect to recognized determinants can be—and should always be—checked, this is not possible for unrecognized determinants. Moreover, the likelihood of randomization equalizing the distribution of unknown determinants depends on whether the number of subjects is sufficiently large. The required size depends on the number of factors determining outcome and their variability between subjects. Random treatment allocation of small numbers of variable subjects serves only to give a false sense of security as it is very unlikely to create equal groups. A trial comparing treatment arms that are initially dissimilar with respect to known determinants of outcome cannot give valid estimates of risk associated with the treatments whether the dissimilarity arose by chance or systematically. Other methods of allocating subjects to treatments exist which work to equalize the distribution of determinants of the outcome between treatment arms. These methods should be used in preference to randomization where there are limited numbers of variable subjects—and people with cerebral palsy are *very* variable. As described in Chapters 2 and 3, the term cerebral palsy encompasses a very wide spectrum of both severity and type of motor disability varying in aetiology and pathology, and the motor disability may be only one of several disabilities.

While the cerebral pathology is static, in the long term the clinical picture of cerebral palsy evolves continuously with the development of the mortor cortex in young people, and we know little about its evolution, particularly of the more severe forms, in older people. The resulting disability derives from the sum not only of primary impairments (*e.g.* weakness, spasticity) but also of impairments secondary to the primary physical impairments (*e.g.* contractures, hip migration, scoliosis), secondary to therapy (*e.g.* pharmacological therapy, surgery, splints or other appliances) and lastly, but probably greatly under-recognized, of psychological impairments secondary to the recognition of one's disability. Depression, for example, sets in as hopes and beliefs in the efficacy of treatment fail to be met. There are also tertiary problems: abnormal motor patterns learnt of necessity to compensate for primary impairments (*e.g.* equinus, crouch gait or internal rotation) are the individual's solution to their motor problems. Secondary and tertiary impairments, whether physical or psychological, tend to increase over time.

The timing of an intervention is therefore frequently a crucial determinant of outcome. Time may be measured chronologically as postconceptional or postnatal age, or in relation to growth or development. For example, reduction of hypertonicity by reversible denervation using botulinum A toxin may confer benefits outlasting its immediate effects when applied at periods of rapid bone growth if it avoids muscle contracture by allowing muscle growth to keep pace with bone growth (Cosgrove and Graham 1994). Alternatively, application of botulinum A toxin at the initiation of a functional skill may allow the acquisition of a normal motor pattern for that skill, rather than a pattern compensating for hypertonicity. For any intervention, it is essential to specify the appropriate timing in the relevant units. If timing differs between subjects then the effects of timing on the outcome must be assessed, for example by stratification. Long term evolution of the clinical picture must also be considered when making comparisons over time, particularly in studies of children.

Clinical picture also varies in the short term, from day to day and even from hour to hour. It varies with *health*, *fatigue* and *mood* in a population that tends to fatigue easily, have significant behavioural issues, and is notorious for its chronic and often serious health problems, in addition to motor impairment. The reproducible assessment of performance may be further hampered if the subject has limited capacity for purposeful intent; if the therapist cannot enlist their cooperation and provide adequate and constant motivation to perform; or if the environment is inappropriate. Variability of performance has implications (i) for the number of assessments required to make a reliable estimate of outcome, and (ii) for choosing conditions under which variability of performance will be minimized. Functional tasks necessarily require the cooperation of the subject and should be inherently motivating. While therapists are trained to continuously adapt the environment to prolong their subject's interest, extrinsic maintenance of motivation is often incompatible with the necessity of maintaining constant conditions. This has implications for choosing appropriate functional goals.

With so much subject variability, huge trials would be needed to generate two equivalent groups of persons with cerebral palsy by chance alone. However, cerebral palsy is so heterogeneous that it is unlikely that *any* management intervention is useful across the entire group. The subgroup most likely to derive benefit must be sought in pilot studies. The commonly used clinical descriptions tend to emphasize topography and the predominant type of movement disorder (Chapter 3); however, two subjects described as having spastic quadriplegia may have very different motor problems, and this type of description is not sufficiently detailed to define target groups for management. The more detailed the descriptions, the greater problems of interobserver reliability are likely to be. Nonetheless, the details of severity (functional abilities), age (chronological and developmental), additional movement disorders (including weakness) and their topographies, secondary impairments and additional impairments may all determine the appropriateness of an intervention. Subject selection for pilot studies is important. Pragmatically it will be dictated by the subjects that are available, but it is important to be aware of the ramifications of characteristics of the sample of subjects to be used. More homogeneous groups of subjects have the likely advantage of more homogeneous outcomes, thereby requiring smaller numbers for a trial of a given power. On the other hand, given that the pool of potential subjects is generally limited, homogeneous samples have the disadvantage that fewer subjects will meet the entry criteria than would be the case with more liberal entry criteria. Furthermore, the more homogeneous the subjects the less potential exists for exploring the generalizability of research observations, that is, the range of subjects to which the conclusions of research may properly be applied. In choosing criteria for subject selection a balance must be found between homogeneity and generalizability, given the number and clinical descriptions of the subjects that are available.

The effect of subject characteristics on outcome can be determined in analysis by stratification or statistical techniques such as multiple regression. If outcome does depend on factors that vary between subjects, and subjects are all pooled, the measured effect of the intervention will be an average for all subjects. In the extreme this means the average of those who derived benefit and of those who did not. Where outcomes are variable it is necessary to scrutinize all subject characteristics to determine whether they could be responsible for outcome variability. Grouping heterogeneous subjects runs the risk of dismissing therapies as unreliable or useless that are in fact useful in limited groups of subjects. In cerebral palsy management research there are never enough locally available patients meeting entry criteria, making multicentre studies desirable. The likely need to explore the effects of patient characteristics makes it very important to record complete and accurate descriptions of patient characteristics with good interobserver agreement about the manner in which those characteristics are described (see Chapter 3).

Interventions
Controlled research requires a comparison of at least two interventions, which must be accurately and completely defined. The intervention of primary interest is compared with *conventional*, *traditional*, *placebo* or *no therapy*. Children and the parents of children with cerebral palsy are very likely to devise their own therapies in the absence of prescribed therapy, and because it is important to be aware of what the control group is exposed to, 'no therapy' does not create a satisfactory control group. Equally, there is seldom a therapeutic equivalent to a pharmaceutical *placebo*, an intervention that can be guaranteed to have no biological/ biomedical effect. It is important that *conventional* or *traditional* therapies be described since very few are adequately standardized and even small variations can be shown to be useful.

Each intervention must be described in sufficient detail for another person to be able to reproduce it. This is difficult for composite therapies based on ill defined theories: for example, conductive education does not have well defined principles, and the application of Bobath therapy has changed over the years. Inadequately defined therapies depend on the interpretation of the provider. This does not mean that they cannot be effective, but it does make them hard to reproduce reliably and thus to evaluate scientifically. Stratification by care providers and identification of provider characteristics associated with desirable outcomes can help to take the art and mystique out of charismatic therapies and put them on a sounder scientific basis. Composite therapies may be split into their more easily defined components. Outcomes following group therapy, for example, can be compared with those following individual therapy; intensive can be compared with less intensive therapy; limited periods with prolonged periods of therapy or individually spoken instructions can be compared with instructions sung by a group as in Conductive Education. This may appear tedious, a slow and unimpressive approach, but the results are more likely to be clear-cut and useable. Failure to split composite interventions into reproducible components has resulted in very expensive and labour intensive intervention research failing to produce any clear answers, largely because no one could be sure as to exactly what the interventions were that were being evaluated (Bairstow *et al.* 1993, Bax 1993).

Changes to an intervention in response to subject characteristics must be documented along with the criteria for making the changes. Only when pilot studies have identified target subjects and optimal techniques, and these are documented in a protocol published in easily available literature, can an intervention be referred to simply by a name. Once the intervention has been defined in this way, the protocol must be adhered to, or the name modified. Currently a single name is sometimes used which may refer to any of a variety of different interventions. For example, the term *physiotherapy* has been used in this field to refer to a huge range of interventions, from passive muscle stretching by a variety of means to education (or re-education) in gross motor skills with or without orthoses or aids, and even early intervention in high risk infants who have not yet demonstrated motor impairment. 'Physiotherapy' therefore does not define any one intervention (Tirosh and Rabino 1989). While it may seem banal to spell out that an ankle was flexed under a certain pressure for a certain duration and that this was repeated a certain number of times within a given period on so many days of the week, this sort of detail enables another physiotherapist to do the same thing. It may be argued that the physiotherapist is the professional and should determine the details of physiotherapy appropriate for each case. That is entirely appropriate provided there is scientifically sound evidence on which the physiotherapist can base her/his decisions. When this is true there is no need for further research.

Outcomes
WHAT ARE APPROPRIATE OUTCOMES?
Prevention or cure?
Traditionally, the lesion(s) responsible for cerebral palsy were considered irreversible. This view has now been challenged by the discovery that in the fetus and newborn at least, brain tissue may grow preferentially into damaged areas (Rutherford *et al.* 1997).

Whether or not the lesion(s) are necessarily irreversible, their impact on motor function may not necessarily be so. Neuronal plasticity, the ability of neurons to take over functions for which they were not originally destined, has been shown to occur in children with hemiplegic cerebral palsy (Carr *et al.* 1993; see also Chapter 6). This plasticity decreased with increasing postconceptional age and was not seen in any of three cases acquired after the postnatal age of 2 years. Neuronal reorganization may be responsible for the imperfect correlation between severity of motor disabilities and extent of cerebral lesions seen with cerebral imaging.

Augmentation of plasticity may reasonably be considered a cure and is the principle aim of early intervention therapies that provide additional stimulation to high risk, primarily very preterm, infants. Early intervention aiming to prevent cerebral palsy has a reasonably self-evident end-point (normal or abnormal motor function) which, together with the increasing numbers of very preterm survivors and their relative homogeneity of clinical presentation, should make rigorous evaluation of early intervention attainable. This has not been and may never be realized on account of the popular perception of its efficacy, which makes some form of early intervention routine for infants born very preterm mandatory in the face of any suggestion of neurological compromise (Bennett and Scott 1997). In Bennett and Scott's study an early intervention programme of additional stimulation was provided to all members of the group randomly selected to receive the intervention, but it was also provided to subjects randomly selected *not* to receive it if and when their assessments indicated deficits. The difference between the intervention and control groups then was not intervention versus none, but prophylactic intervention versus intervention once a need was demonstrated. The study reported no effect on health problems such as cerebral palsy, and a positive effect only on cognitive development and only in children of mothers with less education. The explanation for this observation may be that additional stimulation was less likely to be provided to controls with delayed cognitive development whose mothers had little education than to similar controls with delayed motor development. Therefore all children with motor delay received additional stimulation (either before or at the time the motor delay became apparent), but among children with cognitive delay whose mothers had little education, only the intervention group received any additional stimulation.

It is too late to perform randomized trials of the effects on cerebral palsy outcomes of early intervention versus no intervention, because parents who are prepared not to provide additional stimulation when faced with a child failing to meet motor milestones are no longer representative of all parents. Due to the rapid increase in very preterm survival, these survivors are a new phenomenon: there are no historical controls with which to compare very preterm recipients of early intervention. It is likely that early intervention is here to stay without definitive evaluation as to its efficacy. The results of Bennett and Scott's trial suggest that this may be appropriate if it is correct to assume that there was only one properly controlled comparison of additional stimulation versus none (which was for cognitive development in children of mothers with less education), and this indicated that additional stimulation did improve outcome. The danger of the faulty research design (arising perhaps because it was already too late to perform the trial) is that it might falsely be concluded that early intervention programmes to provide additional stimulation have no effect and should not be funded.

Whether or not early intervention can positively affect motor development, it is seldom considered a cure because it precedes definitive demonstration of the effects of the cerebral lesion(s) on voluntary motor function. It is more likely to be described as prevention. This is because cerebral palsy is defined by deficits of motor function and not by cerebral pathology manifest at birth (see Chapter 4). Better cerebral imaging with more accurate interpretation in conjunction with early intervention programmes may answer whether early intervention programmes (or any other circumstances) can normalize motor function in the presence of cerebral lesions that would normally result in deficits. It should also answer the question as to whether the children who 'outgrow' (Nelson and Ellenberg 1982) their cerebral palsy ever had cerebral lesions generally associated with cerebral palsy. At present, children who demonstrate motor deficits early in life may be labelled as having cerebral palsy, but if the deficits disappear (with or without intervention) they are not considered *cured*. Instead the description is amended, for example, to motor delay. Under these circumstances, cure is not a possible outcome of management for persons described as having cerebral palsy.

Cerebral palsy is not a fatal condition. The increase in mortality risk in children with cerebral palsy comes from congenital anomalies; susceptibility to infection and accidents; poor nutrition resulting from feeding difficulties; epilepsy or other associated impairments; and possibly losing the will to live. Survival is seldom the primary aim of management, although it may be dependent on the quality of care, particularly for the most severely impaired. Thus the two unequivocal epidemiological outcomes, death or cure, are generally inappropriate management outcomes; instead, the aim of management is to increase the *quality of life*.

QUALITY OF LIFE
What this vague term means varies not only with the type and severity of impairments but also with the personalities of individual cases and their carers. Clinical awareness of the individuality of what enhances quality of life is reflected in the increasing use of individualized goals such as those determined using the Canadian Occupation Performance Measure (Law *et al.* 1994), but this awareness tends to be greatest among those concerned with the care of adult patients.

Traditionally the aim of therapy in children with cerebral palsy has been to mimic normal motor development, normalize motor function, reduce neurological signs, and minimize the development of secondary and tertiary impairments. The emphasis on paralleling physical development in the able bodied is often appropriate. For example, maintenance of the head of the femur within the acetabulum is dependent on normal muscular development. Without it there is a high risk of subluxation, which is irreversible, painful and complicates basic patient care. Preventive strategies must be implemented before the effects become apparent, and it is therefore proper that medical caregivers be authoritarian in their insistence on interventions maintaining alignment of the head of the femur, along with a straight spine and adequate muscle length. These preventive activities are becoming increasingly important with the increasing survival of people with moderate or severe cerebral palsy. It is less clear whether it is always in the best interests of the person with cerebral palsy to consider independent ambulation as a necessarily desirable goal, given the existence and community acceptance of satisfactory mobility devices. Similarly, we should question whether therapy should be directed at encouraging the subject to follow the path of unimpaired children in attaining motor skills, particularly since traditional concepts concerning this path may not be accurate (Loria 1980). The human psyche does not respond well to inevitable failure. It is possible that cognitively capable children with severe motor impairments may, provided steps are taken to avoid musculoskeletal deformities, be better served by more cognitive education (for example in computing skills) than by emphasizing physical skills at which they are doomed to fail. Maintenance of self-esteem is of vital importance to avoid psychological impairment.

Quality of life and the placebo effect

Medical trials, particularly of drugs, are often concerned to differentiate *real* from *placebo* effects. This is reasonable in the context of powerful drugs that may have deleterious side-effects because it is necessary to know whether the same somatic effect is as easily obtained with a harmless substance. This has led to an undervaluing of psychological effects and the notion that they are somehow illusory, despite the demonstration that states of mind can dramatically affect bodily health as well as quality of life (which may be considered to be a state of mind). Psychological effects are central to quality of life and are influenced by the subject's beliefs and preferences about therapy, particularly if the intervention requires the subject's active participation. In management trials, then, not only is it often impossible (or unethical) to blind subjects as to which intervention they are receiving, it may be quite inappropriate. Furthermore, the act of randomization might reduce the effectiveness of an intervention that requires subject (or clinician) participation if the subject (or their clinician) has a preference regarding therapy. "It is at least as plausible to assume that experimentation [randomization] reduces the effectiveness of such interventions as to assume, as most researchers have done, that the results of observational [non-randomized] studies are wrong" (Black 1996).

Increasing patient participation in the process of defining therapeutic goals has placed more emphasis on both cosmetic appearance and the achievement of individually desired functional goals by any means available, rather than by copying the means used by the able bodied. Where goals are mutually exclusive, *e.g.* functional versus cosmetic (Rose *et al.* 1985, Fetter 1991), the choice of goal should lie with the patient, provided they are informed of the physical consequences of their choice. Therefore, with the exception of avoiding secondary impairments, there are few unequivocal outcomes by which efficacy may be evaluated, even for subjects of a given clinical description.

Types of outcome: change in impairment, disability, handicap

It is generally appreciated that there are several levels of outcomes, but no standard categorization of these levels. Four categories—technical, functional, patient/carer satisfaction and cost effectiveness—have been described by Pierson (1997). Butler (1995) defined five categories dependent on whether the outcome addresses impairments, disabilities or handicaps (WHO 1980) with three categories addressing impairments:

Impairments: 1. cellular/molecular function
2. organ/organ system function
3. body/body segment function
Disability: 4. role fulfilment at home, school, work
Handicap: 5. participation in society.

There are several parallels between the Butler and Pierson systems, but satisfaction and cost-effectiveness are not specifically addressed by Butler, nor societal participation by Pierson, emphasizing the multifaceted nature of outcomes for people with cerebral palsy.

A *technical outcome* is a physically measurable parameter and parallels outcomes addressing *impairments*. These outcomes can often be measured objectively as they are less dependent on the individual observer or on the cooperation of the subject and therefore tend to be the most often reported. Technical outcomes commonly used in this field include blood concentrations of drugs, range of motion (measured by goniometer), spasticity (measured by the modified Ashworth scale—Bohannon and Smith 1987), muscle strength, weight, height, and increasingly the parameters of gait analysis. Without some change in a technical outcome it is difficult to argue that the intervention has had any physical effect. However, such measurements are usually justified on the grounds that the amelioration of disability and handicap automatically flows from the amelioration of impairments, but this is seldom empirically demonstrated. Normalization of a technical outcome does not necessarily represent a desirable outcome where there is the possibility that the impairment can be used functionally or where one impairment compensates for another. For example, spasticity may be used where strength is lacking or internal rotation may be used to restore abduction capacity (Arnold *et al.* 1997). In such cases reduction of spasticity or internal rotation may decrease functional ability, and subjects are usually more interested in reducing their disability/handicap than their impairments.

A *functional outcome* measures the subject's (or carer's) ability to complete a functional task effectively and largely parallels outcomes addressing *disability* (which the WHO now defines as the inability to perform activities—WHO 1999). They are desirable if the subject wants to perform the task, or if it facilitates a carer's task or relieves the carer of the necessity to assist in any activity of daily living. While effectiveness (task completion) is usually the main criterion, speed, energy expenditure and quality of movement are also frequently considered, because they are associated with satisfaction and social acceptance.

Patient and carer satisfaction
Satisfaction may be associated with outcomes addressing handicap (participation in society) but the overlap is tenuous. Satisfaction is usually assessed by asking patients and carers for their opinion. Another method of assessment available for ongoing therapies is whether the subject stays in the research programme or maintains therapy after the research programme has ended, especially if this involves personal costs. However, it is necessary for the researcher to be aware of other possible explanations of leaving or staying with the therapy. While it may be easier to obtain a measure of satisfaction than one of technical outcome, it is likely to be less objective. For several reasons patients or carers may not give the responses that they genuinely feel, and questions need to be worded and delivered with care.

187

Subjects need to feel safe to express negative feelings. Feelings of satisfaction may change, both in the short and long term, and satisfaction is not quantifiable. The Likert scales (Likert 1932) generally used to assess satisfaction do not have objective end-points: for example, what constitutes *maximum satisfaction* depends on the individual's disposition and the ease with which s/he is satisfied, factors that vary between individuals and may change from day to day within individuals. Furthermore, there is no guarantee of linearity of the scale (equal distances on the scale may not represent equal changes in satisfaction); thus it is inappropriate to treat the distances on the scale quantitatively. The best that can be offered is a representation of the actual distribution of responses (Macnaughton 1996). Satisfaction is very personal because priorities vary between individuals. While some may feel that added flexibility, reduced tremor or the ability to take additional steps is ultimately worth any effort, pain, inconvenience, expense or surgery, others may not.

Cost effectiveness
Evaluation of cost effectiveness is necessary because of limited resources. It is a daunting task because resource expenditure must be weighed against benefit where benefit has to be assessed from the sum of technical outcomes, which tend to be objectively measurable but possibly irrelevant to benefit, and of functional and satisfaction outcomes, which are more relevant to benefit but far more difficult to measure objectively.

In any evaluation, all four types of outcomes need to be considered. It is tempting to measure only technical outcomes. Funding bodies as well as researchers like the security of objectivity, the ease with which statistics may be applied to quantifiable observations and the knowledge that valid measurement of the proposed outcomes is achievable. However, technical outcomes in isolation do not measure benefit to the subjects, and therefore they are not sufficient for evaluation. Technical outcomes are nonetheless essential both in feasibility studies and for the element of objectivity they confer to more subjective end-points.

PURPOSES OF MEASUREMENT
Measurement in therapeutic interventions has three distinct functions. It enables more accurate (1) *description* of the subject, (2) *evaluation* of progress, and/or (3) *prediction* of the future. It may not be possible to use the same measurement instrument to accomplish all three functions.

Descriptive measures
Descriptive measures compare the subject with a recognized group or population and therefore need to be scaled against norms with which the individual's result is compared. The norms remain constant over time or change very slowly, as, for example, with the population distribution of IQ. In contrast, an individual's result may change from day to day, and such variability constitutes part of the description.

Evaluative measures
The primary attribute required of an evaluative measure is sensitivity to small changes

within an individual (responsiveness) and specificity to the factor(s) of interest. Extraneous information, irrelevant to the factor of interest, leads to decreased responsiveness (Law 1987) because there is always random variability around any measurement.

During evaluation of interventions, descriptive measurements are required to measure distributions of subject characteristics that may affect the outcome to assess generalizability of results. The tools for these measurements are very likely to differ from the evaluative tools which should consider *only* those items that the intervention is designed to affect. In some instances it may be appropriate to use a subset of the descriptive tool as the evaluative tool—for example, one dimension of the Gross Motor Function Measure (see below)—but evaluative tools generally require more detail as well as less breadth than descriptive tools.

Predictive measures

A predictive measure predicts a factor that can be measured reliably, but the new (predictive) measurement can be made less invasively, more cheaply or earlier than the *gold standard* against which the result of the predictive measure may be compared. Thus the maintenance of primitive reflexes in late infancy might be used to predict a future description of cerebral palsy, and the accuracy of that prediction can be quantified by observation. A predictive measure should accurately predict the factor and should therefore have good test–retest reliability.

MEASURING OUTCOMES

All measurements should be valid. That is, they should have good interobserver reliability (*i.e.* one observer should get the same result as the next observer). They should have good content and construct reliability; that is, the instrument should measure all aspects of what it purports to measure (content), and give results compatible with all other formal or subjective/intuitive measures of the same thing (construct). The tools for measuring technical outcomes present no inherent difficulty since they attempt to measure factors that are at least theoretically quantifiable, although the techniques for measuring several fundamental factors leave room for improvement; for example, measurements of strength are very dependent on the cooperation of the subject, and the Ashworth Scale, commonly used to assess spasticity, is quite subjective (Bohannon and Smith 1987).

In contrast, functional outcomes may be partially subjective, and satisfaction outcomes are completely subjective. The increasing emphasis on quality of life in all aspects of health care has created an interest in the theory of measuring subjective outcomes which, until recently, was confined to the psychological and educational literature. The theories have been adapted for health outcomes both generally (Kirshner and Guyatt 1985, Streiner and Normal 1989) and specifically for occupational therapy (Law 1987).

Recently much work has gone into the development of outcome measures relevant to cerebral palsy: these are listed and/or discussed in several publications (Haley *et al.* 1991, Campbell 1996, Decker and Foss 1997). A new software package is available that not only describes outcome measures categorized as suitable for impairments, disabilities or handicaps, but also guides selection of the most appropriate measure in any individual, service or programme evaluation (Law *et al.* 1998).

Two norm-referenced measures of function are of particular interest to cerebral palsy management. The Functional Independence Measure (FIM) has an adaptation for children (WeeFIM) and scores activities of daily living under six dimensions including communication and social cognition (Msall *et al.* 1993). The Gross Motor Function Measure (GMFM) (Russell *et al.* 1989) considers five dimensions—lying and rolling; sitting; crawling and kneeling; standing; locomotion—and has recently been applied specifically to children with cerebral palsy (Palisano *et al.* 1997). The process of the development of the GMFM is well documented and demonstrates the enormous effort required to produce a valid, reliable and clinically useful norm-referenced measurement instrument. The rapidity with which the GMFM has been ubiquitously utilized amply demonstrates the need for such instruments. However, even taken in conjunction with a similar tool developed by the same group for measuring fine motor function, the quality of upper extremity skills test (QUEST) (Law *et al.* 1991), these carefully and thoroughly developed measurement tools are not omnipotent measures of motor function in children with cerebral palsy. They are superb norm-referenced descriptive measures against which to assess degree of motor impairment; but, because they cover all aspects of their domain, they take significant time to administer, the activities they assess are not likely to hold intrinsic motivation, and they are insensitive to small changes in motor function which may nonetheless be of sufficient magnitude to represent functionally useful improvements. In addition, there is a ceiling effect making it very difficult to measure improvements in subjects with near-normal function, and they do not address the unusual motor skills, such as fine motor control of the head or foot, sometimes essential for functional attainment in severely impaired persons. As discussed above, the attributes of descriptive and evaluative tools tend to be mutually exclusive, particularly given the time constraints imposed by attention span, which is often limited in the cerebral palsied population. For these reasons the GMFM is seldom the ideal evaluative tool, although it is now frequently being used as such. If no significant changes are measured even when there is a clinical impression of change, using the GMFM as an evaluative tool can be disappointing. More success is obtained when the evaluative component is limited to the GMFM dimension in which the intervention can be anticipated to bring about change (Bower *et al.* 1996). Given the diversity of problems facing people with cerebral palsy, particularly those with severe and multiple impairments, it is likely that there will always be a need to evaluate individually selected functional goals.

Functional goals

Bower *et al.* (1996) have observed that verbalized functional goals that closely specify conditions and degree of performance lead to more rapid improvements in a generalized function than do general aims; thus the goal *to sit on a child's chamber-pot holding onto the sides with both hands for one minute without falling off* leads to more rapid improvement in sitting skills than the general aim *to improve sitting*. As for the able bodied, a series of stepped functional goals with increasing levels of skill must be set one after the other. Functional goals must be chosen carefully, considering the following:

• *Motivation.* The goal should be intrinsically motivating. The subject or, where that is impossible, the carer must be involved in the choice of goal to ensure that it holds a personal interest and benefit. Such goals will usually be dynamic rather than static. Few people want to maintain sitting or standing for the sake of it. Motivation must be obtained by choosing an activity of interest for which sitting or standing is necessary. Sitting, for example, may be required to play a computer game. If a subject cannot nominate such an activity, achievement of the static goal is unlikely to improve their quality of life. Intrinsic motivation removes the need for extrinsic motivation which is a major incentive to vary test conditions. These goals should also be attainable. Ideally the subject should already be able to attempt the goal but desires improvement. This avoids the frustration of repeated total failure or the later discovery that the goal holds no intrinsic interest for the subject.

• *Validity.* Ensure that you understand what determines goal attainment and that degree of attainment assesses what you are interested in assessing—for example, the time taken to eat something may not measure fine motor function if the child is feeling nauseous.

• *Valid and unambiguous measurement.* Measure a single, specified and quantifiable outcome—for example, specify an assessment duration and measure the number of repetitions achieved *or* specify a number of repetitions and measure the time it takes to do them, whichever is more relevant to daily living. Try not to allow more than one factor to vary between assessments.

Goals must have unambiguous and objectively observable end-points. For example, if measuring the duration of task, the point of initiation must be clearly identifiable. It may not be sufficient, especially for younger or intellectually impaired children, simply to say, 'Go'.

It is easier to devise valid methods of measurement for static goals than for dynamic ones, but relevance and motivation must not be sacrificed for ease of assessment. In the assessment of a dynamic proximal stability splint (Blair *et al.* 1995), disagreement concerning the effects of the splint between community observers and formal goal testing often arose because community observers assessed dynamic activities chosen by the children which they were highly motivated to attain while formal tests assessed static goals which held no intrinsic interest for the children.

Introducing objectivity to the assessment of subjective and unquantifiable factors
Use may be made of interobserver reliability to introduce a measure of objectivity when measuring nebulous and subjective outcomes such as changes in quality of life, satisfaction, temperament and overall function. Interobserver reliability measures the variation in measurement obtained by different observers measuring the same thing and is often used to assess observer reliability. Two statistics are commonly used. Kappa is used for categorical variables (Holman *et al.* 1983), while the intra-class correlation (ICC) is used for continuous variables (Armitage 1994). The numerical value, which can vary between zero and one, depends on the numbers of subjects, categories and observers as well as how much they agree, so values can strictly be compared only within a study. However, a high value indicates that the different observers agree on the direction of change more than can be anticipated by chance alone. Provided there are a reasonable number of independent observers, non-chance agreement strongly suggests that there has been a genuine change in the factor even if individual assessments appear subjective and unquantifiable. Thus

TABLE 13.1
Agreement/disagreement between three classes of observers on the presence of involuntary movement in 24 subjects with cerebral palsy*

	No. of subjects	Paediatricians	Therapists	Community observers
Complete agreement	5	–	–	–
	10	+	+	+
Pediatricians disagree	1[1]	+	–	–
	1	–	+	+
Therapists disagree	6	+	–	+
Community observers disagree	1[2]	+	+	–
Number of disagreements		2	6	1

Key: – denotes that involuntary movement was not reported;
    + denotes that involuntary movement was reported.
[1]Very subtle involuntary movement that did not noticeably affect function.
[2]Subject had only one community observer
*Previously unpublished data from E. Blair (1995).

even without a quantifiable outcome, measuring the amount of agreement between independently made subjective opinions allows us to quantify the degree of faith we can have in the validity of those opinions.

Whose subjective opinions should be considered?
Realistic assessments of how a child behaves in her/his normal environment may best be made by a frequent observer with an ongoing commitment to the child who can place that child's observations in a long term perspective. Such observers are the most likely to be able to choose times when the child is in typical states under reproducible conditions, and these times will be difficult to schedule (to obtain a professional assessment). The most frequent observers are also those most likely to be able to observe less frequent behaviours. In our study of the proximal stability splint (Blair *et al.* 1995) reports of the existence of involuntary movement were compared between three classes of observers (Table 13.1). Two developmental paediatricians completed neurodevelopmental assessments during a one hour examination specifically to describe movement disorder. The therapists were the occupational therapists or physiotherapists administering weekly therapy, and the community observers were parents and other caregivers in frequent regular contact who had not been asked specifically to look for involuntary movement. While there is broad agreement, there is some variation, and it is not clear which group should be considered the gold standard. However, while the paediatricians making the formal assessments disagreed with the other two groups for two children and therapists disagreed for six children, community observers disagreed for only one child, and this child was also the only subject to have only one community observer. We concluded that community observers, who saw the children most often, were uniquely placed to be accurate observers and that greater weight should be placed on their reports, particularly when they exhibited interobserver reliability.

Implications for study design

RANDOMIZED CONTROLLED CLINICAL TRIALS

The heterogeneous clinical descriptions of cerebral palsy, the rarity of each description of cerebral palsy, the varying nature of the subjects and the numerous outcomes of primary interest may singly or together render randomized, blinded, controlled clinical trials practically impossible and/or inappropriate for evaluating management in people with cerebral palsy. While the randomized controlled trial design embodies scientific principles that are necessary for valid research, it is not the only possible way to avoid or minimize systematic bias, to avoid the possibility of mistaking association for causation, or to deal with random error. In addition, randomized trials have their own ethical problems. Researchers can only ethically randomize patients if they are genuinely uncertain (*equipoised*) as to which is the better intervention. As the research progresses, the relative benefits of the interventions being compared become clearer. At some point there will be, for example, a 70 per cent chance that one intervention is superior. Equipoise is destroyed, but the prespecified desirable level of confidence in this conclusion is not yet attained—there remains a 30 per cent chance that it is not superior. Is it ethical to continue randomization? Is it ethical not to continue randomization? To blind the researcher to the results sidesteps the issue. Fundamentally more patients must be randomized to definitively answer the question than are needed to destroy equipoise (Burton *et al.* 1997).

OTHER CONTROLLED STUDY DESIGNS

Crossover trial design overcomes the problem of individual heterogeneity because it compares each subject only with her/himself. The classic design allocates subjects to each intervention (generally termed A for the baseline intervention and B for the experimental intervention) at random (Ottenbacher 1986). This design needs both (i) a larger sample size than obligatory alternation of interventions, and (ii) interventions with finite and preferably known 'wash-out' times. Thus they are not appropriate for interventions with long lasting or permanent effects. If such effects are anticipated it is necessary to remove the random allocation and stipulate that A must precede B. This may lead to systematic bias if there are time-ordered effects. For example, the outcome may be improved by the novelty or increased attention of being a research subject, which would tend to improve outcomes in earlier periods to a greater extent than in later periods. Alternatively, outcomes may improve as a result of learning how to do the assessments, which would tend to improve outcomes in later periods. If time ordering due to seasonal effects is anticipated, trial entry can be staggered. This assumes that subjects are homogeneous with respect to seasonal effects. While this may be a valid assumption, it is important to be constantly aware of what assumptions are being made. Pilot studies may be required to ascertain whether the assumptions are met.

Crossover trial analysis is complicated by studying children who are developing at a significant rate compared with the time frame of the trial. The baseline outcome is then constantly shifting. While it is possible to measure how the outcome changes during the baseline period, it has to be assumed that the outcome would change in the same way as was observed during the baseline period during the intervention period if the intervention had not been applied. This may not be valid as development does not always proceed in a smooth continuous manner, but might, for example, proceed in a series of irregular jumps.

Given the diversity of problems facing people with cerebral palsy, it is frequently appropriate to ask: What is the optimal therapy for *this* subject? The so-called *N-of-one* study (a crossover study with a single subject) has been designed to answer it, but the results from such a design are not generalizable. Should several subjects with similar problems present over the course of time, it is reasonable to perform a series of N-of-one studies in which the results are pooled and stratified by patient characteristics. This is then a crossover trial with sequential entry.

Research design must be tailored to fit the problem, both scientifically and practically. Crossover designs offer a lot of scope (Ottenbacher 1986), but adequate control must be ensured, and assumptions must constantly be sought. When assumptions are recognized they must be checked, or, where this is not possible, it must be questioned whether conclusions would be invalidated or generalizability changed if the assumptions were not true. The evaluation of each therapeutic modality must be tackled individually. There is no prototype research design applicable to all situations. There is nonetheless an essential outline common to all scientific medical research. It consists of careful and systematic documentation of unselected observations of all relevant outcomes following different management options, which have been applied under comparable conditions so that valid comparisons can be made and conclusions drawn for specified groups of patients. The principles are no different from any other scientific research, but they may be hard to follow using templates created to suit circumstances that differ from those in the management of cerebral palsy. Bower *et al.* (1996) noted the extreme difficulties of conducting a randomized controlled trial of 44 subjects, 11 in each of four intervention arms, a sample size of distinctly unimpressive proportions by the standards of other fields of epidemiological research.

Conclusions

Much good work in evaluating interventions for the management of cerebral palsy is in progress, but even more remains to be done. The cerebral palsy group needs to be divided into accurately described subgroups according to the problems that are amenable to therapy. More effort needs to go into the means of identifying the outcomes most important to each individual, to match the current progress in developing valid and reliable means of measuring them. More effort needs to go into identifying cause-and-effect relationships between individual elements of interventions and specific elements of outcome.

Given the highly individual and complex nature of some problems facing individuals with cerebral palsy, randomized controlled trials may not always be the optimal research design to assess efficacy even when all the components of an intervention are well characterized. While it is too early for randomized controlled trials for some interventions, for some it is already too late. For many interventions, practical considerations may create insurmountable barriers to conducting randomized trials. Other research designs will have to be tailored to fit the practical problems while still maintaining the scientific requirements of avoiding or minimizing systematic bias, avoiding mistaking association for causation, and dealing with random error. While the management of cerebral palsy may always remain something of an art, in the interests of all concerned it is an art that needs a sound scientific basis.

14
TOWARDS A NEW ERA IN CEREBRAL PALSY EPIDEMIOLOGY?

"The present era of epidemiology is coming to a close. The focus on risk factors at the individual level—the hallmark of this era—will no longer serve. We need to be concerned equally with causal pathways at the societal level and with pathogenesis and causality at the molecular level."

(Susser and Susser 1996b)

Whereas this book follows our previous one of a similar title (Stanley and Alberman 1984), it has been completely rewritten to include new research and new thinking about epidemiological research in the cerebral palsies. The most important messages are firstly to think in causal pathways and secondly to seek the best evidence when choosing interventions to either prevent or treat the cerebral palsies. Other suggestions relate to the pragmatic aspects of what the cerebral palsies are and how best to classify and describe the various types. These latter approaches, covered in Chapters 2 and 3, are crucial if we are to compare and contrast our epidemiological data in more powerful ways than we have done in the past (see recommendations below). Research aimed at identifying the health and social needs of children and adults with cerebral palsy must be based on prevalent cases, classified by their functional capacity. Aetiological studies must be based on incident cases, whether alive or dead, and grouped by likely causal pathway.

In spite of intensive efforts in perinatal care in developed countries, overall rates of cerebral palsies in birth cohorts since 1984 have not fallen (Chapter 4). Indeed there is evidence that cerebral palsy rates increased in preterm and very preterm births in the 1980s but now seem to have levelled out. We are intensely curious as to how these rates will respond to the various social and medical influences in the variety of possible causal pathways over the next decade. The strong interest in these trends illustrates the enormous importance of cerebral palsy data collections (see recommendations below) to monitor trends, to provide samples of cases for observational research and, we strongly suggest, as outcomes for randomized trials of interventions, for which they are rarely used. In response to these needs for good data, many new cerebral palsy registers have been established, a list of which is given in the Appendix.

We hope that this book will encourage more useful and productive ways of thinking about causes of the cerebral palsies and of other perinatal outcomes. More multidisciplinary research is needed. We want to encourage thinking in causal pathways, getting away from simplistic consideration of single sufficient causes and multivariate analyses (Chapter 5).

We feel that the earlier a causal pathway can be interrupted the less the fetus is likely to be compromised and the greater the likelihood of successful prevention. Intervening earlier may also be cheaper and more cost effective. Whilst we have been enthusiastic about causal pathways, the development of statistical methods to recognize them is in its infancy. Thus we need to devise methods of statistical analysis that identify and investigate interactions between factors rather than 'controlling' for them and thus disregarding what may be their significant contribution along a pathway.

In Chapters 6 to 10 we interpret our current knowledge of important risk factors for the cerebral palsies using the model of causal pathways.

We suggest that, in terms of discovering effective interventions of early causal paths, it is better to think about maldevelopment globally rather than attempting to categorize factors, for example, as strictly genetic or as early teratogens (Chapter 6). Influences throughout pregnancy such as infections, inflammation, vascular complications and toxic effects can cause major defects of the brain both by interrupting early organogenesis and by later disruptions and interruptions of brain development. The role of neuroimaging may be critical here in elucidating how many term infants without any recognized risk factors or perinatal problems may have had major interferences during development.

Chapter 7 suggests several possible causal pathways to white matter damage in very preterm newborns. Whilst this is the most important brain anomaly in these children with cerebral palsy, it is unlikely to be the only one. More studies of the origins of very preterm birth are needed as well as of the ways in which they may influence the risk of brain pathology.

Chapter 8 discusses the ways in which intrauterine growth restriction should be considered and measured for epidemiological studies. Our challenge here is to identify and measure pathological fetal growth. As well, in following our causal pathway approach, it is interesting that the most common causes of intrauterine growth restriction such as maternal smoking and pre-eclampsia do not seem to be common causal pathways to cerebral palsy. This suggests that the hypothesis that poor growth *per se* results in an inherently 'vulnerable fetus' does not explain the very significant risk of cerebral palsy observed in those infants classified as small for gestational age; it remains a mystery.

Given the interest in birth asphyxia and brain damage over recent decades, it was important to thoroughly review the attempts to measure birth asphyxia, what the underlying cellular mechanisms are thought to be and what pathways could explain the considerable association observed with cerebral palsy. Pathways to cerebral palsy from major intrapartum hypoxic events always include immediate neonatal encephalopathy. Although there is considerable aetiological heterogeneity in all parts of the pathway, our challenge is still accurate attribution. It is important to remember that antenatal, as well as intrapartum, causes of brain pathology can give the classic 'birth asphyxia – neonatal encephalopathy – cerebral palsy' sequence. The antenatal antecedents of signs associated with birth asphyxia remain poorly understood.

As infertility treatments have increased the occurrence of multiple births, more pathways to cerebral palsy involving multiples now occur than in 1984, particularly those with triplets and higher orders (Chapter 10). The risks of cerebral palsy are high due to a variety of possible causal pathways including those associated with preterm delivery, low birthweight, and the sharing of placentae, blood supply and a confined space.

Postneonatally acquired cerebral palsy is reviewed in Chapter 11 where we note a worrying increase in 'social' causes of this most preventable group of the cerebral palsies. The impact of vaccination for *Haemophilus influenzae* type b has not yet been seen in registers and sadly may well be offset by an increase in child abuse.

A major revolution in the evaluation of medical care since the 1984 book stimulated Chapters 12 and 13. Chapter 12 attempts to use systematic reviews of the evidence for any antenatal, perinatal or postneonatal intervention influencing the occurrence of cerebral palsy via any of the pathways mentioned in the earlier chapters. Tables 12.7 and 12.8 (p. 155) summarize these interventions and suggest those for which there is good evidence of effectiveness, those which demand more research and those which are not effective in reducing cerebral palsy rates. Such an exercise is as useful to indicate what research needs to be done as to develop guidelines for prevention (see recommendations below). Chapter 13 outlines the practical problems of, and some solutions to, evaluating therapies for children with cerebral palsy.

The future of cerebral palsy research

The importance of cerebral palsy in terms of parental concerns, costs to the community (*Morbidity and Mortality Weekly Review* 1995), and increasingly of expensive and damaging litigation demands a better research response than it has had so far. Despite the problems of working with a heterogeneous group of disorders that represent only a part of the spectrum of adverse perinatal outcomes, we must respond to the challenges outlined in this book. Some interventions, such as those that increase survival, may be so important that a slight increase in cerebral palsy is an acceptable price to pay. But we must recognize the fact that most randomized trials of expensive perinatal interventions have ignored the quality of life of the survivors.

WHERE DO WE GO FROM HERE?

We are excited about the evolution in epidemiology in response to the revolution in bio-medical research. We must acknowledge the enormous complexity of the social, physical and chemical environments in which we live and of the air, water and food we ingest, and the huge variability in individual genetic influences which result in the diverse range of inherent biological and psychosocial responses to these environments (Fig. 14.1). There are a plethora of factors associated with the development of complex diseases like cerebral palsy and other neurodevelopmental problems.

The 'black box' approach to epidemiology in which an exposure is related to an outcome without any obligation to interpolate either intervening factors or even pathogenesis (although many epidemiologists do try) has now been found wanting (McMichael 1994; Koopman 1996; Susser and Susser 1996a,b; Khoury and Yang 1998). Following the fall in infectious disease rates in developed countries, epidemiologists were challenged by epidemics of chronic disease of completely unknown aetiology. This led to the rise in multivariate analysis and more sophisticated handling of individual risk factors. However, these current

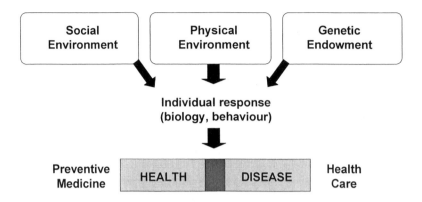

Fig. 14.1. The determinants of health and disease.

epidemiological approaches which identify immediate biological causes have not been overly successful in reducing the incidence of chronic disease nor indeed in stemming the worldwide spread of infections such as HIV. This may be because models that ignore broader contexts are often too simplistic.

ECOLOGICAL AND SOCIAL CONTEXTS IN CAUSAL PATHWAYS

There is now concern that the current epidemiological focus on risk factors and disease outcomes in individuals ignores the ecological and social contexts of the societal or individual behaviours in which such risk factors occur. As we have argued, full knowledge of causal pathways takes into account these early and important stimuli to the sequence and opens up early and more effective strategies (see Table 12.1, p. 139). Epidemiology thus also must link up with the ecological and social context in which data collection and analysis occur, realizing that the overall system in which pathways commence is as crucial to the solution as the underlying biological mechanisms.

EPIDEMIOLOGY IN THE NEW BIOMEDICAL REVOLUTION

There have been several biomedical and technological discoveries in genetics, biochemistry, immunology and radiology which may change epidemiology and medical research for all time. How best can we use these to elucidate causal pathways and interrupt them to avoid complex diseases like cerebral palsy?

Many authors have written about molecular epidemiology (*e.g.* McMichael 1994, Ambrosone and Kadlubar 1997). We believe that there is an exciting future for epidemiologists arising from new techniques in genetics and biomedical science (including imaging) to improve on current methods which use questionnaire, record review or interviews to: (i) measure exposures; (ii) measure the effects of exposures; (iii) measure individual susceptibility; and (iv) identify specific outcomes.

Interest in toxicology and carcinogenesis has resulted in a greater capacity to measure environmental exposures accurately both outside and inside the body. Acknowledging the enormous heterogeneity in response to environmental and pharmaceutical compounds has spawned a whole new approach and capacity to measure individual susceptibility to exposures. We should use these new techniques to identify vulnerable subgroups. For example, there may be genes for poor fetal growth, or metabolic, immunological or placental markers which correlate with responses to asphyxia or infection or the capacity of the fetus to resist or be susceptible to other influences.

Using such techniques may increase our chances of identifying aetiology, as causal pathways will be more obvious in those who are susceptible than in those more resistant to a particular exposure or situation. Tissue changes which indicate exposure or a response to it have been studied extensively in relation to carcinogenesis and may well bear fruit in relation to other exposures such as infections and other teratogens. Imaging techniques that are being developed now show promise in terms of cerebral structures and metabolism. They have already made an enormous difference to how we view brain damage in the very preterm infant (Chapter 7). Identification of underlying biological mechanisms or pathogenesis will be enhanced by such rigorous data, which were often not available to the frustrated epidemiologist of the past. The new genetics, biomedical markers and imaging are starting to offer epidemiologists a window into disease pathogenesis in organs, cells and even molecules.

EPIDEMIOLOGISTS NEED TO COLLABORATE

These are exciting times for epidemiologists but demanding ones too. Truly collaborative studies are required to ensure the best use of these technological advances with cross-training and interdisciplinary groups being developed. As Susser and Susser (1996b) have written, "The potential contribution of these advances to epidemiology is an exquisite refinement of the definition and measurement of susceptibility, exposure, and outcome. Such refinement also clarifies the intervening pathways and so elucidates with precision causal processes and not merely causal factors. We can be confident that new techniques, properly applied, can help dig epidemiology out of the slough of marginally significant risk estimates." What epidemiologists can bring to other disciplines is the excitement of using their science in human populations and putting it to work for the public's health in preventions that are really effective. Nor should the contribution of epidemiology to those sciences be under-estimated. For example, epidemiology brings concepts of sample size and power, confounding, effect modification and gene–environment interactions to the study of genetics to create the relatively new field of genetic epidemiology. This is bringing powerful new methods to identify the genetic factors in complex diseases (such as asthma, heart disease and cancer). These diseases tend to be far more numerous and hence a greater burden to society than the single gene disorders (Khoury and Yang 1998).

TECHNOLOGICAL REVOLUTION IN INFORMATION SYSTEMS

The third arena in which change is upon us is in information systems technology. Not only does this mean that epidemiological, biostatistical and computing scientists bring powerful and sophisticated methods from chronic disease epidemiology to the collaborative table, but large amounts of data on large populations are collectable and readily accessible to many of us all over the world. There is now the capacity for rapid exchange of ideas and of information; international collaborations to share data and to conduct multicentre studies and trials; and record-linked data bases bringing together biological, genetic, epidemiological and social data on large numbers of people. The development of generally accessible electronic data bases of systematic reviews of the effects of medical care, such as the Cochrane data base, can start to change the way we practice and the research we do.

Recommendations for future research
In the face of this information revolution, what should the international community of those committed to researching cerebral palsy (and allied disorders) be contemplating?

NETWORKS OF CEREBRAL PALSY REGISTERS
As most possible causes of the cerebral palsies are individually rare, multicentre studies are needed to be able to identify them. We suggest that the individual groups of researchers in each country who run cerebral palsy registers, or who are interested in the cerebral palsies, should work together to establish collaborative research and monitoring activities.

Long-standing international cooperation between centres conducting research in cerebral palsy has resulted in ongoing benefits. An outstanding example is the 'standard form for recording clinical findings in children with a motor deficit of central origin' (Evans *et al.* 1989), an initiative of UK researchers in the 1980s developed in consultation with the international community as a means of minimizing interobserver variation in the classification of cerebral palsy and now used by many registers. The Little Foundation promoted collaboration by organizing international meetings to discuss such crucial issues as a research definition of birth asphyxia and the future directions in cerebral palsy registers and research. A direct outcome was the collaborative study of cerebral palsy in multiple births involving 11 centres in Australia, UK, Sweden and USA, data from which which are currently being analysed.

Increasing interest in monitoring the occurrence of cerebral palsy is reflected in the growing number of cerebral palsy registers worldwide. Register methodology and sources of differences are being closely scrutinized and discussed (Ens-Dokkum *et al.* 1994, Johnson 1995, Pharoah *et al.* 1997a, Topp *et al.* 1997b, Hutchison and Harpin 1998, Parkes *et al.* 1998a). Consequently, new registers are emerging in the light of wide consultation and with a view to more accurate comparisons and collaborative research.

Another recent development is the collaborative effort between five UK registers to coordinate and develop cerebral palsy research in the UK (Pharoah *et al.* 1997a, Parkes *et al.* 1998b), which is in turn part of a larger programme of Surveillance of Cerebral Palsy in Europe (SCPE) supported by the European Commission. This has been established with the objectives of (1) harmonizing cerebral palsy data collection using a standard definition and an agreed minimum data set; (2) comparing cerebral palsy prevalence rates over time, between populations, and within subgroups, and examining the extent to which variations can be associated with differences in prevalence of risk factors; and (3) providing protocols for future collaborative studies (http://europath.imag.fr). Australia, also, is progressing to national collaboration with the addition of a cerebral palsy register in South Australia which has adopted the same basic methods as the Western Australian Register, including computer software, to further simplify pooling of data. This move to align methodologies between registers will minimize differences in reported rates, and true variations may begin to emerge. Various characteristics and basic rates of existing cerebral palsy data collections, not all of which are ongoing, are shown in the Appendix (pp. 208–211).

Registers which concentrate only on cerebral palsy have some limitations. For example, specific aetiologies or antecedents, such as excessive alcohol intake, intrauterine growth restriction or very preterm birth, can have a variety of outcomes, and the proportions of survivors with developmental problems other than cerebral palsy may be much higher than earlier studies would suggest and are thus of considerable concern. Some registers collect information on a broader group (Johnson *et al.* 1993, Boyle *et al.* 1996), and others are part of a record-linked total population data base of various childhood diseases and conditions (Stanley *et al.* 1997) which enables not only descriptions of the variety of outcomes from various perinatal antecedents but also linkage to all births ensuring accurate and complete denominators.

NETWORKS OF NEONATAL INTENSIVE CARE UNITS/PERINATAL CENTRES
There is an urgent need to ensure that new and existing perinatal interventions are evaluated in relation to the quality of life of the survivors. This is not only to guide cost-effective decision making about the provision of perinatal care but also to help quantify for parents, caregivers and support services for the disabled the load resulting from the increased survival of very preterm infants.

There are several neonatal networks which exist to conduct multicentre trials, to monitor the introduction of technologies and to pool follow-up figures (Donoghue 1997, Wright and Papile 1997, Parry *et al.* 1998). A recent review of the US networks described how such multicentre collaborations with common data and computer systems with their external links to industry, agencies and institutes could provide much better information than any one unit or centre working on its own (Wright and Papile 1997). However, few of the networks are population based and funding is not assured. Figure 14.2 summarizes the breadth of activities, both observational studies and randomized trials, of the US neonatal data bases.

Jerold Lucey went further in a recent editorial in *Pediatrics* entitled 'Neuroprotection and perinatal brain care: The field of the future, currently going nowhere!?" (Lucey 1997), written in response to an article by Vannucci and Perlman (1997) on 'Interventions for perinatal hypoxic–ischaemic encephalopathy'. He alluded to the very successful networks established by the National Cancer Institute which result in 95 per cent of *all* children <18 years of age with cancer in the USA being enrolled in randomized controlled trials. Excellent linkages to basic science laboratories ensures knowledge and technology transfer both to laboratory and from it to clinical research and care. He lists several excellent reasons why such an approach is necessary to overcome the present problems and inertia in the area of brain research. He acknowledged the neonatal networks mentioned above but only to comment on how poorly resourced they were and to suggest that more of us needed to work together. He suggests that now is the time to try to set up a system that would facilitate cooperation between basic neuroscientists, clinical neuroscientists, obstetricians, neonatologists as well as relevant

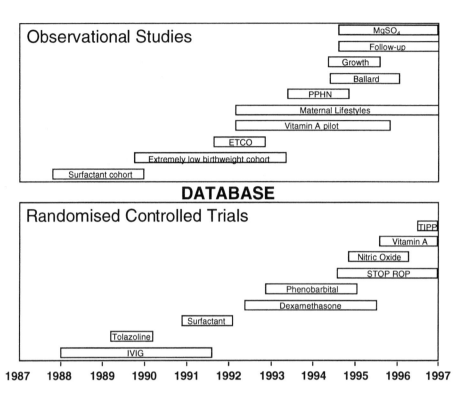

Fig. 14.2. Summary of the large randomized controlled trials and observational studies conducted by the NICHD Neonatal Research Network. (Reproduced by permission from Wright and Papile 1997.) PPHN = persistent pulmonary hypertension of the newborn; ETCO = end-tidal CO concentration to predict jaundice in term infants; TIPP = trial of indomethacin prphylaxis in preterm infants; STOP ROP = supplemental therapeutic oxygen for pre-threshold retinopathy of prematurity.

national institutes and foundations, neonatal networks and industry. He is proposing a large federally funded US programme of coordinated, multidisciplinary research. It will need intellectual and political leadership. We strongly support his statements and although he limits them to asphyxiated infants, the same groups should be interested in all pathways to poor neurological outcomes. He suggests that this should be a US driven activity and again that seems sensible given the recent commitment to increased NIH funding and the relatively greater capacity to raise private funds in the US. Given the costs of long term disabilities such as the cerebral palsies, we can think of no better investment.

ISSUES PERTAINING TO RANDOMIZED TRIALS
It is vital that cerebral palsy (and other neurodevelopmental problems) are included as outcomes in randomized controlled trials of pregnancy and perinatal care by following up subjects well into childhood to an age when cerebral palsy (and other disabilities) can be recognized. Such trials should consider using registers of cerebral palsy to provide a

complete ascertainment of the condition. Randomized trials must be large enough to be able to analyse the effects of the interventions on cerebral palsy. This may need to be done in multicentre studies as suggested above. If enough trials are done which meet these criteria then we recommend also that they be systematically reviewed to summarize the effects of medical and public health care to prevent cerebral palsy and to determine effective management.

The advantages of all these recommendations would include more high quality multi-centre studies including trials of new management strategies which have been neglected in the past (see Chapter 13). Linkages to those working in the Cochrane Collaboration would ensure that the most important trials would be done and that meta-analyses could underpin the development of the most appropriate hypotheses to test in relation to new managements.

We earnestly hope that the coming years will see an exciting acceleration in the progress of cerebral palsy research. This research should explore causal pathways and possibilities for prevention, evaluate therapies, adopt evidence-based practice, and secure a sound knowledge of the prevalence and distribution of cerebral palsy to enable planning for long term needs.

APPENDIX

CEREBRAL PALSY REGISTERS WORLDWIDE, WITH CONTACT DETAILS

REGISTER	CONTACT DETAILS
AUSTRALIA	

(1) Western Australian Cerebral Palsy Register
    PI: Prof. Fiona Stanley
        Dr Eve Blair
    TVW Telethon Institute for Child Health
    PO Box 855
    West Perth, WA 6872
    Australia
	Ms Linda Watson
	Tel: +61 8 9340 8418
	Fax: +61 8 9388 3414
	E-mail: linda@ichr.uwa.edu.au

(2) South Australian Cerebral Palsy Register
    PI: Dr Peter Flett
        Dr Eric Haan
    Women's and Children's Hospital
    72 King William Road
    North Adelaide, SA 5006
    Australia
	Marie Gilbert, Coordinator
	Tel: +61 8 8204 7242
	Fax: +61 8 8204 6088
	E-mail: cpregister@wch.sa.gov.au

(3) Victorian Cerebral Palsy Register
    PI: Dr Dinah Reddihough
        Mrs Lynn Robert
        Ms Janet Walstab
    Dept of Child Development & Rehabilitation
    Royal Children's Hospital
    Flemington Road
    Parkville, VIC 3052
    Australia
	Ms Janet Walstab
	Tel: +61 3 9345 5095
	Fax: +61 3 9345 5871
	E-mail: reddihod@cryptic.rch.unimelb.edu.au

DENMARK	

(4) Cerebral Palsy Register in Eastern Denmark
    PI: Dr Peter Uldall, Child Neurologist
        Dr Monica Topp, Obstetrician
    The Cerebral Palsy Register, DIKE
    Svanemøellevej 25
    DK-2100 Copenhagen
    Denmark
	Dr Monica Topp
	Tel: +45 39 20 7777
	Fax: +45 39 20 8010
	E-mail: mot@dike.dk

FRANCE	

(5) RHEOP (Registre des Handicaps de l'Enfant et
    Observatoire Perinatal)
    PI: Dr Christine Cans
        Dr Pascale Guillem
        Dr Claire Ambrico
    RHEOP
    23 Avenue Albert 1er de Belgique
    38100 Grenoble
    France
	Dr Christine Cans
	Tel: +33 4 76 87 6240 (poste 3111)
	Fax: +33 4 76 46 8106
	E-mail: christine@imag.fr

FRANCE (continued)

(6) Toulouse Population-based CP Survey
    PI: Dr Florence Baille, Epidemiologist
        Dr Hélène Grandjean, Researcher
    INSERM CJF 94 06
    Hôpital La Grave
    31052 Toulouse
    FRANCE

Dr Florence Baille
Tel: +33 5 6177 7808
Fax: +33 5 6159 2483
E-mail: baille@cict.fr

GERMANY

(7) Bilateral Spastic Cerebral Palsy in SW-Germany
    PI: Prof. Ingeborg Krägeloh-Mann
        Prof. Richard Michaelis
    Eberhard Karls University, Pediatric Hospital
    Department of Child Neurology
    Hoppe-Seyler-Straße 1
    D-72076 Tübingen
    or Rümelinstraße 23
        D-72070 Tübingen

Prof. Dr Ingeborg Krägeloh-Mann
Tel: +49 7071-29-84737
Fax: +49 7071-44-0359
E-mail: igkraege@med.uni-tuebingen.de

REPUBLIC OF IRELAND

(8) CRC Cerebral Palsy Register, Eastern Ireland
    PI: Dr Valerie Dowding, Epidemiologist
        Dr Owen Hensey, Medical Director, CRC
    Central Remedial Clinic
    Vernon Avenue
    Clontarf
    Dublin 3
    Ireland

Dr Valerie Dowding
Dr Owen Hensey
Tel: +353 1 833 2206
Fax: +353 1 833 5496

(9) Southern Ireland Cerebral Palsy Register
    PI: Prof. Gerald Cussen, Neonatologist
        Dr Janet Barry, Paediatrician
        Ms Anne Moloney, Clinical Psychologist
        Dr Michael Crowley, Epidemiologist/IT
    Shanakiel House
    Rose Hill
    Sundays Well
    Cork
    Ireland

Prof. Gerald Cussen
Dr Michael Crowley
Tel: +353 21 542052
Fax: +353 21 542055
E-mail: crowleym@tinet.ie

ITALY

(10) Central Italy Cerebral Palsy Register
    PI: (1) Dr M. Giulia Torrioli
    Universita Cattolica S. Cuore
    Via della Pineta Sacchetti, 526
    Rome
    Italy
       (2) Dr Maria Miccli
    Osservatorio Epidemiologico Regione Lazio
    Via de S. Costanza, 53
    00198 – Rome
    Italy

Dr M. Giulia Torrioli
Tel: +39 6 3015 4901
Fax: +39 6 338 3211
E-mail: mc8682@mclink.it

Dr Maria Miccli
Tel: +39 6 5168 6407
Fax: +39 6 5168 6463
Email   matinf@sirio.regione.lazio.it

NORWAY

(11) Cerebral Palsy in the County of Vestfold, Norway
     PI: Dr Alf Meberg
        Dr Harald Broch
     Vestfold Central Hospital
     3117 Tønsberg
     Norway

Dr Alf Meberg
Tel: +47 333 42000
Fax: +47 333 43963

SLOVENIA

(12) National Cerebral Palsy Register
     PI: Prof. Dr Milivoj Velickovic Perat
     University Paediatric Hospital
     Dept of Developmental Neurology
     SI-1525 Ljubljana
     Slovenia

Prof. Dr Milivoj Velickovic Perat
Tel: +386 61 324297
Fax: +386 61 324293
E-mail: milivoj.velickovic@mf.uni-lj.si

SWEDEN

(13) Western Sweden Cerebral Palsy Register
     PI: Prof. Bengt Hagberg
        Dr Gudrun Hagberg
     Department of Pediatrics
     East Hospital
     S-416 85 Göteborg
     Sweden

Prof. Bengt Hagberg
Dr Gudrun Hagberg
Tel: +46 31 37 5168
Fax: +46 31 25 7960
E-mail: hagberg@pediat.gu.se

UK

(14) NE Thames Cerebral Palsy Register
     PI: Prof. Eva Alberman
     Wolfson Institute of Preventive Medicine
     The Medical College
     St Bartholomew's Hospital
     Charterhouse Square
     London EC1 6BQ
     England

Prof. Eva Alberman
Tel: +44 (0)208 340 3122
Fax: +44 (0)208 341 2593
E-mail: kenevalb@compuserve.com

Dr Katrina Williams
E-mail: KatrinaW@nch.edu.au

(15) Oxford Register of Early Childhood Impairments
     PI: Dr Ann Johnson, Medical Coordinator
     National Perinatal Epidemiology Unit
     Radcliffe Infirmary
     Woodstock Road
     Oxford OX2 6HE
     England

Ms Jenny Sayer, Administrative Coordinator
Tel: +44 (0)1865 224 172
Fax: +44 (0)1865 792 270
E-mail: oreci@perinat.ox.ac.uk

(16) Mersey Region Cerebral Palsy Register
     PI: Prof. P.O.D. Pharoah
        Dr M.J. Platt
     Department of Public Health
     Muspratt Building
     University of Liverpool
     Liverpool L69 3GB
     England

Prof. P.O.D. Pharoah
Tel: +44 (0)151 794 5577
Fax: +44 (0)151 794 5272
E-mail: p.o.d.pharoah@liverpool.ac.uk

UK (continued)

(17) North of England Collaborative Cerebral Palsy
Survey

(18) North-East England Retrospective Cerebral Palsy
Survey
PI: Prof. Steve Jarvis
       Dr Allan Colver
Donald Court House
13 Walker Terrace
Gateshead NE8 3EB
England

Prof. Steve Jarvis
Dr Allan Colver
Tel: +44 (0)191 477 6000
Fax: +44 (0)191 477 0370
E-mail: Allan.Colver@ncl.ac.uk

(19) Scottish Register of Children with a Motor Deficit
of Central Origin
PI: Dr James Chalmers
Information and Statistics Division
Trinity Park House
South Trinity Road
Edinburgh EH5 3SQ
Scotland

Dr James Chalmers
Tel: +44 (0)131 551 8662
Fax: +44 (0)131 551 1392
E-mail: Jim.Chalmers@isd.csa.scot.nhs.uk

(20) Northern Ireland Cerebral Palsy Project
PI: Ms Jackie Parkes
       Dr Helen Dolk
       Dr Nan Hill
Mulhouse Building
Institute of Clinical Science
Grosvenor Road
Belfast BT12 6BJ
N. Ireland

Ms Jackie Parkes
Tel: +44 (0)1232 331 463
Fax: +44 (0)1232 320 664
E-mail: j.parkes@qub.ac.uk

USA

(21) California Cerebral Palsy Project
PI: Judith Grether, PhD
California Birth Defects Monitoring Program
1900 Powell Street, Suite 1050
Emeryville
CA 94608
USA

Dr Judith Grether
Tel: +1 510 597 2334
Fax: +1 510 653 1678
E-mail: jgrether@hw1.cahwnet.gov

(22) Metropolitan Atlanta Developmental Disabilities
Surveillance Program
PI: Coleen Boyle, PhD
       Marshalyn Yeargin-Allsopp, MD
Centres for Disease Control and Prevention (CDC)
Mailstop F-15
Atlanta
GA 30334
USA

Dr Coleen Boyle
Tel: +1 770 488 7366
Fax: +1 770 488 7361
E-mail: cab3@cdc.gov

TABLE A.1
Cerebral palsy and low birthweight rates amongst live births in each of the cerebral palsy registers

Register	Study period	Live births/year	CP* rate/1000 live births	CP* rate/1000 neonatal survivors <1500 g	% Postneonatal
(1) Western Australian CP Register	1956– (ongoing)	25,000	2.15 (1975–92)	54.2 (1975–92)	15.7% (1975–92)
(2) South Australian CP Register	1993– (ongoing)	19,000	N/A	N/A	N/A
(3) Victorian CP Register (Dite et al. 1995)	1970– (ongoing)	65,000	1.31[1] (1970–89)	N/A	11.5% (1970–95)
(4) CP Register in East Denmark (Topp et al. 1997c)	1971– (ongoing)	30,000	2.8 (1979–86)	104[2] (1979–86)	Not collected
(5) RHEOP, France	1980– (ongoing)	14,000	Approx. 1.8 (1980–89)	N/A	Approx. 7.4% (1980–89)
(6) Toulouse Population-based CP Survey	1976–1985	11,000	2.1 (1976–85)	N/A	N/A
(7) Bilateral Spastic CP in SW-Germany	1973–1986	17,000	1.2[3] (1975–86)	39.4[3] (1975–86)	Not collected
(8) CRC CP Register, Eastern Ireland (Dowding et al. 1988)	1976– (ongoing)	18–25,000	2.1 (1976–87)[4]	N/A	10.7% (1976–81)
(9) Southern Ireland CP Register	1966– (ongoing)	8–10,000	2.07	105.3[5]	9.1%
(10) Central Italy CP Register	1983– (ongoing)	3,800	N/A	N/A	N/A
(11) CP in County of Vestfold, Norway (Meberg and Broch 1995)	1970– (ongoing)	2,500	2.31 (1970–94)	77.9 (1970–94)	Not collected
(12) National CP Register of Slovenia (Kavcic and Perat 1998)	1988– (ongoing)	28,000	3.0 (1981–90)	57.5 (1987–90)	Not collected
(13) Western Sweden CP Register (Hagberg et al. 1989a,1993, 1996)	1954– (ongoing)	20,000	1.85 (1959–90)	74.6 (1975–90)	6.3% (1979–90)

(14) NE Thames CP Register (Williams et al. 1996)	1980–1986	50,000	1.16 (1985–86)	32.7[6] (1985–86)	5.4% (1985–86)
(15) ORECI, Oxford (Johnson et al. 1998b)	1984– (ongoing)	35,000	2.4 (1984–92)	69.9 (1984–92)	7.3% (1984–92)
(16) Mersey Region CP Register (Pharoah et al. 1990, 1989)	1966– (ongoing)	25–30,000	1.91 (1967–89)	68.4 (1975–89)	18% (1966–77)
(17) N England Collaborative CP Survey	1991– (ongoing)	34,000	2.25 (1991–94)	N/A	2.8% (1991–94)
(18) NE England Retrospective CP Survey	1960–1990	9,000	1.92 (1964–90)	65.0 (1974–93)	N/A
(19) Scottish Register of Central Motor Deficit	1984– (ongoing)	60,000	1.92 (1985–89)	60.9 (1985–89)	6% (1985–89)
(20) Northern Ireland CP Register (Parkes et al. 1998b)	1981– (ongoing)	25–28,000	2.2 (1977–91)	83.7[7] (1987–91)	7.5% (1977–92)
(21) California CP Project (Cummins et al. 1993)	1983–1985	50,000	1.23[8] (1983–85)	51.0[8] (1983–85)	Not collected
(22) Atlanta DD Surveillance Program	1981– (ongoing)	27–39,000	1.79 (1981–90)	52.3[8] (1981–90)	10.5% (1981–90)

N/A = not available.
*Excluding cases due to postneonatal causes.
[1]Moderate and severe spastic cerebral palsy.
[2]<31 week rate per 1000 live births.
[3]Bilateral spastic cerebral palsy.
[4]Includes provisional rate for 1985–87.
[5]<1500 g rate per 1000 7-day survivors.
[6]Rate per 1000 one-year survivors.
[7]<1500 g rate per 1000 live births.
[8]Rate per 1000 three-year survivors.

TABLE A.2
Age limits applied in each of the cerebral palsy registers and availability of comparable population data

Register	Age at complete ascertainment	Age limits for postnatal cases	Minimum age of survival	Availability of population data			
				$LB^1 \times BW^2$	Survivors $\times BW^2$	$LB^1 \times GA^3$	Survivors $\times GA^3$
(1) Western Australian CP Register	5 years	28 days–<5 years	None	1968→	1968→	1980→	1980→
(2) South Australian CP Register	5 years	28 days– (undecided)	None	1993→	1993→	1993→	1993→
(3) Victorian CP Register (Dite et al. 1995)	5 years	1 month–<6 years	None	1982→	1982→	1982→	1982→
(4) CP Register in East Denmark (Topp et al. 1997c)	5 years	Not collected	1 year	1971→	1971→	1979→	1979→
(5) RHEOP, France	7 years	28 days–7 years	2 years	1980→	1980→	N/A	N/A
(6) Toulouse Population-based CP Survey	8 years	28 days–8 years	None	N/A	N/A	N/A	N/A
(7) Bilateral Spastic CP in SW-Germany	5 years	Not collected	2 years	1973→	1973→	N/A	N/A
(8) CRC CP Register, Eastern Ireland (Dowding et al. 1988)	4 years	28 days–<4 years	None	1976–81	N/A	1976–81	N/A
(9) Southern Ireland CP Register	6 years	8 days–3 years	2 years	1984→	1984→	1984→	1984→
(10) Central Italy CP Register	2 years	Birth–5 years	None	1983→	1983→	1983→	1983→
(11) CP in County of Vestfold, Norway (Meberg and Broch 1995)	4 years	Not collected	1 year	1970→	1970→	1970→	1970→
(12) National CP Register of Slovenia (Kavcic and Perat 1998)	3 years	Not routinely collected	1 year	1988→	1988→	1988→	1988→

(13) Western Sweden CP Register (Hagberg et al. 1989a,1993, 1996)	4 years	1 month–<2 years	2 years	1954→	1954→	1973→	1973→
(14) NE Thames CP Register (Williams et al. 1996)	Not relevant	2 months– (not specified)	None	1980–86	1980–86	1984–86	N/A
(15) ORECI, Oxford (Johnson et al. 1998b)	5 years	28 days–2 years	1 year	1984→	1984→	N/A	N/A
(16) Mersey Region CP Register (Pharoah et al. 1990, 1989)	Not specified	28 days–5 years	None	1967→	1967→	N/A	N/A
(17) N England Collaborative CP Survey	5 years	1 month–5 years	None	1991→	1991→	1991→	1991→
(18) NE England Retrospective CP Survey	5 years	1 month–5 years	None	1960→	1960→	1960→	1960→
(19) Scottish Register of Central Motor Deficit	Not specified	Not specified	None	1984→	1984→	1984→	1984→
(20) Northern Ireland CP Register (Parkes et al. 1998b)	5 years	1 month–<5 years	3 years	1987→	N/A	N/A	N/A
(21) California CP Project (Cummins et al. 1993)	Not relevant	Not collected	3 years	1983–85	N/A	N/A	N/A
(22) Atlanta DD Surveillance Program	3 years	>28 days–10 years	3 years	1981→	1981→	1981[4]→	1981[4]→

N/A = not available.

[1]LB = live births.

[2]BW = birthweight.

[3]GA = gestational age at delivery.

[4]From birth certificates—of limited value.

REFERENCES

Ackermann-Liebrich, U., Alberman, E., Moessinger, A., Paneth, N., Reynolds, O., Schneider, H., Stanley, F., Wigglesworth, J. (1996) 'Perinatal epidemiology meeting: The Epidemiology of Cerebral Palsies held in Berne, Switzerland, 14–15 March 1996.' *Paediatric and Perinatal Epidemiology*, **10**, 355–357.

Adamson, S.J., Alessandri, L.M., Badawi, N., Burton, P.R., Pemberton, P.J., Stanley, F. (1995) 'Predictors of neonatal encephalopathy in full term infants.' *British Medical Journal*, **311**, 598–602.

Addor, V., Santos-Eggimann, B., Fawer, C-L., Paccaud, F., Calame, A. (1998) 'Impact of infertility treatments on the health of newborns.' *Fertility and Sterility*, **69**, 210–215.

Adinolfi, M. (1993) 'Infectious diseases in pregnancy, cytokines and neurological impairment: an hypothesis.' *Developmental Medicine and Child Neurology*, **35**, 549–558.

Alberman, E. (1984) 'Describing the cerebral palsies: methods of classifying and counting.' *In:* Stanley, F., Alberman, E. (Eds.) *The Epidemiology of the Cerebral Palsies. Clinics in Developmental Medicine No. 87.* London: Spastics International Medical Publications, pp. 27–31.

—— Creasy, M.R. (1977) 'Frequency of chromosomal abnormalities in miscarriages and perinatal deaths.' *Journal of Medical Genetics*, **14**, 313–315.

—— Benson, J., Kani, W. (1985) 'Disability in survivors of low birthweight.' *Archives of Disease in Childhood*, **60**, 913–919.

Allan, W.C., Vohr, B., Makuch, R.W., Katz, K.H., Ment, L.R. (1997) 'Antecedents of cerebral palsy in a multicenter trial of indomethacin for intraventricular hemorrhage.' *Archives of Pediatrics and Adolescent Medicine*, **151**, 580–585.

Allen, M.C. (1984) 'Developmental outcome and follow up of the small for gestational age infant.' *Seminars in Perinatology*, **8**, 123–156.

—— Amiel-Tison, C., Alexander, G.R. (1998) 'Measurement of gestational age and maturity.' *Prenatal and Fetal Medicine*, **3**, 56–59.

Allen, U.D., Navas, L., King, S.M. (1993) 'Effectiveness of intrapartum penicillin prophylaxis in preventing early onset group B streptococcal infection: results of a meta-analysis.' *Canadian Medical Association Journal*, **149**, 1659–1665.

Al-Rajeh, S., Bademosi, O., Awada, A., Ismail, H., Al-Shammasi, S., Dawodu, A. (1991) 'Cerebral palsy in Saudi Arabia: a case–control study of risk factors.' *Developmental Medicine and Child Neurology*, **33**, 1048–1052.

Ambrosone, C.B., Kadlubar, F.F. (1997) 'Toward an integrated approach to molecular epidemiology.' *American Journal of Epidemiology*, **146**, 912–918.

American College of Obstetrics and Gynecology Committee on Obstetric Practice (1994) 'Utility of umbilical cord blood acid-base assessment. Number 138 – April 1994.' *International Journal of Gynecology and Obstetrics*, **45**, 303–304.

Amiel-Tison, C., Pettigrew, A.G. (1991) 'Adaptive changes in the developing brain during intrauterine stress.' *Brain and Development*, **13**, 67–76.

Amini, S.B., Catalano, P.M., Hirsch, V., Mann, L.I. (1994) 'An analysis of birth weight by gestational age using a computerized perinatal data base, 1975–1992.' *Obstetrics and Gynecology*, **83**, 342–352.

Ananth, C.V., Savits, D.A., Luther, E.R., Bowes, W.A.J. (1997) 'Preeclampsia and preterm birth subtypes in Nova Scotia, 1986 to 1992.' *American Journal of Perinatology*, **14**, 17–23.

Anderson, R.L., Golbus, M.S., Curry, C.J.R., Cullen, P.W., Hastrup, W.H. (1990) 'Central nervous system damage and other anomalies in surviving fetus following second trimester antenatal death of co-twin.' *Prenatal Diagnosis*, **10**, 513–518.

Arens, L.J., Molteno, C.D. (1989) 'A comparative study of postnatally-acquired cerebral palsy in Cape Town.' *Developmental Medicine and Child Neurology*, **31**, 246–254.

Armitage, P. (1994) 'Intraclass correlation.' *In:* Armitage, P., Berry, G. (Eds.) *Statistical Methods in Medical Research, 3rd Edn.* Oxford: Blackwell Scientific, pp. 273–276.

Arnold, A.S., Komattu, A.V., Delp, S.L. (1997) 'Internal rotation gait: a compensatory mechanism to restore abduction capacity decreased by bone deformity?' *Developmental Medicine and Child Neurology*, **39**, 40–44.

Badawi, N., Kurinczuk, J.J., Hall, D., Field, D., Pemberton, P.J., Stanley, F.J. (1997) 'Newborn encephalopathy in term infants: three approaches to population-based investigation.' *Seminars in Neonatology*, **2**, 181–188.

———— Keogh, J.M., Alessandri, L.M., O'Sullivan, F., Burton, P.R., Pemberton, P.J., Stanley, F.J. (1998a) 'Antepartum risk factors for newborn encephalopathy: the results of the Western Australian case control study.' *British Medical Journal*, **317**, 1549–1553.

———— Keogh, J.M., Alessandri, L.M., O'Sullivan, F., Burton, P.R., Pemberton, P.J., Stanley, F.J. (1998b) 'Intrapartum risk factors for newborn encephalopathy: the Western Australian case–control study.' *British Medical Journal*, **317**, 1554–1558.

—— Watson, L., Petterson, B., Blair, E., Slee, J., Haan, E., Stanley, F. (1998c) 'What constitutes cerebral palsy?' *Developmental Medicine and Child Neurology*, **40**, 520–527.

Bairstow, P., Cochrane, R., Hur, J. (1993) *Evaluation of Conductive Education for Children with Cerebral Palsy. Final Report (Parts I and II)*. London: HMSO.

Bale, J.F., Murph, J.R. (1992) 'Congenital infections and the nervous system.' *Pediatric Clinics of North America*, **39**, 669–690.

Baley, J.E., Fanaroff, A.A. (1992a) 'Neonatal infections, Part 1: Infection related to nursery care practices.' *In:* Sinclair, J.C., Bracken, M.B. (Eds.) *Effective Care of the Newborn Infant*. Oxford: Oxford University Press, pp. 454–476.

—— (1992b) 'Neonatal infections, Part 2: Specific infectious diseases and therapies.' *In:* Sinclair, J.C., Bracken, M.B. (Eds.) *Effective Care of the Newborn Infant*. Oxford: Oxford University Press, pp. 477–506.

Bancalari, E., Sinclair, J.C. (1992) 'Mechanical ventilation.' *In:* Sinclair, J.C., Bracken, M.B. (Eds.) *Effective Care of the Newborn Infant*. Oxford: Oxford University Press, pp. 200–220.

Barkovich, A.J., Gressens, P., Evrard, P. (1992) 'Formation, maturation, and disorders of brain neocortex.' *American Journal of Neuroradiology*, **13**, 423–446.

—— Rowley, H., Bollen, A. (1995) 'Correlation of prenatal events with the development of polymicrogyria.' *American Journal of Neuroradiology*, **16**, 822–827.

—— Kuzniecky, R.I., Dobyns, W.B., Jackson, G.D., Becker, L.E., Evrard, P. (1996) 'A classification scheme for malformations of cortical development.' *Neuropediatrics*, **27**, 59–63.

Barth, P.G. (1984) 'Prenatal clastic encephalopathies.' *Clinical Neurology and Neurosurgery*, **86**, 65–75.

—— (1987) 'Disorders of neuronal migration.' *Canadian Journal of Neurological Sciences*, **14**, 1–16.

Bauer, C.R., Morrison, J.C., Poole, W.K., Korones, S.B., Boehm, J.J., Rigatto, H., Zachman, R.D. (1984) 'A decreased incidence of necrotizing enterocolitis after prenatal glucocorticoid therapy.' *Pediatrics*, **73**, 682–688.

Bax, M. (1993) 'Conductive education assessed.' *Developmental Medicine and Child Neurology*, **35**, 659–660. *(Editorial.)*

—— Nelson, K.B. (1993) 'Birth asphyxia: a statement.' *Developmental Medicine and Child Neurology*, **35**, 1022–1024.

Beebe, L.A., Cowan, L.D., Altshuler, G. (1996) 'The epidemiology of placental features: associations with gestational age and neonatal outcome.' *Obstetrics and Gynecology*, **87**, 771–778.

Bekedam, D., Visser, G., de Vries, J., Prechtl, H. (1985) 'Motor behaviour in the growth retarded fetus.' *Early Human Development*, **12**, 155–165.

Bénichou, J., Zupan, V., Fernandez, H., Marpeau, L., Marret, S. (1998) 'Tocolytic magnesium sulphate and paediatric mortality.' *Lancet*, **351**, 290–291. *(Letter.)*

Benirschke, K. (1994) 'Placenta pathology: questions to the perinatologist.' *Journal of Perinatology*, **14**, 371–375.

Bennett, F.C., Scott, D.T. (1997) 'Long term perspective on premature infant outcome and contemporary intervention issues.' *Seminars in Perinatology*, **21**, 190–201.

Berg, A.T. (1988) 'Childhood neurological morbidity and its association with gestational age, intrauterine growth retardation and perinatal stress.' *Paediatric and Perinatal Epidemiology*, **2**, 229–239.

—— (1989) 'Indices of fetal growth-retardatation, perinatal hypoxia-related factors and childhood neurological morbidity.' *Early Human Development*, **19**, 271–283.

Berger, R., Bender, S., Sefkow, S., Klingmueller, V., Kuenzel, W., Jensen, A. (1997) 'Peri/intraventricular haemorrhage: a cranial ultrasound study on 5286 neonates.' *European Journal of Obstetrics, Gynecology, and Reproductive Biology*, **75**, 191–203.

Berkowitz, G.S., Blackmore-Prince, C., Lapinski, R.H., Savitz, D.A. (1998) 'Risk factors for preterm birth subtypes.' *Epidemiology*, **9**, 279–285.

213

Berkowitz, R.L., Stone, J.L., Eddleman, K.A. (1997) 'One hundred consecutive cases of selective termination of an abnormal fetus in a multifetal gestation.' *Obstetrics and Gynecology*, **90**, 606–610.

Bernal, J., Nunez, J. (1995) 'Thyroid hormones and brain development.' *European Journal of Endocrinology*, **133**, 390–398.

Bernstein, P.S., Divon, M.Y. (1997) 'Etiologies of fetal growth restriction.' *Clinical Obstetrics and Gynecology*, **40**, 723–729.

Bessis, R. (1995) 'Ultrasound scanning techniques.' *In:* Keith, L.G., Papiernik, E., Keith, D.M., Luke, B. (Eds.) *Multiple Pregnancy: Epidemiology, Gestation and Perinatal Outcome.* New York: Parthenon, pp. 195–204.

Bhuta, T., Henderson-Smart, D.J. (1998) 'Elective high frequency oscillatory ventilation vs. conventional ventilation in preterm infants with acute pulmonary dysfunction (Cochrane Review).' *In: Cochrane Library. Issue 4.* Oxford: Update Software. (http://www.update-software.com/cochrane.htm)

Black, N. (1996) 'Why we need observational studies to evaluate the effectiveness of health care.' *British Medical Journal*, **312**, 1215–1218.

Blair, E. (1993) 'A research definition for 'birth asphyxia'?' *Developmental Medicine and Child Neurology*, **35**, 449–455.

—— (1994) 'Cerebral palsy and intrapartum care: wrong denominator used.' *British Medical Journal*, **309**, 1229. *(Letter.)*

—— (1996a) 'Model to identify potentially preventable cerebral palsy of intrapartum origin.' *Archives of Disease in Childhood*, **75**, F143. *(Letter.)*

—— (1996b) 'Obstetric antecedents of cerebral palsy.' *Fetal and Maternal Medicine Review*, **8**, 199–215.

—— (1996c) 'The undesirable consequences of controlling for birth weight in perinatal epidemiological studies.' *Journal of Epidemiology and Community Health*, **50**, 559–563.

—— (1996d) 'Why do Aboriginal newborns weigh less? Determinants of birthweight for gestation.' *Journal of Paediatrics and Child Health*, **32**, 498–503.

—— (1999) 'Paediatric implications of IUGR with special reference to cerebral palsy.' *In:* Baker, P., Kingdom, J. (Eds.) *Intra-uterine Growth Restriction.* London: Springer-Verlag. *(In press.)*

—— Stanley, F. (1985) 'Interobserver agreement in the classification of cerebral palsy.' *Developmental Medicine and Child Neurology*, **27**, 615–622.

—— —— (1982) 'An epidemiological study of cerebral palsy in Western Australia, 1956–1975. III: Postnatal aetiology.' *Developmental Medicine and Child Neurology*, **24**, 575–585.

—— —— (1988) 'Intrapartum asphyxia: A rare cause of cerebral palsy.' *Journal of Pediatrics*, **112**, 515–519.

—— —— (1990) 'Intrauterine growth and spastic cerebral palsy. I. Association with birth weight for gestational age.' *American Journal of Obstetrics and Gynecology*, **162**, 229–237.

—— —— (1992) 'Intrauterine growth and spastic cerebral palsy. II. The association with morphology at birth.' *Early Human Development*, **28**, 91–103.

—— —— (1993a) 'Aetiological pathways to spastic cerebral palsy.' *Paediatric and Perinatal Epidemiology*, **7**, 302–317.

—— —— (1993b) 'When can cerebral palsy be prevented? The generation of causal hypotheses by multivariate analysis of a case–control study.' *Paediatric and Perinatal Epidemiology*, **7**, 272–301.

—— —— (1997) 'Issues in the classification and epidemiology of cerebral palsy.' *Mental Retardation and Developmental Disabilities Research Reviews*, **3**, 184–193.

—— Ballantyne, J., Horsman, S., Chauvel, P. (1995) 'A study of a dynamic proximal stability splint in the management of children with cerebral palsy.' *Developmental Medicine and Child Neurology*, **37**, 544–554.

—— Palmer, L., Stanley, F. (1996) 'Cerebral palsy in very low birth weight infants, pre-eclampsia and magnesium sulphate.' *Pediatrics*, **97**, 780–781. *(Letter.)*

Blondel, B., Bréart, G. (1995) 'Home visits during pregnancy: consequences on pregnancy outcome, use of health services and women's situations.' *Seminars in Perinatology*, **19**, 263–271.

Bloom, R.S., Cropley, C. (1994) *Textbook of Neonatal Resuscitation.* Dallas, TX: American Heart Association.

Bohannon, R.W., Smith, M.B. (1987) 'Interrater reliability of a modified Ashworth scale of muscle spasticity.' *Physical Therapy*, **67**, 206–207.

Bomsel-Helmreich, O., Al Mufti, W. (1995) 'The mechanism of monozygosity and double ovulation.' *In:* Keith, L.G., Papiernik, E., Keith, D., Luke, B. (Eds.) *Multiple Pregnancy: Epidemiology, Gestation and Perinatal Outcome.* New York: Parthenon, pp. 25–40.

Bower, C., Condon, R., Payne, J., Burton, P., Watson, C., Wild, B. (1998) 'Measuring the impact of conjugate vaccines on invasive *Haemophilus influenzae* type b infection in Western Australia.' *Australian and New Zealand Journal of Public Health*, **22**, 67–72.

Bower, E., McLellan, D.L., Arney, J., Campbell, M.J. (1996) 'A randomised controlled trial of different intensities of physiotherapy and different goal-setting procedures in 44 children with cerebral palsy.' *Developmental Medicine and Child Neurology*, **38**, 226–237.

Boyle, C.A., Yeargin-Allsopp, M., Doernberg, N.S., Holmgreen, P., Murphy, C.C., Schendel, D.E. (1996) 'Prevalence of selected developmental disabilities in children 3–10 years of age: the Metropolitan Atlanta Developmental Disabilities Surveillance Program, 1991.' *Morbidity and Mortality Weekly Report*, **45** (SS-2), 1–14.

Bozynski, M.E., Nelson, M.N., Matalon, T.A., Genaze, D.R., Rosati-Skertich, C., Naughton, P.M., Meier, W.A. (1985) 'Cavitary periventricular leukomalacia: incidence and short-term outcome in infants weighing less than or equal to 1200 grams at birth.' *Developmental Medicine and Child Neurology*, **27**, 572–577.

Breart, G., Blondel, B., Tuppin, P., Grandjean, H., Kaminski, M. (1995) 'Did preterm deliveries continue to decrease in France in the 1980s?' *Paediatric and Perinatal Epidemiology*, **9**, 296–306.

Bruce, I.C., Rawson, J.A. (1994) 'Development of motor functions in the fetus.' *In:* Thorburn, G.D., Harding, R. (Eds.) *Textbook of Fetal Physiology.* Oxford: Oxford University Press, pp. 301–309.

Bundey, S. (1997) 'Prevalence and type of cerebral palsy.' *Developmental Medicine and Child Neurology*, **39**, 568. *(Letter.)*

Burke, C.J., Tannenberg, A.E., Payton, D.J. (1997) 'Ischaemic cerebral injury, growth retardation, and placental infarction.' *Developmental Medicine and Child Neurology*, **39**, 726–730.

Burn, J. (1995) 'The spectrum of genetic disorders in twins.' *In:* Ward, H., Whittle, M. (Eds.) *Multiple Pregnancy.* London: RCOG Press, pp. 74–82.

Burton, P.R., Gurrin, L.C., Hussey, M.H. (1997) 'Interpreting the clinical trials of extracorporeal membrane oxygenation in the treatment of persistent pulmonary hypertension of the newborn.' *Seminars in Neonatology*, **2**, 69–79.

Butler, C. (1995) 'Outcomes that matter.' *Developmental Medicine and Child Neurology*, **37**, 753–754.

Callahan, T.L., Hall, J.E., Ettner, S.L., Christiansen, C.L., Greene, M.F., Crowley, W.F.J. (1994) 'The economic impact of multiple-gestation pregnancies and the contribution of assisted-reproduction techniques to their incidence.' *New England Journal of Medicine*, **331**, 244–249.

Calvert, S.A., Hoskins, E.M., Fong, K.W., Forsyth, S.C. (1987) 'Etiological factors associated with the development of periventricular leukomalacia.' *Acta Paediatrica Scandinavica*, **76**, 254–259.

Campbell, S.K. (1996) 'Quantifying the effects of interventions for movement disorders resulting from cerebral palsy.' *Journal of Child Neurology*, **11**, S61–S70.

Carr, L.J. (1996) 'Development and reorganization of descending motor pathways in children with hemiplegic cerebral palsy.' *Acta Paediatrica*, **85** (Suppl. 416), 53–57.

Carr, L.J., Harrison, L.M., Evans, A.L., Stephens, J.A. (1993) 'Patterns of central motor reorganization in hemiplegic cerebral palsy.' *Brain*, **116**, 1223–1247.

Carroli, G., Belizan, J., Stamp, G. (1998) 'Episiotomy policies in vaginal births (Cochrane Review).' *In: Cochrane Library. Issue 4.* Oxford: Update Software. (http://www.update-software.com/cochrane.htm)

Ceesay, S.M., Prentice, A.M., Cole, T.J., Foord, F., Weaver, L.T., Poskitt, E.M.E., Whitehead, R.G. (1997) 'Effects on birth weight and perinatal mortality of maternal dietary supplements in rural Gambia: 5 year randomised controlled trial.' *British Medical Journal*, **315**, 786–790.

Centers for Disease Control (1997) 'Rubella and congenital rubella syndrome – United States, 1994–1997.' *Morbidity and Mortality Weekly Report*, **46**, 350–354.

—— (1998) 'Measles, mumps, and rubella – vaccine use and strategies for elimination of measles, rubella, and congenital rubella syndrome and control of mumps: Recommendations of the Advisory Committee on Immunization Practices (ACIP).' *Morbidity and Mortality Weekly Report*, **47** (RR-8), 1–57.

Chalmers, I. (1989) 'Inquiry into stillbirths and infant deaths.' *British Medical Journal*, **299**, 339–340.

—— Enkin, M., Keirse, M.J.N.C. (Eds.) (1989) *Effective Care in Pregnancy and Childbirth. Vol. I: Pregnancy, Parts I–V.* Oxford: Oxford University Press.

Chang, G.Y., Leuder, F.L., Di Michele, D.M., Radkowski, M.A., McWilliams, L.J., Jansen, R.D. (1997) 'Heparin and the risk of intraventricular hemorrhage in premature infants.' *Journal of Pediatrics*, **131**, 362–366.

Chien, P.F.W., Khan, K.S., Arnott, N. (1996) 'Magnesium sulphate in the treatment of eclampsia and pre-eclampsia: an overview of the evidence from randomised trials.' *British Journal of Obstetrics and Gynaecology*, **103**, 1085–1091.

Chiswick, M.L. (1986) 'Commentary on current World Health Organization definitions used in perinatal statistics.' *British Journal of Obstetrics and Gynaecology*, **93**, 1236–1238.

Cincotta, R., Oldham, J., Sampson, A. (1996) 'Antepartum and postpartum complications of twin–twin transfusion.' *Australian and New Zealand Journal of Obstetrics and Gynaecology*, **36**, 303–308.

Clarke, C.A., Donohoe, W.T.A., McConnell, J.C., Finn, R., Krevans, J.R., Kulke, W., Lehane, D., Sheppard, P.M. (1963) 'Future experimental studies on the prevention of Rh haemolytic disease.' *British Medical Journal*, **2**, 979–984.

Clarren, S.K., Alvord, E.C., Sumi, S.M., Streissguth, A.P., Smith, D.W. (1978) 'Brain malformations related to prenatal exposure to ethanol.' *Journal of Pediatrics*, **92**, 64–67.

Cochrane, A.L. (1979) *A Critical Review with Particular Reference to the Medical Profession. Medicines for the Year 2000.* London: Office of Health Economics.

Cochrane Collaboration (1997) *Cochrane Collaboration Brochure.* Oxford: Cochrane Collaboration.

—— (1998) *Cochrane Pregnancy and Childbirth Data Base.* Oxford: Cochrane Collaboration.

—— (1998) *Review Manager (Revman). Version 3.1 for Windows.* Oxford: The Cochrane Collaboration. *(Computer program.)*

Coetzee, E.J., Dommisse, J., Anthony, J. (1998) 'A randomised controlled trial of intravenous magnesium sulphate versus placebo in the management of women with severe pre-eclampsia.' *British Journal of Obstetrics and Gynaecology*, **105**, 300–303.

Collins, M., Paneth, N. (1998) 'Pre-eclampsia and cerebral palsy: are they related?' *Developmental Medicine and Child Neurology*, **40**, 207–211.

Cooke, R.W. (1987) 'Early and late cranial ultrasonographic appearances and outcome in very low birthweight infants.' *Archives of Disease in Childhood*, **62**, 931–937.

—— (1990) 'Cerebral palsy in very low birthweight infants.' *Archives of Disease in Childhood*, **65**, 201–206.

—— (1994) 'Survival and cerebral palsy morbidity in preterm infants.' *Lancet*, **343**, 1578. *(Letter.)*

Coorssen, E.A., Msall, M.E., Duffy, L.C. (1991) 'Multiple minor malformations as a marker for prenatal etiology of cerebral palsy.' *Developmental Medicine and Child Neurology*, **33**, 730–736.

Cosgrove, A.P., Graham, H.K. (1994) 'Botulinum toxin A prevents the development of contractures in the hereditary spastic mouse.' *Developmental Medicine and Child Neurology*, **36**, 379–385.

Cowan, L.D., Hudson, L.S. (1991) 'The epidemiology and natural history of infantile spasms.' *Journal of Child Neurology*, **6**, 355–364.

Crichton, J.U., Mackinnon, M., White, C.P. (1995) 'The life-expectancy of persons with cerebral palsy.' *Developmental Medicine and Child Neurology*, **37**, 567–576.

Crowley, P. (1989) 'Promoting pulmonary maturity.' *In:* Chalmers, I., Enkin, M., Keirse, M.J.N.C. (Eds.) *Effective Care in Pregnancy and Childbirth. Vol. 1: Pregnancy, Parts I–V.* Oxford: Oxford University Press, pp. 746–764.

—— (1998) 'Corticosteroids prior to preterm delivery (Cochrane Review).' *In: Cochrane Library. Issue 4.* Oxford: Update Software. (http://www.update-software.com/cochrane.htm)

Crowther, C.A., Moore, V. (1998) 'Magnesium maintenance therapy after threatened preterm labour for prevention of preterm birth (Cochrane Review).' *In: Cochrane Library. Issue 4.* Oxford: Update Software. (http://www.update-software.com/cochrane.htm)

—— Hiller, J.E., Haslam, R.R., Robinson, J.S., Giles, W., Gill, A., Walters, W., Rowley, M., Evans, C., *et al.* (1997) 'Australian Collaborative Trial of Antenatal Thyrotropin-Releasing Hormone: Adverse effects at 12-month follow-up.' *Pediatrics*, **99**, 311–317.

—— Alfirevic, Z., Haslam, R.R. (1998a) 'Antenatal thyrotropin-releasing hormone (TRH) prior to preterm delivery (Cochrane Review).' *In: Cochrane Library. Issue 4.* Oxford: Update Software. (http://www.update-software.com/cochrane.htm)

—— Hiller, J., Doyle, L., Lumley, J., Carlin, J. (1998b) 'Tocolytic magnesium sulphate and paediatric mortality.' *Lancet*, **351**, 291. *(Letter.)*

Cummins, S.K., Nelson, K.B., Grether, J.K., Velle, E.M. (1993) 'Cerebral palsy in four northern California counties, births 1983 through 1985.' *Journal of Pediatrics*, **123**, 230–237.

Dammann, O., Leviton, A. (1997a) 'Does prepregnancy bacterial vaginosis increase a mother's risk of having a preterm infant with cerebral palsy?' *Developmental Medicine and Child Neurology*, **39**, 836–840.

—— —— (1997b) 'Maternal intrauterine infection, cytokines, and brain damage in the preterm newborn.' *Pediatric Research*, **42**, 1–8.

—— —— Du, E. (1997) 'The role of perinatal brain damage in developmental disabilities – an epidemiologic perspective.' *Mental Retardation and Developmental Disabilities Research Reviews*, **3**, 13–21.

216

Darling, M. (1998) 'Low-dose aspirin not for pre-eclampsia.' *Lancet*, **352**, 342.

Debus, O., Koch, H.G., Kurlemann, G., Strater, R., Vielhaber, H., Weber, P., Nowak-Gottl, U. (1998) 'Factor V Leiden and genetic defects of thrombophilia in childhood porencephaly.' *Archives of Disease in Childhood*, **78**, F121–F124.

Decker, B.R., Foss, J.J. (1997) 'Pediatrics: Assessment of specific functions.' *In:* Van Deusen, J., Brunt, D. (Eds.) *Assessment in Occupational Therapy and Physical Therapy*. Philadelphia: W.B. Saunders, pp. 375–400.

Delgado-Rodríguez, M., Gomez-Olmedo, M., Bueno-Cavanillas, A., García-Martín, M., Gálvez-Vargas, R. (1995) 'Recall bias in a case–control study of low birth weight.' *Journal of Clinical Epidemiology*, **48**, 1133–1140.

De Lia, L.E., Kulmann, R.S., Harstad, T.W. (1995) 'Fetoscopic laser ablation of placental vessels in severe previable twin–twin transfusion syndrome.' *American Journal of Obstetrics and Gynecology*, **172**, 1202–1211.

DeLong, G.R. (1993) 'Effect of nutrition on brain development in humans.' *American Journal of Clinical Nutrition*, **57**, 286S–290S.

—— Robbins, J., Condliffe, P.G. (1989) 'Iodine and the brain.' *In: Proceedings of the International Conference on Iodine and the Brain, Bethesda, Maryland, March 21–23, 1988*. New York: Plenum.

DeLong, R. (1987) 'Neurological involvement in iodine deficiency disorders.' *In:* Hetzel, B.S., Dunn, J.T., Stanbury, J.B. (Eds.) *The Prevention and Control of Iodine Deficiency Disorder*. Amsterdam: Elsevier, pp. 49–63.

den Ouden, L., van de Bor, M., van Bel, F., Janssen, H., Brand, R., Ruys, J.H. (1990) 'Serum CK-BB activity in the preterm infant and outcome at two and four years of age.' *Developmental Medicine and Child Neurology*, **32**, 509–514.

de Onis, M., Villar, J., Gülmerzoglu, M. (1998) 'Nutritional interventions to prevent intrauterine growth retardation: evidence from randomized controlled trials.' *European Journal of Clinical Nutrition*, **52**, Suppl. 1, S83–S93.

D'Ercole, C., Girard, N., Cravello, L., Boubli, L., Potier, A., Raybaud, C., Blanc, B. (1998) 'Prenatal diagnosis of fetal corpus callosum agenesis by ultrasound and magnetic resonance imaging.' *Prenatal Diagnosis*, *18*, 247–253.

Derom, C., Derom, R., Vlietinck, R. (1987) 'Increased monozygotic twinning rate after ovulation induction.' *Lancet*, **1**, 1236.

Derom, R., Orlebeke, J., Eriksson, A., Thierry, M. (1995) 'The epidemiology of multiple births in Europe.' *In:* Keith, L.G., Papiernik, E., Keith, D.M., Luke, B. (Eds.) *Multiple Pregnancy: Epidemiology, Gestation and Perinatal Outcome*. New York: Parthenon, pp. 145–162.

de Vries, L.S., Dubowitz, L.M., Dubowitz, V., Kaiser, A., Lary, S., Silverman, M., Whitelaw, A., Wigglesworth, J.S. (1985) 'Predictive value of cranial ultrasound in the newborn baby: a reappraisal.' *Lancet*, **2**, 137–140.

—— Eken, P., Groenendaal, F., van Haastert, I.C., Meiners, L.C. (1993) 'Correlation between degree of periventricular leukomalacia diagnosed using cranial ultrasound and MRI later in infancy in children with cerebral palsy.' *Neuropediatrics*, **24**, 263–268.

—— Groenendaal, F., Eken, P., van Haastert, I.C., Rademaker, K.J., Meiners, L.C. (1997) 'Infarcts in the vascular distribution of the middle cerebral artery in preterm and fullterm infants.' *Neuropediatrics*, **28**, 88–96.

—— Eken, P., Groenendaal, F., Rademaker, K.J., Hoogervorst, B., Bruinse, H.W. (1998a) 'Antenatal onset of haemorrhagic and/or ischaemic lesions in preterm infants: prevalence and associated obstetric variables.' *Archives of Disease in Childhood*, **78**, F51–F56.

—— Rademaker, K.J., van Haastert, I.C., Vandertop, W.P., Gooskens, R., Meiners, L.C. (1998b) 'Correlation between neonatal cranial ultrasound, MRI in infancy and outcome in infants with a large haemorrhage with or without unilateral parenchymal involvement.' *Neuropediatrics*, **29**, 180–188.

DiGiacomo, J.E., Hay, W.W.J. (1992) 'Abnormal glucose homeostasis.' *In:* Sinclair, J.C., Bracken, M.B. (Eds.) *Effective Care of the Newborn Infant*. Oxford: Oxford University Press, pp. 590–601.

Dijxhoorn, M.J., Visser, G.H.A., Touwen, B.C.L., Huisjes, H.J. (1987) 'Apgar score, meconium and acidaemia at birth in small-for-gestational age infants born at term and their relation to neonatal neurological morbidity.' *British Journal of Obstetrics and Gynaecology*, **94**, 873–879.

Di Renzo, G., Romero, R., Cockburn, F. (Eds.) (1998) *Prenatal and Neonatal Medicine*. Carnforth, Lancs: Parthenon.

Dite, G.S., Reddihough, D.S., Robert, L.A. (1995) *Second Report of the Victorian Cerebral Palsy Register*. Parkville, Victoria: Department of Child Development and Rehabilitation.

217

Dobyns, W.B., Elias, E.R., Newlin, A.C., Pagon, R.A., Ledbetter, D.H. (1992) 'Causal heterogeneity in isolated lissencephaly.' *Neurology*, **42**, 1375–1388.

—— Andermann, E., Andermann, F., Czapansky-Beilman, D., Dubeau, F., Dulac, O., Guerrini, R., Hirsh, B., Ledbetter, D.H., *et al.* (1996) 'X-linked malformations of neuronal migration.' *Neurology*, **47**, 331–339.

Dolk, H., Parkes, K., Hill, A.E. (1996) 'Cerebral palsy prevalence in relation to socio-economic deprivation in Northern Ireland.' *Paediatric and Perinatal Epidemiology*, **10**, A4. *(Abstract.)*

Donoghue, D.A. (1997) *Australian and New Zealand Neonatal Network, 1995.* Sydney: Australian Institute of Health and Welfare, National Perinatal Statistics Unit.

Dowding, V.M., Barry, C. (1988) 'Cerebral palsy: changing patterns of birthweight and gestational age (1976/81).' *Irish Medical Journal*, **81**, 25–29.

—— —— (1990) 'Cerebral palsy: social class differences in prevalence in relation to birthweight and severity of disability.' *Journal of Epidemiology and Community Health*, **44**, 191–195.

Duc, G., Sinclair, J.C. (1992) 'Oxygen administration.' *In:* Sinclair, J.C., Bracken, M.B. (Eds.) *Effective Care of the Newborn Infant.* Oxford: Oxford University Press, pp. 178–199.

Duggan, M.B., Ogala, W. (1982) 'Cerebral palsy in Nigeria—a report from Zaria.' *Annals of Tropical Paediatrics*, **2**, 7–11.

Duley, L., Gülmezoglu, A.M., Henderson-Smart, D.J. (1998) 'Anticonvulsants for women with pre-eclampsia (Cochrane Review).' *In: Cochrane Library. Issue 4.* Oxford: Update Software. (http://www.update-software.com/cochrane.htm)

Dunn, A., Macfarlane, A. (1996) 'Recent trends in the incidence of multiple births and associated mortality in England and Wales.' *Archives of Disease in Childhood*, **75**, F10–F19.

du Plessis, A.J., Johnston, M.V. (1997) 'Hypoxic–ischemic brain injury in the newborn – Cellular mechanisms and potential strategies for neuroprotection.' *Clinics in Perinatology*, **24**, 627–654.

Dwyer, T., Ponsonby, A-L.B., Newman, N.M., Gibbons, L.E. (1991) 'Prospective cohort study of prone sleeping position and sudden infant death syndrome.' *Lancet*, **337**, 1244–1247.

—— —— Blizzard, L., Newman, N.M., Cochrane, J.A. (1995) 'The contribution of changes in the prevalence of prone sleeping position to the decline in sudden infant death syndrome in Tasmania.' *Journal of the American Medical Association*, **273**, 783–789.

Dyer, S. (1997) 'Appropriate intervention – treating cerebral palsy in Zambia.' *Appropriate Technology*, **23**, 21–24.

Edwards, A.D., Mehmet, H. (1996) 'Apoptosis in perinatal hypoxic–ischaemic cerebral damage.' *Neuropathology and Applied Neurobiology*, **22**, 494–498.

—— Wyatt, J.S., Thoresen, M. (1998) 'Treatment of hypoxic–ischaemic brain damage by moderate hypothermia.' *Archives of Disease in Childhood*, **78**, F85–F91.

Eken, P., de Vries, L.S., van der Graaf, Y., Meiners, L.C., van Nieuwenhuizen, O. (1995) 'Haemorrhagic–ischaemic lesions of the neonatal brain: correlation between cerebral visual impairment, neurodevelopmental outcome and MRI in infancy.' *Developmental Medicine and Child Neurology*, **37**, 41–55.

Ellenberg, J.H., Nelson, K.B. (1979) 'Birth weight and gestational age in children with cerebral palsy or seizure disorders.' *American Journal of Diseases of Children*, **133**, 1044–1048.

—— —— (1988) 'Cluster of perinatal events identifying infants at high risk for death or disability.' *Journal of Pediatrics*, **113**, 546–552.

Ellis, M.I. (1980) 'Follow-up study of survivors after intra-uterine transfusion.' *Developmental Medicine and Child Neurology*, **22**, 48–54.

Ellis, R.F., Berger, G.S., Keith, L., Depp, R. (1979) 'The Northwestern University Multihospital Twin Study. II. Mortality of first versus second twins.' *Acta Geneticae Medicae et Gemellologiae*, **28**, 347–352.

Emond, A., Golding, J., Peckham, C. (1989) 'Cerebral palsy in two national cohorts.' *Archives of Disease in Childhood*, **64**, 848–852.

Encha-Razavi, F. (1995) 'Fetal neuropathology.' *In:* Duckett, S. (Ed.) *Pediatric Neuropathology.* Baltimore: Williams & Wilkins, pp. 108–122.

Ens-Dokkum, M., Johnson, A., Schreuder, A.M., Veen, S., Wilkinson, A.R., Brand, R., Ruys, J.H., Verloove-Vanhorick, S.P. (1994) 'Comparison of mortality and rates of cerebral palsy in two populations of very low birthweight infants.' *Archives of Disease in Childhood*, **70**, F96–F100.

Ergander, U., Eriksson, M., Zetterstrom, R. (1983) 'Severe neonatal asphyxia.' *Acta Paediatrica Scandinavica*, **72**, 321–325.

Ernst, E. (1995) 'What is wrong with anecdotal evidence?' *Physical Medicine and Rehabilitation*, **5**, 145–146.

Eronen, M., Pesonen, E., Kurki, T., Ylikorkala, O., Hallman, M. (1994) 'Increased incidence of bronchopulmonary dysplasia after antenatal administration of indomethacin to prevent preterm labor.' *Journal of Pediatrics*, **124**, 782–788.

Eschenbach, D.A. (1997) 'Amniotic fluid infection and cerebral palsy: Focus on the fetus.' *Journal of the American Medical Association*, **278**, 247–248.

Escobar, G.J., Littenberg, B., Petitti, D.B. (1991) 'Outcome among among surviving very low birthweight infants: a meta-analysis.' *Archives of Disease in Childhood*, **66**, 204–211.

Evans, P.M., Alberman, E. (1985) 'Recording motor defects of children with cerebral palsy.' *Developmental Medicine and Child Neurology*, **27**, 404–406.

—— Elliot, M., Alberman, E., Evans, S. (1985) 'Prevalence and disabilities in 4 to 8 year olds with cerebral palsy.' *Archives of Disease in Childhood*, **60**, 940–945.

—— Johnson, A., Mutch, L., Alberman, E. (1986) 'Report of a meeting on the Standardisation of the Recording and Reporting of Cerebral Palsy.' *Developmental Medicine and Child Neurology*, **28**, 547–548.

—— —— —— —— (1989) 'A standard form for recording clinical findings in children with a motor deficit of central origin.' *Developmental Medicine and Child Neurology*, **31**, 117–129.

Evrard, P., Marret, S., Gressens, P. (1997) 'Environmental and genetic determinants of neural migration and postmigratory survival.' *Acta Paediatrica*, **86**, Suppl. 422, 20–26.

Ewigman, B.G., Crane, J.P., Frigoletto, F.D., LeFevre, M.L., Bain, R.P., McNellis, D., RADIUS Study Group (1993) 'Effect of prenatal ultrasound screening on perinatal outcome.' *New England Journal of Medicine*, **329**, 821–827.

Fawer, C.L., Diebold, P., Calame, A. (1987) 'Periventricular leucomalacia and neurodevelopmental outcome in preterm infants.' *Archives of Disease in Childhood*, **62**, 30–36.

Fenichel, G.M. (1983) 'Hypoxic–ischemic encephalopathy in the newborn.' *Archives of Neurology*, **40**, 261–266.

Ferrari, F., Cioni, G., Prechtl, H.F.R. (1990) 'Qualitative changes of general movements in preterm infants with brain lesions.' *Early Human Development*, **23**, 193–231.

Fetter, L. (1991) 'Measurement and treatment in cerebral palsy. An argument for a new approach.' *Physical Therapy*, **71**, 244–247.

Finer, N.N., Robertson, C.M., Richards, R.T., Pinnell, L.E., Peters, K.L. (1981) 'Hypoxic–ischemic encephalopathy in term neonates: Perinatal factors and outcome.' *Journal of Pediatrics*, **98**, 112–117.

Fitzhardinge, P.M., Steven, E.M. (1972) 'The small-for-date infant. I. Later growth patterns.' *Pediatrics*, **49**, 671–681.

Fletcher, N.A., Foley, J. (1993) 'Parental age, genetic mutation, and cerebral palsy.' *Journal of Medical Genetics*, **30**, 44–46.

Fooks, J., Mutch, L., Yudkin, P., Johnson, A., Elbourne, D. (1997) 'Comparing two methods of follow up in a multicentre randomised trial.' *Archives of Disease in Childhood*, **76**, 369–376.

Forssberg, H., Tedroff, K.B. (1997) 'Botulinum toxin treatment in cerebral palsy: intervention with poor evaluation.' *Developmental Medicine and Child Neurology*, **39**, 635–640.

Foulon, W., Van Liedekerke, D., Demanet, C., Decatte, L., Dewaele, M., Naessens, A. (1995) 'Markers of infection and their relationship to preterm delivery.' *American Journal of Perinatology*, **12**, 208–211.

Fowler, K.B., Pass, R.F. (1991) 'Sexually transmitted diseases in mother of neonates with congenital cytomegalovirus infection.' *Journal of Infectious Diseases*, **164**, 259–264.

Freda, V.J., Gorman, J.G., Pollack, W. (1964) 'Successful prevention of experimental Rh sensitization in man with an anti-Rh gamma-2-globulin antibody preparation: a preliminary report.' *Transfusion*, **4**, 26–32.

Freeman, J.M., Freeman, A.D. (1992) 'Cerebral palsy and the 'bad baby' malpractice crisis: New York State shines light toward the end of the tunnel.' *American Journal of Diseases of Children*, **146**, 725–727.

Freeman, R. (1990) 'Intrapartum fetal monitoring – a disappointing story.' *New England Journal of Medicine*, **322**, 624–626.

French, N.P., Hagan, R., Evans, S., Benninger, H., Mullan, A., Snowball, L., Palmer, L. (1996) 'A geographic outcome study: Disabilities below 33 weeks gestation.' *Pediatric Research*, **39**, A1572.

Fujikura, T., Froehlich, L.A. (1974) 'Mental and motor development in monozygotic co-twins with dissimilar birth weights.' *Pediatrics*, **53**, 884–889.

Fusi, L., McParland, P., Fisk, N., Wigglesworth, J. (1991) 'Acute twin–twin transfusion: A possible mechanism for brain-damaged survivors after intrauterine death of a monochorionic twin.' *Obstetrics and Gynecology*, **78**, 517–520.

Gaffney, G., Sellers, S., Flavell, V., Squier, M., Johnson, A. (1994a) 'Case–control study of intrapartum care, cerebral palsy, and perinatal death.' *British Medical Journal*, **308**, 743–750.

—— Squier, M., Johnson, A., Flavell, V., Sellers, S. (1994b) 'Clinical associations of prenatal ischaemic white matter injury.' *Archives of Disease in Childhood*, **70**, F101–F106.

Gardosi, J., Chang, A., Kalyan, B., Sahota, D., Symonds, E.M. (1992) 'Customised antenatal growth charts.' *Lancet*, **339**, 283–287.

Geva, E., Lerner-Geva, L., Stavorovsky, Z., Modan, B., Freedman, L., Amit, A., Yovel, I., Lessing, J.B. (1998) 'Multifetal pregnancy reduction: a possible risk factor for periventricular leukomalacia in premature newborns.' *Fertility and Sterility*, **69**, 845–850.

Gibbs, J.M., Weindling, A.M. (1994) 'Neonatal intracranial lesions following placental abruption.' *European Journal of Pediatrics*, **153**, 195–197.

Gilbert, G.L. (1996) 'Congenital fetal infections.' *Seminars in Neonatology*, **1**, 91–105.

Ginsberg, H.G., Goldsmith, J.P. (1998) 'Controversies in neonatal resuscitation.' *Clinics in Perinatology*, **25**, 1–15.

Glass, P., Bulas, D.I., Wagner, A.E., Rajasingham, S.R., Civitello, L.A., Papero, P.H., Coffman, C.E., Short, B.L. (1997) 'Severity of brain injury following neonatal extracorporeal membrane oxygenation and outcome at age 5 years.' *Developmental Medicine and Child Neurology*, **39**, 441–448.

Gluckman, P.D. (1997) 'Endocrine and nutritional regulation of prenatal growth.' *Acta Paediatrica*, Suppl. 423, 153–157.

—— Williams, C. E. (1992) 'When and why do brain cells die?' *Developmental Medicine and Child Neurology*, **34**, 1010–1014.

Godfrey, K.M. (1998) 'Maternal regulation of fetal development and health in adult life.' *European Journal of Obstetrics, Gynecology, and Reproductive Biology*, **78**, 141–150.

Goldenberg, R.L., Andrews, W.W. (1996) 'Intrauterine infection and why preterm prevention programs have failed.' *American Journal of Public Health*, **86**, 781–783. *(Editorial.)*

Golding, J., Paterson, M., Kinlen, L.J. (1990) 'Factors associated with childhood cancer in a national cohort study.' *British Journal of Cancer*, **62**, 304–308.

—— Greenwood, R., Birmingham, K., Mott, M. (1992) 'Childhood cancer, intramuscular vitamin K, and pethidine given during labour.' *British Medical Journal*, **305**, 341–346.

Goodlin, R.C. (1996) 'Determining the time before birth when ischemia and hypoxemia initiated cerebral palsy.' *Obstetrics and Gynecology*, **87**, 477–478. *(Letter.)*

Govaert, P., de Vries, L.S. (1997) 'Pathology: antenatal brain damage.' *In: An Atlas of Neonatal Brain Sonography. Clinics in Developmental Medicine No. 141/142.* London: Mac Keith Press, pp. 109–163.

Graham, M., Levene, M.I., Trounce, J.Q., Rutter, N. (1987) 'Prediction of cerebral palsy in very low birth-weight infants: prospective ultrasound study.' *Lancet*, **2**, 593–596.

Grant, A. (1998) 'Elective versus selective Caesarean delivery of the small baby (Cochrane Review).' *In: Cochrane Library. Issue 4.* Oxford: Update Software. (http://www.update-software.com/cochrane.htm)

—— O'Brien, N., Joy, M-T., Hennessy, E., MacDonald, D. (1989) 'Cerebral palsy among children born during the Dublin randomized trial of intrapartum monitoring.' *Lancet*, **2**, 1233–1235.

Grant, P.E., Barkovich, A.J. (1997) 'Neuroimaging in CP – Issues in pathogenesis and diagnosis.' *Mental Retardation and Developmental Disabilities Research Reviews*, **3**, 118–128.

Gravenhorst, J.B. (1989) 'Rhesus isoimmunization.' *In:* Chalmers, I., Enkin, M., Keirse, M.J.N.C. (Eds.) *Effective Care in Pregnancy and Childbirth, Vol. I: Pregnancy. Parts I–V.* Oxford: Oxford University Press, pp. 565–577.

Gray, P.H., Hurley, T.M., Rogers, Y.M., O'Callaghan, M.J., Tudehope, D.I., Burns, Y.R., Mohay, H.A. (1997) 'Survival and neonatal and neurodevelopmental outcome of 24–29 week gestation infants according to primary cause of preterm delivery.' *Australian and New Zealand Journal of Obstetrics and Gynaecology*, **37**, 1161–1168.

Graziani, L.J., Pasto, M., Stanley, C., Pidcock, F., Desai, H., Desai, S., Branca, P., Goldberg, B. (1986) 'Neonatal neurosonographic correlates of cerebral palsy in preterm infants.' *Pediatrics*, **78**, 88–95.

—— Gringlas, M., Baumgart, S. (1997) 'Cerebrovascular complications and neurodevelopmental sequelae of neonatal ECMO.' *Clinics in Perinatology*, **24**, 655–675.

Greer, F.R. (1995) 'Vitamin K deficiency and hemorrhage in infancy.' *Clinics in Perinatology*, **22**, 759–777.

Grether, J.K., Nelson, K.B. (1996) 'Placental infection and risk of cerebral palsy in very low birth weight infants. Reply.' *Journal of Pediatrics*, **129**, 777–778. *(Letter.)*

—— —— (1997) 'Maternal infection and cerebral palsy in infants of normal birth weight.' *Journal of the American Medical Association*, **278**, 207–211.

—— —— Cummins, S.K. (1993) 'Twinning and cerebral palsy: Experience in four northern California counties, births 1983 through 1985.' *Pediatrics*, **92**, 854–858.

—— —— Emery, E.S., Cummins, S.K. (1996) 'Prenatal and perinatal factors and cerebral palsy in very low birth weight infants.' *Journal of Pediatrics*, **128**, 407–414.

—— Hoogstrate, J., Selvin, S., Nelson, K.B. (1998) 'Magnesium sulfate tocolysis and risk of neonatal death.' *American Journal of Obstetrics and Gynecology*, **178**, 1–6.

GRIT Study Group (1996) 'When do obstetricians recommend delivery for a high-risk preterm growth-retarded fetus? Growth Restriction Intervention Trial.' *European Journal of Obstetrics, Gynecology, and Reproductive Biology*, **67**, 121–126.

Gross, S.J. (1997) 'Intrauterine growth restriction – a genetic perspective.' *Clinical Obstetrics and Gynecology*, **40**, 730–739.

—— Bifano, E.M., D'Eugenio, D.B., Hakanson, D.O., Hingre, R.V. (1994) 'Prospective randomized controlled trial of conventional treatment or transport for ECMO in infants with severe persistent pulmonary hypertension (PPHN): Two year follow up.' *Pediatric Research*, **36**, 17A.

Gülmezoglu, A.M., Hofmeyr, G.J. (1998) 'Hospitalisation for bed rest for suspected impaired fetal growth (Cochrane Review).' *In: Cochrane Library. Issue 4.* Oxford: Update Software. (http://www.update-software.com/cochrane.htm)

—— de Onis, M., Villar, J. (1997) 'Effectiveness of interventions to prevent or treat impaired fetal growth.' *Obstetrical and Gynecological Survey*, **52**, 139–148.

Gustavson, K-H., Hagberg, B., Sanner, G. (1969) 'Identical syndromes of cerebral palsy in the same family.' *Acta Paediatrica Scandinavica*, **58**, 330–340.

Guyer, B., Martin, J.A., MacDorman, M.F., Anderson, R.N., Strobino, D.M. (1997) 'Annual summary of vital statistics – 1996.' *Pediatrics*, **100**, 905–918.

Haerer, A.F., Anderson, D.W., Schoenbergh, B.S. (1984) 'Prevalence of cerebral palsy in the biracial population of the Copiah County, Mississippi.' *Developmental Medicine and Child Neurology*, **26**, 195–199.

Hagberg, B., Hagberg, G. (1989) 'The changing panorama of infantile hydrocephalus and cerebral palsy over forty years – a Swedish survey.' *Brain and Development*, **11**, 368–373.

—— —— (1993) 'The origins of cerebral palsy.' *In:* David, T.J. (Ed.) *Recent Advances in Paediatrics, Vol. 11.* Edinburgh: Churchill Livingstone, pp. 67–83.

—— Hagberg, G., Olow, I. (1984) 'The changing panorama of cerebral palsy in Sweden. IV. Epidemiological trends 1959–78.' *Acta Paediatrica Scandinavica*, **73**, 433–440.

—— —— —— Von Wendt, L. (1989a) 'The changing panorama of cerebral palsy in Sweden. V. The birth year period of 1979–82.' *Acta Paediatrica Scandinavica*, **78**, 283–290.

—— —— Zetterstrom, R. (1989b) 'Decreasing perinatal mortality – increase in cerebral palsy morbidity?' *Acta Paediatrica Scandinavica*, **78**, 664–670.

—— Olow, I., (1993) 'The changing panorama of cerebral palsy in Sweden. VI. Prevalence and origin during the birth year period 1983–1986.' *Acta Paediatrica*, **82**, 387–393.

—— —— —— von Wendt, L. (1996) 'The changing panorama of cerebral palsy in Sweden. VII. Prevalence and origin in the birth year period 1987–90.' *Acta Paediatrica*, **85**, 954–960.

Halac, E., Halac, J., Begue, E.F., Casanas, J.M., Indiveri, D.R., Petit, J.K., Figueroa, M.J., Olmas, J.M., Rodriguez, L.A., Obregon, R.J. (1990) 'Prenatal and postnatal corticosteroid therapy to prevent neonatal necrotizing enterocolitis: a controlled trial.' *Journal of Pediatrics*, **117**, 132–138.

Haley, S.M., Coster, W.J., Ludlow, L.H. (1991) 'Pediatric functional outcome measures.' *Physical Medicine and Rehabilitation Clinics of North America*, **2**, 689–723.

Hanna, J., Wild, B.E. (1991) 'Bacterial meningitis in children under five years of age in Western Australia.' *Medical Journal of Australia*, **155**, 160–164.

Haque, K.N. (1986) 'Cerebral palsy in Riyadh, Saudi Arabia.' *Pakistan Paediatric Journal*, **10**, 1–12.

Harding, J.E., Bauer, M.K., Kimble, R.M. (1997) 'Antenatal therapy for intrauterine growth retardation.' *Acta Paediatrica*, Suppl. 423, 196–200.

Hawdon, J.M., Hey, E., Kolvin, I., Fundudis, T. (1990) 'Born too small—is outcome still affected?' *Developmental Medicine and Child Neurology*, **32**, 943–953.

Henderson, J.P., Beattie, C.P., Hale, E.G., Wright, T. (1984) 'The evaluation of new services: possibilities for preventing congenital toxoplasmosis.' *International Journal of Epidemiology*, **13**, 65–72.

Henderson-Smart, D. (1991) 'Throwing the baby out with the fetal monitoring? Obstetric care, birth asphyxia and brain damage.' *Medical Journal of Australia*, **154**, 576–578.

—— (1995) 'Postnatal consequences of chronic intrauterine compromise.' *Reproduction, Fertility, and Development*, **7**, 559–565.

—— Crowther, C.A. (1997) 'The Cochrane databases of randomized controlled trials and systematic reviews in pregnancy, childbirth and neonatal care.' *Seminars in Neonatology*, **2**, 211–219.

Hetts, S.W. (1998) 'To die or not to die – An overview of apoptosis and its role in disease.' *Journal of the American Medical Association*, **279**, 300–307.

Hetzel, B. (1994a) 'Historical development of the concepts of the brain – Thyroid relationships.' *In:* Stanbury, J.B. (Ed.) *The Damaged Brain of Iodine Deficiency: Cognitive, Behavioral, Neuromotor, Educative Aspects.* New York: Cognizant Communication Corporation, pp. 1–7.

—— (1994b) 'Iodine deficiency and fetal brain damage.' *New England Journal of Medicine*, **331**, 1770–1771.

—— Pandav, C.S. (1996) *S.O.S. for a Billion – the Conquest of Iodine Deficiency Disorders.* New Delhi: Oxford University Press.

—— Dunn, J.T., Stanbury, J.B. (Eds.) (1987) *The Prevention and Control of Iodine Deficiency Disorder.* Amsterdam: Elsevier.

—— Zimmet, P., Seeman, E. (1997) 'Endocrine and metabolic disorders.' *In:* Detels, R., Holland, W.W., McEwen, J., Omenn, G. S. (Eds.) *Oxford Textbook of Public Health, 3rd Edn.* Oxford: Oxford University Press, pp. 1113–1142.

Hey, E. (1985) 'Fetal hypoxia and subsequent handicap: the problem of establishing a causal link.' *In:* Chamberlain, G., Orr, C.J.B., Sharp, F. (Eds.) *Litigation and Obstetrics and Gynaecology: Proceedings of the 14th Study Group of the Royal College of Obstetrics and Gynaecology.* London: Royal College of Obstetrics and Gynaecology, pp. 233–242.

Hill, A.B., Hill, I.D. (1991) 'Statistical evidence and inference.' *In:* Hill, A.B., Hill, I.D. (Eds.) *Bradford Hill's Principles of Medical Statistics, 12th Edn.* London: Edward Arnold, pp. 272–276.

Hodnett, E.D. (1995) 'Support from caregivers during childbirth (Cochrane Review).' *In: Cochrane Library. Issue 4.* Oxford: Update Software. (http://www.update-software.com/cochrane.htm)

—— (1998) 'Support from caregivers during at risk pregnancy (Cochrane Review).' *In: Cochrane Library. Issue 4.* Oxford: Update Software. (http://www.update-software.com/cochrane.htm)

—— Roberts, I. (1998) 'Home based social support for socially disadvantaged mothers (Cochrane Review).' *In: Cochrane Library. Issue 4.* Oxford: Update Software. (http://www.update-software.com/cochrane.htm)

Hofmeyr, G.J. (1998a) 'Amnioinfusion for intrapartum umbilical cord compression (Cochrane Review).' *In: Cochrane Library. Issue 4.* Oxford: Update Software. (http://www.update-software.com/cochrane.htm)

—— (1998b) 'Amnioinfusion prophylactically versus therapeutically for intrapartum oligohydramnios (Cochrane Review).' *In: Cochrane Library. Issue 4.* Oxford: Update Software. (http://www.update-software.com/cochrane.htm)

—— (1998c) ''Fetal distress' in labour managed operatively versus conservatively (Cochrane Review).' *In: Cochrane Library. Issue 4.* Oxford: Update Software. (http://www.update-software.com/cochrane.htm)

—— (1998d) 'Tocolysis with intravenous betamimetics prophylactically in the second stage of labour (Cochrane Review).' *In: Cochrane Library. Issue 4.* Oxford: Update Software. (http://www.update-software.com/cochrane.htm)

Holman, C.D.J., James, I.R., Heenan, P.J., Matz, L.R., Blackwell, J.B., Kelsall, G.R.H., Singh, A., Ten Seldam, R.E.J. (1983) 'An improved method of analysis of observer variation between pathologists.' *Histopathology*, **6**, 581–589.

—— English, D.R., Bower, C., Kurinczuk, J.J. (1996) 'NHMRC recommendations on abstinence from alcohol in pregnancy.' *Medical Journal of Australia*, **164**, 699. *(Letter.)*

Holmes, G.E., Hassanein, R.S. (1988) 'Significance of minor abnormalities in children.' *American Family Physician*, **38**, 185–189.

Horbar, J.D. (1992) 'Prevention of periventricular–intraventricular hemorrhage.' *In:* Sinclair, J.C., Bracken, M.B. (Eds.) *Effective Care of the Newborn Infant.* Oxford: Oxford University Press, pp. 562–589.

Howell, C.J. (1998) 'Epidural vs non-epidural anaethesia in labour (Cochrane Review).' *In: Cochrane Library. Issue 4.* Oxford: Update Software. (http://www.update-software.com/cochrane.htm)

Hughes, I., Newton, R. (1992) 'Genetic aspects of cerebral palsy.' *Developmental Medicine and Child Neurology*, **34**, 80–86.

Hutchison, T., Harpin, V. (1998) 'Survey of UK computerised special needs registers.' *Archives of Disease in Childhood*, **78**, 312–315.

Hutton, J.L., Cooke, T., Pharoah, P.O.D. (1994) 'Life expectancy in children with cerebral palsy.' *British Medical Journal*, **309**, 431–435.

Ingram, T.T.S. (1984) 'A historical view of the definition and classification of the cerebral palsies.' *In:* Stanley, F., Alberman, E. (Eds.) *The Epidemiology of the Cerebral Palsies. Clinics in Developmental Medicine No. 87.* London: Spastics International Medical Publications, pp. 1–11.

Ipata, A.E., Cioni, G., Bottai, P., Fazzi, B., Canapicchi, R., Van Hof-Van Duin, J. (1994) 'Acuity card testing in children with cerebral palsy related to magnetic resonance images, mental levels and motor abilities.' *Brain and Development*, **16**, 195–203.

Jacobs, P.A. (1990) 'The role of chromosome abnormalities in reproductive failure.' *Reproduction, Nutrition, and Development*, **30**, Suppl. 1, 63S–74S.

James, W.H. (1997) 'Recent secular trends in multiple birth rates.' *Archives of Disease in Childhood*, **77**, F77. *(Letter.)*

Jarvis, S., Hey, E. (1984) 'Measuring disability and handicap due to cerebral palsy.' *In:* Stanley, F., Alberman, E. (Eds.) *The Epidemiology of the Cerebral Palsies. Clinics in Developmental Medicine No. 87.* London: Spastics International Medical Publications, pp. 35–45.

Jeffery, H.E., Lahra, M.M. (1998) 'Eight-year outcome of universal screening and intrapartum antibiotics for maternal group B streptococcal carriers.' *Pediatrics*, **101**, E21–E26.

Johanson, R.B., Menon, V.J. (1998) 'Vacuum extraction vs forceps delivery (Cochrane Review).' *In: Cochrane Library. Issue 4.* Oxford: Update Software. (http://www.update-software.com/cochrane.htm)

Johnson, A. (1995) 'Use of registers in child health.' *Archives of Disease in Childhood*, **72**, 474–477.

—— (1997) 'Randomised controlled trials in perinatal medicine: 3. Identifying and measuring endpoints in randomised controlled trials.' British Journal of Obstetrics and Gynaecology, 104, 768–771.

—— Townshend, P., Yudkin, P., Bull, D., Wilkinson, A.R. (1993) 'Functional abilities at age 4 years of children born before 29 weeks of gestation.' *British Medical Journal*, **306**, 1715–1718.

—— Field, D., Elbourne, D., Grant, A., Davis, D., Greenough, A., Hale, P., Hamilton, L., Levene, M., *et al.* (1998a) 'The collaborative UK ECMO trial: Follow-up to 1 year of age.' *Pediatrics*, **101**, E11–E110.

—— King, R., Sayer, J., Ashurst, H., Macfarlane, A., Berridge, G. (1998b) 'Oxford Register of Early Childhood Impairments: a regional register (ORECI).' *In:* Pilcher, L., Kumiega, L. (Eds.) *National Perinatal Epidemiology Unit Annual Report 1997.* Oxford: National Perinatal Epidemiology Unit.

Jones, K.L., Smith, D.W. (1975) 'The fetal alcohol syndrome.' *Teratology*, **12**, 1–10.

Jordens, C.F.C., Hawe, P., Irwig, L.M., Henderson-Smart, D.J., Ryan, M., Donoghue, D.A., Gabb, R.G., Fraser, I.S. (1998) 'Use of systematic reviews of randomised trials by Australian neonatologists and obstetricians.' *Medical Journal of Australia*, **168**, 267–270.

Kaczorowski, J., Levitt, C., Hanvey, L., Avard, D., Chance, G. (1998) 'A national survey of use of obstetric procedures and technologies in Canadian hospitals: routine or based on existing evidence.' *Birth*, **25**, 11–18.

Kari, M.A., Hallman, M., Eronen, M., Teramo, K., Virtanen, M., Koivisto, M., Ikonen, R.S. (1994) 'Prenatal dexamethasone treatment in conjunction with rescue therapy of human surfactant: a randomized placebo-controlled multicenter study.' *Pediatrics*, **93**, 730–736.

Kavcic, A., Perat, M.V. (1998) 'Prevalence of cerebral palsy in Slovenia: birth years 1981 to 1990.' *Developmental Medicine and Child Neurology*, **40**, 459–463.

Keeling, J.W. (1995) 'Anomalous development in twins.' *In:* Whittle, H., Ward, M. (Eds.) *Multiple Pregnancy.* London: RCOG Press, pp. 83–99.

Keirse, M.J.N.C., Grant, A., King, J.F. (1989) 'Preterm labour.' *In:* Chalmers, I., Enkin, M., Keirse, M.J.N.C. (Eds.) *Effective Care in Pregnancy and Childbirth. Vol. 1: Pregnancy. Parts I–V.* Oxford: Oxford University Press, pp. 694–745.

Khoury, M.J., Yang, Q.H. (1998) 'The future of genetic studies of complex human diseases: An epidemiologic perspective.' *Epidemiology*, **9**, 350–354.

King, J., Flenady, V. (1998) 'Antibiotics in preterm labour with intact membranes (Cochrane Review).' *In: Cochrane Library. Issue 4.* Oxford: Update Software. (http://www.update-software.com/cochrane.htm)

King, R., Johnson, A. (1995) *Oxford Register of Early Childhood Impairments: Annual Report 1995.* Oxford: Women's Centre, Radcliffe Hospital.

Kingdom, J., Baker, P., Blair, E. (1999) 'Definitions of intrauterine growth restriction.' *In:* Baker, P., Kingdom, J. (Eds.) *Intra-uterine Growth Restriction.* London: Springer-Verlag. *(In press.)*

Kinsella, J.P., Abman, S.H. (1998) 'Controversies in the use of inhaled nitric oxide therapy in the newborn.' *Clinics in Perinatology*, **25**, 203–217.

Kirshner, B., Guyatt, G. (1985) 'A methodological framework for assessing health indices.' *Journal of Chronic Diseases*, **38**, 27–36.

Kitchen, W.H., Doyle, L.W., Ford, G.W., Rickards, A.L., Lissenden, J.V., Ryan, M.M. (1987) 'Cerebral palsy in very low birthweight infants surviving to 2 years with modern perinatal intensive care.' *American Journal of Perinatology*, **4**, 29–35.

223

Kjellmer, I., Liedholm, M., Sultan, B., Wennergren, M., Götborg, C.W., Thordstein, M. (1997) 'Long-term effects of intrauterine growth retardation.' *Acta Paediatrica*, **86**, Suppl. 422, 83–84.

Klassen, T.P., Jadad, A.R., Moher, D. (1998) 'Guides for reading and interpreting systematic reviews. I. Getting started.' *Archives of Pediatrics and Adolescent Medicine*, **152**, 700–704.

Kliegman, R.M. (1995) 'Neonatal technology, perinatal survival, social consequences, and the perinatal paradox.' *American Journal of Public Health*, **85**, 909–913.

Kline, J., Stein, Z., Susser, M. (1989) *Conception to Birth: Epidemiology of Prenatal Development*. New York: Oxford University Press.

Koopman, J.S. (1996) 'Comment: emerging objectives and methods in epidemiology.' *American Journal of Public Health*, **86**, 630–632.

Korst, L.M., Phelan, J.P., Ahn, M.O., Martin, G.I. (1996) 'Nucleated red blood cells: An update on the marker for fetal asphyxia.' *American Journal of Obstetrics and Gynecology*, **175**, 843–846.

Krägeloh-Mann, I., Petersen, D., Hagberg, B., Michaelis, R. (1994) 'MRI in the timing of pathological events – a study in bilateral spastic cerebral palsy children.' *In:* Lou, H.C., Greisen, G., Larsen, J.F. (Eds.) *Brain Lesions in the Newborn, Alfred Benzon Symposium No. 37*. Copenhagen: Munksgaard Press, pp. 178–191.

—— —— Hagberg, G., Vollmer, B., Hagberg, B., Michaelis, R. (1995) 'Bilateral spastic cerebral palsy--MRI pathology and origin. Analysis from a representative series of 56 cases.' *Developmental Medicine and Child Neurology*, **37**, 379–397.

Kramer, M.S. (1987) 'Determinants of low-birth weight: Methodological assessment and meta-analysis.' *Bulletin of the World Health Organization*, **65**, 663–737.

Kramer, M.S. (1998) 'High protein supplementation in pregnancy (Cochrane Review).' *In: Cochrane Library. Issue 4*. Oxford: Update Software. (http://www.update-software.com/cochrane.htm)

—— Olivier, M., McLean, F.H., Willis, D.M., Usher, R.H. (1990) 'Impact of intrauterine growth retardation and body proporionality on fetal and neonatal outcome.' *Pediatrics*, **86**, 707–713.

Kraus, F.T. (1997) 'Cerebral palsy and thrombi in placental vessels of the fetus: Insights from litigation.' *Human Pathology*, **28**, 246–248.

Kuban, K.C.K., Leviton, A. (1994) 'Cerebral palsy.' *New England Journal of Medicine*, **330**, 188–195.

—— —— Pagano, M., Fenton, T., Strassfeld, R., Wolff, M. (1992) 'Maternal toxemia is associated with reduced incidence of germinal matrix hemorrhage in premature babies.' *Journal of Child Neurology*, **7**, 70–76.

Kulier, R., Hofmeyr, G.J. (1998) 'Tocolytics for suspected intrapartum fetal distress (Cochrane Review).' *In: Cochrane Library. Issue 4*. Oxford: Update Software. (http://www.update-software.com/cochrane.htm)

Kurki, T., Hallman, M., Zilliacus, R., Teramo, K., Ylikorkala, O. (1992) 'Premature rupture of the membranes: Effect of penicillin prophylaxis and long-term outcome of the children.' *American Journal of Perinatology*, **9**, 11–16.

Kurland, L.T., Faro, S.N., Siedler, H. (1960) 'Minamata disease. The outbreak of a neurologic disorder in Minamata, Japan, and its relationship to the ingestion of seafood contaminated by mercuric compounds.' *World Neurology*, **1**, 370–395.

Kyllerman, M. (1982) 'Dyskinetic cerebral palsy. II. Pathogenetic risk factors and intra-uterine growth.' *Acta Paediatrica Scandinavica*, **71**, 551–558.

—— Bager, B., Bensch, J., Bille, B., Lolw, I., Voss, H. (1982) 'Dyskinetic cerebral palsy. I. Clinical categories, associated neurological abnormalities and incidences.' *Acta Paediatrica Scandinavica*, **71**, 543–550.

Läärä, E., Olsén, P., Muhli, A., Hartikainen, A-L., Rantakallio, P., Järvelin, M-R. (1997) 'The occurrence of preterm delivery associated with some maternal and fetal conditions in two birth cohorts from northern Finland with an interval of 20 years.' *In:* Olsén, P. (Ed.) *Preterm Birth and Preterm Children – a Study of the Northern Finland One-Year Birth Cohorts for 1966 and 1985/6*. Oulu: Oulu University Press, pp. 1–11.

Laisram, N., Srivastava, V.K., Srivastava, R.K. (1992) 'Cerebral palsy – an etiological study.' *Indian Journal of Pediatrics*, **59**, 723–728.

Landy, H.J., Nies, B.M. (1995) 'The vanishing twin.' *In:* Keith, L.G., Papiernik, E., Keith, D.M., Luke, B. (Eds.) *Multiple Pregnancy: Epidemiology, Gestation and Perinatal Outcome*. New York: Parthenon, pp. 59–71.

Law, M. (1987) 'Measurement in occupational therapy: scientific criteria for evaluation.' *Canadian Journal of Occupational Therapy*, **54**, 133–138.

—— Cadman, D., Rosenbaum, P., Walter, S., Russell, D., DeMatteo, C. (1991) 'Neurodevelopmental therapy and upper extremity casting for children with cerebral palsy.' *Developmental Medicine and Child Neurology*, **33**, 379–387.

—— Polatajko, H., Pollock, N., McColl, M.A., Carswell, A., Baptiste, S. (1994) 'Pilot testing of the Canadian Occupational Performance Measure: clinical and measurement issues.' *Canadian Journal of Occupational Therapy*, **61**, 191–197.

—— King, G., MacKinnon, E., Russell, D., Murphy, C., Hurley, P., Bosch, E. (1998) *All About Outcomes: A Program to Help You Understand, Evaluate, and Choose Pediatric Outcome Measures.* Thorofare, NJ: Slack Professional. *(Computer software.)*

Lebeer, J. (1998) 'How much brain does a mind need? Scientific, clinical, and educational implications of ecological plasticity.' *Developmental Medicine and Child Neurology*, **40**, 352–357.

Lee, S.H., Ewert, D.P., Frederick, P.D., Mascola, L. (1992) 'Resurgence of congenital rubella syndrome in the 1990s.' *Journal of the American Medical Association*, **267**, 2616–2620.

Leitich, H., Egarter, C., Reisenberger, K., Kaider, A., Berghammer, P. (1998) 'Concomitant use of glucocorticoids: A comparison of two metaanalyses on antibiotic treatment in preterm premature rupture of membranes.' *American Journal of Obstetrics and Gynecology*, **178**, 899–908.

Levene, M.I. (1990) 'Cerebral ultrasound and neurological impairment: telling the future.' *Archives of Disease in Childhood*, **65**, 469–471.

—— (1992) 'The impact of intensive neonatal care on the frequency of mental and motor handicap.' *Current Opinion in Neurology and Neurosurgery*, **5**, 333–338.

—— Kornberg, J., Williams, T.H.C. (1985) 'The incidence and severity of post-asphyxial encephalopathy in full-term infants.' *Early Human Development*, **11**, 21–26.

—— Grindulis, H., Sands, C., Moore, J.R. (1986) 'Comparison of two methods of predicting outcome in perinatal asphyxia.' *Lancet*, **1**, 67–69.

—— Dowling, S., Graham, M., Fogelman, K., Galton, M., Phillips, M. (1992) 'Impaired motor function (clumsiness) in 5 year old children: correlation with neonatal ultrasound scans.' *Archives of Disease in Childhood*, **67**, 687–690.

Leviton, A. (1987) 'Single-cause attribution.' *Developmental Medicine and Child Neurology*, **29**, 805–807. *(Annotation.)*

—— (1993) 'Preterm birth and cerebral palsy: is tumor necrosis factor the missing link?' *Developmental Medicine and Child Neurology*, **35**, 553–558.

—— (1995) 'The perinatal paradox.' *American Journal of Public Health*, **85**, 906–907. *(Editorial.)*

—— Gilles, F. (1996) 'Ventriculomegaly, delayed myelination, white matter hypoplasia, and "periventricular" leukomalacia: How are they related?' *Pediatric Neurology*, **15**, 127–136.

—— Nelson, K.B. (1992) 'Problems with definitions and classifications of newborn encephalopathy.' *Pediatric Neurology*, **8**, 85–90.

—— Paneth, N. (1990) 'White matter damage in preterm newborns – an epidemiologic perspective.' *Early Human Development*, **24**, 1–22.

—— Pagano, M., Kuban, K.C.K., Krishnamoorthy, K.S., Sullivan, K.F., Allred, E.N. (1991) 'The epidemiology of germinal matrix hemorrhage during the first half-day of life.' *Developmental Medicine and Child Neurology*, **33**, 138–145.

—— Kuban, K.C., Pagano, M., Allred, E.N., Van Marter, L. (1993) 'Antenatal corticosteroids appear to reduce the risk of postnatal germinal matrix hemorrhage in intubated low birth weight newborns.' *Pediatrics*, **91**, 1083–1088.

—— Paneth, N., Susser, M., Reuss, M.L., Allred, E.N., Kuban, K., Sanocka, U., Hegyi, T., Hiatt, M., *et al.* (1997) 'Maternal receipt of magnesium sulfate does not seem to reduce the risk of neonatal white matter damage.' *Pediatrics*, **99**, E21–E25.

Likert, R. (1932) 'A technique for the measurement of attitudes.' *Archives of Psychology*, **140**, 1–55.

Little, W.J. (1862) 'On the influence of abnormal parturition, difficult labours, premature birth, and asphyxia neonatorum, on the mental and physical condition of the child, especially in relation to deformities.' (Reprinted 1958 in *Cerebral Palsy Bulletin*, **1**, 5–36.)

Liu, K., Boag, G., Costello, S., Daneman, A., Kirpalani, H., Whyte, H. (1990) 'Widened subarachnoid space in pre-discharge cranial ultrasound: evidence of cerebral atrophy in immature infants?' *Developmental Medicine and Child Neurology*, **32**, 882–887.

Lorenz, J.M., Wooliever, D.E., Jetton, J.R., Paneth, N. (1998) 'A quantitative review of mortality and developmental disability in extremely premature newborns.' *Archives of Pediatrics and Adolescent Medicine*, **152**, 425–435.

Loria, C. (1980) 'Relationship of proximal to distal function in motor development.' *Physical Therapy*, **60**, 167–172.

Low, J.A. (1997) 'Intrapartum fetal asphyxia: Definition, diagnosis, and classification.' *American Journal of Obstetrics and Gynecology*, **176**, 957–959.

—— Galbraith, R.S., Muir, D., Killen, H., Pater, B., Karchmar, J. (1982) 'Intrauterine growth retardation: A study of long-term morbidity.' *American Journal of Obstetrics and Gynecology*, **142**, 670–677.

—— Panagiotopoulos, C., Derrick, E.J. (1994) 'Newborn complications after intrapartum asphyxia with metabolic acidosis in the term fetus.' *American Journal of Obstetrics and Gynecology*, **170**, 1081–1087.

Lucas, A., Morley, R., Cole, T.J. (1988) 'Adverse neurodevelopmental outcome of moderate neonatal hypo-glycaemia.' *British Medical Journal*, **297**, 1304–1308.

Lucey, J.F. (1997) 'Neuroprotection and perinatal brain care: The field of the future, currently going nowhere!?' *Pediatrics*, **100**, 1030–1031. *(Editorial.)*

Lumey, J.H. (1992) 'Decreased birthweights in infants after maternal *in utero* exposure to the Dutch famine of 1944–1945.' *Paediatric and Perinatal Epidemiology*, **6**, 240–253.

—— Ravelli, A.C.J., Wiessing, L.G., Koppe, J.G., Treffers, P.E., Stein, Z.A. (1993) 'The Dutch famine birth cohort study: design, validation of exposure, and selected characteristics of subjects after 43 years follow-up.' *Paediatric and Perinatal Epidemiology*, **7**, 354–367.

Lumley, J. (1988) 'Does continuous intrapartum fetal monitoring predict long-term neurological disorders?' *Paediatric and Perinatal Epidemiology*, **2**, 299–307.

—— Astbury, J. (1989) 'Advice for pregnancy.' *In:* Chalmers, I., Enkin, M., Keirse, M.J.N.C. (Eds.) *Effective Care in Pregnancy and Childbirth. Vol. I: Pregnancy. Parts I–V.* Oxford: Oxford University Press, pp. 237–254.

—— Correy, J.F., Newman, N.M. (1985a) 'Cigarette smoking, alcohol consumption and fetal outcome in Tasmania 1981–82.' *Australian and New Zealand Journal of Obstetrics and Gynaecology*, **25**, 33–40.

—— Lester, A., Renou, P., Wood, C. (1985b) 'A failed RCT to determine the best method of delivery for very low birth weight infants.' *Controlled Clinical Trials*, **6**, 120–127.

MacDonald, D. (1996a) 'Cerebral palsy and intrapartum fetal monitoring.' *New England Journal of Medicine*, **335**, 659–660. *(Editorial.)*

—— (1996b) 'Electronic fetal monitoring in predicting cerebral palsy' *New England Journal of Medicine*, **335**, 288. *(Letter.)*

Macfarlane, A., Johnson, A., Bower, P. (1990) 'Disabilities and health problems in childhood.' *In:* Botting, B.J., Macfarlane, A.J., Price, F.V. (Eds.) *Three, Four or More: A Study of Triplet and Higher Order Births.* London: HMSO, pp. 153–160.

MacGillivray, I., Campbell, D.M. (1995) 'The changing pattern of cerebral palsy in Avon.' *Paediatric and Perinatal Epidemiology*, **9**, 146–155.

Machin, G.A., Still, K. (1995) 'The twin–twin transfusion syndrome.' *In:* Keith, L.G., Papiernik, E., Keith, D.M., Luke, B. (Eds.) *Multiple Pregnancy: Epidemiology, Gestation and Perinatal Outcome.* New York: Parthenon, pp. 367–394.

Mac Keith, R.C., Polani, P.E. (1958) 'Cerebral palsy.' *Lancet*, **1**, 61. *(Letter.)*

MacLennan, A. (1984) 'Clinical characteristics of multiple gestation: Mortality and morbidity.' *In:* Creasy, R.K., Resnik, R. (Eds.) *Maternal–Fetal Medicine: Principles and Practice.* Philadelphia: W.B. Saunders, pp. 527–528.

—— for the International Cerebral Palsy Task Force (1999) 'A template for defining a causal relationship between acute intrapartum events and cerebral palsy: international consensus statement.' *British Medical Journal*, **319**, 1054–1059.

—— Stanley, F., Blair, E., Rice, G., Stone, P., Robinson, J., Henderson-Smart, D., Yu, V., Harbord, M., *et al.* (1995) 'Consensus statement on the origins of cerebral palsy.' *Australian and New Zealand Journal of Obstetrics and Gynaecology*, **35**, 126–131.

Macnaughton, R. J. (1996) 'Numbers, scales and qualitative research.' *Lancet*, **347**, 1099–1100.

Mahadevan, N., Pearce, M., Steer, P. (1994) 'The proper measure of intrauterine growth retardation is function, not size.' *British Journal of Obstetrics and Gynaecology*, **101**, 1032–1035.

Maisels, M.J. (1992) 'Neonatal jaundice.' *In:* Sinclair, J.C., Bracken, M.B. (Eds.) *Effective Care of the New-born Infant.* Oxford: Oxford University Press, pp. 507–561.

Makwabe, C.M., Mgone, C.S. (1984) 'The pattern and aetiology of cerebral palsy as seen in Dar es Salaam, Tanzania.' *East African Medical Journal*, **12**, 896–899.

Mallard, E.C., Williams, C.E., Johnston, B.M., Gluckman, P.D. (1994) 'Increased vulnerability to neuronal damage after umbilical cord occlusion in fetal sheep with advancing gestation.' *American Journal of Obstetrics and Gynecology*, **170**, 206–214.

Manning, F.A., Bondaji, N., Harman, C.R., Casiro, O., Menticoglou, S., Morrison, I., Berck, D.J. (1998) 'Fetal assessment based on fetal biophysical profile scoring. VIII. The incidence of cerebral palsy in tested and untested perinates.' *American Journal of Obstetrics and Gynecology*, **178**, 696–706.

Marsál, K., Persson, P-H., Larsen, T., Lilja, H., Selbing, A., Sultan, B. (1996) 'Intrauterine growth curves based on ultrasonically estimated foetal weights.' *Acta Paediatrica*, **85**, 843–848.

McMichael, A.J. (1994) 'Invited commentary – "Molecular epidemiology": New pathway or new travelling companion?' *American Journal of Epidemiology*, **140**, 1–11.

Meberg, A., Broch, H. (1995) 'A changing pattern of cerebral palsy. Declining trend for incidence of cerebral palsy in the 20-year period 1970–89.' *Journal of Perinatal Medicine*, **23**, 395–402.

Mercer, B.M., Miodovnik, M., Thurnau, G.R., Goldenberg, R.L., Das, A.F., Ramsey, R.D., Rabello, Y.A., Meis, P.J., Moawad, A.H., *et al.* (1997) 'Antibiotic therapy for reduction of infant morbidity after preterm premature rupture of the membranes – A randomized controlled trial.' *Journal of the American Medical Association*, **278**, 989–995.

Mercuri, E., Dubowitz, L., Paterson-Brown, S., Cowan, F. (1998) 'Incidence of cranial ultrasound abnormalities in apparently well newborns on a post-natal ward: correlation with antenatal and perinatal factors and neurological status.' *Archives of Disease in Childhood*, **79**, F185–F189.

Miller, E., Cradock-Watson, J.E., Pollock, T.M. (1982) 'Consequences of confirmed maternal rubella at successive stages of pregnancy.' *Lancet*, **2**, 781–784.

—— Marshall, R., Vurdien, J. (1993) 'Epidemiology, outcome and control of varicella-zoster infection.' *Reviews in Medical Microbiology*, **4**, 222–230.

Miller, G. (1988) 'Ataxic cerebral palsy and genetic predisposition.' *Archives of Disease in Childhood*, **63**, 1260–1261.

—— (1989) 'Minor congenital anomalies and ataxic cerebral palsy.' *Archives of Disease in Childhood*, **64**, 557–562.

—— (1991) 'Cerebral palsy and minor congenital anomalies.' *Clinical Pediatrics*, **30**, 97–98.

—— (1994) 'Dyskinetic cerebral palsy and birth asphyxia.' *Developmental Medicine and Child Neurology*, **36**, 928–929. *(Letter.)*

Mistry, R.T., Neilson, J.P. (1998) 'Intrapartum fetal ECG plus heart rate recording (Cochrane Review).' *In: Cochrane Library. Issue 4.* Oxford: Update Software. (http://www.update-software.com/cochrane.htm)

Mitchell, E.A., Brunt, J.M., Everard, C. (1994) 'Reduction in mortality from sudden infant death syndrome in New Zealand: 1986–92.' *Archives of Disease in Childhood*, **70**, 291–294.

Mittendorf, R. (1994) 'Does cesarean delivery prevent cerebral palsy or other neurologic problems of childhood?' *Obstetrics and Gynecology*, **84**, 481–482. *(Letter.)*

—— Covert, R., Boman, J., Khoshnood, B., Lee, K-S., Siegler, M. (1997) 'Is tocolytic magnesium sulphate associated with increased total paediatric mortality?' *Lancet*, **350**, 1517–1518.

Mongelli, M., Gardosi, J. (1996) 'Reduction of false-positive diagnosis of intrauterine growth restriction by application of customised fetal growth standards.' *Obstetrics and Gynecology*, **88**, 844–848.

—— Chung, T.K.H., Chang, A.M.Z. (1997) 'Obstetric intervention and benefit in conditions of very low prevalence.' *British Journal of Obstetrics and Gynaecology*, **104**, 771–774.

Monreal, F.J. (1985) 'Consideration of genetic factors in cerebral palsy.' *Developmental Medicine and Child Neurology*, **27**, 325–330.

Morbidity and Mortality Weekly Report (1995) 'Economic costs of birth defects and cerebral palsy – United States, 1992.' *Morbidity and Mortality Weekly Report*, **44**, 694–699.

Morgane, P.J., Austin-LaFrance, R.J., Bronzino, J.D., Tonkiss, J., Galler, J.R. (1992) 'Malnutrition and the developing central nervous system.' *In:* Isaacson, R.L., Jensen, K.F. (Eds.) *The Vulnerable Brain and Environmental Risks.* New York: Plenum Press, pp. 3–44.

Morikawa, S., Itakura, A., Hayakawa, F., Mizutani, S., Matsuzawa, K., Kurauchi, O. (1997) 'Timing of insults causing abnormal outcome in preterm infants 1989–1992.' *International Journal of Gynecology and Obstetrics*, **59**, 1–6.

Morton, D.H., Bennett, M.J., Seargeant, L.E., Nichter, C.A., Kelley, R.I. (1991) 'Glutaric aciduria type I: Common cause of episodic encephalopathy and spastic paralysis in the Amish of Lancaster County, Pennsylvania.' *American Journal of Medical Genetics*, **41**, 89–95.

Msall, M.E., DiGaudio, K.M., Duffy, L.C. (1993) 'Use of functional assessment in children with developmental disabilities.' *Physical Medicine and Rehabilitation Clinics of North America*, **4**, 517–527.

227

Mul, T., Mongelli, M., Gardosi, J. (1996) 'A comparative analysis of second-trimester ultrasound dating formulae in pregnancies conceived with artificial reproductive techniques.' *Ultrasound in Obstetrics and Gynecology*, **8**, 397–402.

Mulrow, C.D., Oxman, A.D. (Eds.) (1997) *Cochrane Collaboration Handbook. In: Cochrane Library. Issue 4.* Oxford: Update Software. (http://www.update-software.com/cochrane.htm)

Murph, J.R., Souza, I.E., Dawson, J.D., Benson, P., Petheram, S.J., Pfab, D., Gregg, A., O'Neill, M.E., Zimmerman, B., Bale, J.F. (1988) 'Epidemiology of congenital cytomegalovirus infection. Maternal risk factors and molecular analysis of cytomegalovirus strains.' *American Journal of Epidemiology*, **147**, 940–947.

Murphy, C.C., Yeargin-Allsopp, M., Decouflé, P., Drews, C.D. (1993) 'Prevalence of cerebral palsy among ten-year-old children in metropolitan Atlanta, 1985 through 1987.' *Journal of Pediatrics*, **123**, S13–S19.

Murphy, D.J. (1996) 'Placental infection and risk of cerebral palsy in very low birth weight infants.' *Journal of Pediatrics*, **129**, 776–777. *(Letter.)*

—— MacKenzie, I.A. (1995) 'The mortality and morbidity associated with umbilical cord prolapse.' *British Journal of Obstetrics and Gynaecology*, **102**, 826–830.

—— Sellers, S., MacKenzie, I.Z., Yudkin, P.L., Johnson, A.M. (1995) 'Case–control study of antenatal and intrapartum risk factors for cerebral palsy in very preterm singleton babies.' *Lancet*, **346**, 1449–1454.

—— Hope, P.L., Johnson, A. (1996a) 'Ultrasound findings and clinical antecedents of cerebral palsy in very preterm infants.' *Archives of Disease in Childhood*, **74**, F105–F109.

—— Squier, M.V., Hope, P.L., Sellers, S., Johnson, A. (1996b) 'Clinical associations and time of onset of cerebral white matter damage in very preterm babies.' *Archives of Disease in Childhood*, **75**, F27–F32.

—— Hope, P.L., Johnson, A. (1997) 'Neonatal risk factors for cerebral palsy in very preterm babies – case–control study.' *British Medical Journal*, **314**, 404–408.

Murphy, P.A. (1993) 'Preterm birth prevention programs: a critique of current literature.' *Journal of Nurse-Midwifery*, **38**, 324–335.

Mutch, L.W., Alberman, E., Hagberg, B., Kodama, K., Perat, M.V. (1992) 'Cerebral palsy epidemiology: where are we now and where are we going?' *Developmental Medicine and Child Neurology*, **34**, 547–555.

Myers, R.E. (1972) 'Two patterns of perinatal brain damage and their conditions of occurrence.' *American Journal of Obstetrics and Gynecology*, **112**, 246–276.

Myrianthopoulos, N.C. (1976) 'Congenital malformations in twins.' *Acta Geneticae Medicae et Gemellologiae*, **25**, 331–335.

National Perinatal Epidemiology Unit (1996) *Report 1996.* Oxford: National Perinatal Epidemiology Unit.

—— (1997) *Oxford Register of Early Childhood Impairments: Annual Report 1997.* Oxford: National Perinatal Epidemiology Unit.

Nehgme, R.A., O'Connor, T.Z., Lister, G., Bracken, M.B. (1992) 'Patent ductus arteriosus.' *In:* Sinclair, J.C., Bracken, M.B. (Eds.) *Effective Care of the Newborn Infant.* Oxford: Oxford University Press, pp. 281–324.

Neilson, J.P. (1998) 'Routine ultrasound in early pregnancy (Cochrane Review).' *In: Cochrane Library. Issue 4.* Oxford: Update Software. (http://www.update-software.com/cochrane.htm)

—— Alfirevic, Z. (1998) 'Doppler ultrasound in high risk pregnancies (Cochrane Review).' *In: Cochrane Library. Issue 4.* Oxford: Update Software. (http://www.update-software.com/cochrane.htm)

—— Levene, M. I. (1997) 'The Cochrane Collaboration: progress in perinatal medicine.' *Archives of Disease in Childhood*, **77**, F176–F177.

Neligan, G.A., Kolvin, I., Scott, D.McL., Garside, R.F. (1976) *Born Too Soon or Born Too Small. Clinics in Developmental Medicine No. 61.* London: Spastics International Medical Publications.

Nelson, K.B. (1986) 'Cerebral palsy: what is known regarding cause?' *Annals of the New York Academy of Sciences*, **477**, 22–26.

—— (1988) 'What proportion of cerebral palsy is related to birth asphyxia?' *Journal of Pediatrics*, **112**, 572–574.

—— (1989) 'Relationship of intrapartum and delivery room events to long-term neurologic outcome.' *Clinics in Perinatology*, **14**, 995–1007.

—— (1991) 'Prenatal origin of hemiparetic cerebral palsy: How often and why?' *Pediatrics*, **88**, 1059–1061.

—— (1994) 'Timing the onset of cerebral palsy and other developmental disorders.' *In:* Lou, H., Greisen, G., Larsen, J.F. (Eds.) *Brain Lesions in the Newborn: Hypoxic and Haemodynamic Pathogenesis.* Copenhagen: Munksgaard, pp. 136–148.

—— (1997) 'Magnesium sulfate and risk of cerebral palsy in very low-birth-weight infants.' *Journal of the American Medical Association*, **276**, 1843–1844.

—— Ellenberg, J.H. (1982) 'Children who 'outgrew' cerebral palsy.' *Pediatrics*, **69**, 529–536.

—— —— (1984) 'Obstetric complications as risk factors for cerebral palsy or seizure disorders.' *Journal of the American Medical Association*, **251**, 1843–1848.

—— —— (1985a) 'Antecedents of cerebral palsy. I. Univariate analysis of risks.' *American Journal of Diseases of Children*, **139**, 1031–1038.

—— —— (1985b) 'Predictors of low and very low birth weight and the relation of these to cerebral palsy.' *Journal of the American Medical Association*, **253**, 1473–1479.

—— —— (1986a) 'Antecedents of cerebral palsy. Multivariate analysis of risk.' *New England Journal of Medicine*, **315**, 81–86.

—— —— (1986b) 'Antecedents of seizure disorders in early childhood.' *American Journal of Diseases of Children*, **140**, 1053–1061.

—— —— (1995) 'Childhood neurological disorders in twins.' *Paediatric and Perinatal Epidemiology*, **9**, 135–145.

—— Emery, E.S.I. (1993) 'Birth asphyxia and the neonatal brain: What do we know and when do we know it?' *Clinics in Perinatology*, **20**, 327–344.

—— Grether, J.K. (1995) 'Can magnesium sulfate reduce the risk of cerebral palsy in very low birthweight infants?' *Pediatrics*, **95**, 263–269.

—— —— (1996) 'Cerebral palsy in very low birth weight infants, pre-eclampsia and magnesium sulfate. Reply.' *Pediatrics*, **97**, 781–782. *(Letter.)*

—— —— (1997) 'Cerebral palsy in low-birthweight infants – Etiology and strategies for prevention.' *Mental Retardation and Developmental Disabilities Research Reviews*, **3**, 112–117.

—— —— (1998) 'Potentially asphyxiating conditions and spastic cerebral palsy in infants of normal birthweight.' *American Journal of Obstetrics and Gynecology*, **179**, 507–513.

—— Leviton, A. (1991) 'How much of neonatal encephalopathy is due to birth asphyxia?' *American Journal of Diseases of Children*, **145**, 1325–1331.

—— Dambrosia, J.M., Ting, T.Y., Grether, J.K. (1996) 'Uncertain value of electronic fetal monitoring in predicting cerebral palsy.' *New England Journal of Medicine*, **334**, 613–618.

Newacheck, P.W., Taylor, W.R. (1992) 'Childhood chronic illness: Prevalence, severity and impact.' *American Journal of Public Health*, **82**, 364–371.

Newman, N. (1986) 'Alcohol.' *In:* Chamberlain, G., Lumley, J. (Eds.) *Prepregnancy Care: A Manual for Practice*. Chichester: John Wiley, pp. 183–208.

Newnham, J. (1998) 'Consequences of fetal growth restriction.' *Current Opinion in Obstetrics and Gynecology*, **10**, 145–149.

Nicoll, A., Elliman, D., Ross, E. (1998) 'MMR vaccination and autism 1998: Déja vu – pertussis and brain damage 1974?' *British Medical Journal*, **316**, 715–716.

Niswander, K.R. (1991) 'EFM and brain damage in term and post-term infants.' *Contemporary Ob/Gyn*, **25**, 39–50.

Nixon, J. (1994) 'Swimming pools and drowning.' *Australian Journal of Public Health*, **18**, 3. *(Editorial.)*

Ohlsson, A., Myhr, T.L. (1994) 'Intrapartum chemoprophylaxis of prenatal group B streptococcal infections: A critical review of randomized controlled trials.' *American Journal of Obstetrics and Gynecology*, **173**, 910–917.

Okan, N., Okan, M., Eralp, Ö., Aytekin, A.H. (1995) 'The prevalence of neurological disorders among children in Gemlik (Turkey).' *Developmental Medicine and Child Neurology*, **37**, 597–603.

Olds, D.L., Eckenrode, J., Henderson, C.R., Kitzman, H., Powers, J., Cole, R., Sidora, K., Morris, P., Pettitt, L.M., Luckey, D. (1997) 'Long-term effects of home visitation on maternal life course and child abuse and neglect – Fifteen-year follow-up of a randomized trial.' *Journal of the American Medical Association*, **278**, 637–643.

Olegård, R., Sabel, K-G., Aronsson, M., Sandin, B., Johansson, P.R., Carlsson, C., Kyllerman, M., Iversen, K., Hrbek, A. (1979) 'Effects on the child of alcohol abuse during pregnancy: retrospective and prospective studies.' *Acta Paediatrica Scandinavica*, **68**, Suppl. 275, 112–121.

Olsén, P., Pääkkö, E., Vainionpää, L., Pyhtinen, J., Järvelin, M-R. (1997) 'Magnetic resonance imaging of periventricular leukomalacia and its clinical correlation in children.' *Annals of Neurology*, **41**, 754–761.

O'Reilly, D.E., Walentynowicz, J.E. (1981) 'Etiological factors in cerebral palsy: an historical review.' *Developmental Medicine and Child Neurology*, **23**, 633–642.

O'Shea, T.M., Klinepeter, K.L., Dillard, R.G. (1998a) 'Prenatal events and the risk of cerebral palsy in very low birth weight infants.' *American Journal of Epidemiology*, **147**, 362–369.

—— —— Meis, P.J., Dillard, R.G. (1998b) 'Intrauterine infection and the risk of cerebral palsy in very low-birthweight infants.' *Paediatric and Perinatal Epidemiology*, **12**, 72–83.

229

—— Preisser, J.S., Klinepeter, K.L., Dillard, R.G. (1998c) 'Trends in mortality and cerebral palsy in a geographically based cohort of very low birth weight neonates born between 1982 to 1994.' *Pediatrics*, **101**, 624–627.

Ottenbacher, K.J. (1986) *Evaluating Clinical Change: Strategies for Occupational and Physical Therapists.* Baltimore, MD: Williams & Wilkins.

Ottman, R., Annegars, J.F., Risch, N., Hauser, W.A., Susser, E. (1996) 'Relations of genetic and environmental factors in the etiology of epilepsy.' *Annals of Neurology*, **39**, 442–449.

Ounsted, M. (1987) 'Causes, continua, and other concepts. II. Risks are not causes.' *Paediatric and Perinatal Epidemiology*, **1**, 130–135.

—— Moar, V., Scott, W.A. (1981) 'Perinatal morbidity and mortality in small-for-dates babies: the relative importance of some maternal factors.' *Early Human Development*, **5**, 367–375.

Özmen, M., Çaliskan, M., Apak, S., Gökçay, G. (1993) '8-year clinical experience in cerebral palsy.' *Journal of Tropical Medicine*, **39**, 52–54.

Ozminkowski, R.J., Wortman, P.M., Roloff, D.W. (1988) 'Inborn/outborn status and neonatal survival: a meta-analysis of non-randomized studies.' *Statistics in Medicine*, **7**, 1207–1221.

Palisano, R., Rosenbaum, P., Walter, S., Russell, D., Wood, E., Galuppi, B. (1997) 'Development and reliability of a system to classify gross motor function in children with cerebral palsy.' *Developmental Medicine and Child Neurology*, **39**, 214–223.

Palmer, L., Petterson, B., Blair, E., Burton, P. (1994) 'Family patterns of gestational age at delivery and growth *in utero* in moderate and severe cerebral palsy.' *Developmental Medicine and Child Neurology*, **36**, 1108–1119.

—— Blair, E., Petterson, B., Burton, P. (1995) 'Antenatal antecedents of moderate and severe cerebral palsy.' *Paediatric and Perinatal Epidemiology*, **9**, 171–184.

Paneth, N. (1993) 'The causes of cerebral palsy. Recent evidence.' *Clinical and Investigative Medicine*, **16**, 95–102.

—— (1998) 'Prenatal ultrasound – safe or sinister?' *Lancet*, **352**, 5–6.

—— Kiely, J. (1984) 'The frequency of cerebral palsy: a review of population studies in industrialised nations since 1950.' *In:* Stanley, F.J., Alberman, E. (Eds.) *The Epidemiology of the Cerebral Palsies. Clinics in Developmental Medicine No. 87.* London: Spastics International Medical Publications, pp. 46–56.

—— Stark, R.I. (1983) 'Cerebral palsy and mental retardation in relation to indicators of perinatal asphyxia.' *American Journal of Obstetrics and Gynecology*, **147**, 960–966.

—— Pinto-Martin, J., Gardiner, J., Wallenstein, S., Katsikiotis, V., Hegyi, T., Hiatt, I.M., Susser, M. (1993) 'Incidence and timing of germinal matrix/intraventricular hemorrhage in low birth weight infants.' *American Journal of Epidemiology*, **137**, 1167–1176.

—— Rudelli, R., Kazam, E., Monte, W. (1994) *Brain Damage in the Preterm Infant.* Cambridge: Cambridge University Press.

—— Jetton, J., Pinto-Martin, J., Susser, M., Clark, C., Gardiner, J., Holzman, C., Lorenz, J.M., Reuss, M.L. (1997) 'Magnesium sulfate in labor and risk of neonatal brain lesions and cerebral palsy in low birth weight infants.' *Pediatrics*, **99**, E11–E16.

Papiernik, E. (1993) 'Prevention of preterm labour and delivery.' *Baillière's Clinical Obstetrics and Gynaecology*, **7**, 499–521.

Parkes, J., Dolk, H., Hill, N. (1998a) 'Does the child health computing system adequately identify children with cerebral palsy?' *Journal of Public Health Medicine*, **20**, 102–104.

—————— (1998b) *The Northern Ireland Cerebral Palsy Research Project, 1997 Report.* Belfast: Queen's University.

Parkinson, C., Wallis, S., Harvey, D. (1981) 'School achievement and behaviour of children who were small-for-dates at birth.' *Developmental Medicine and Child Neurology*, **23**, 41–50.

Parry, G.J., Gould, C.R., McCabe, C.J., Tarnow-Mordi, W.O., International Neonatal Network, Scottish Neonatal Consultants, Nurses Collaborative Study Group (1998) 'Annual league tables of mortality in neonatal intensive care units: longitudinal study.' *British Medical Journal*, **316**, 1931–1935.

Patel, N.B., Owen, P. (1995) 'Fetal assessment in the third trimester: biophysical methods.' *In:* Chamberlain, G. (Ed.) *Turnbull's Obstetrics, 2nd Edn.* Edinburgh: Churchill Livingstone, pp. 231–251.

Pearlman, M., Faix, R. (1997) 'No rush to obliterate genital tract colonisation in pregnant women.' *Lancet*, **350**, 531–532.

Peliowski, A., Finer, N. (1992) 'Birth asphyxia in the term infant.' *In:* Sinclair, J.C., Bracken, M.B. (Eds.) *Effective Care of the Newborn Infant.* Oxford: Oxford University Press, pp. 249–280.

Perinatal Trials Group (1998) *Perinatal Trials Group Newsletter*. Oxford: British Association of Perinatal Medicine.

Perlman, J.M., Risser, R.C., Gee, J.B. (1997) 'Pregnancy-induced hypertension and reduced intraventricular hemorrhage in preterm infants.' *Pediatric Neurology*, **17**, 29–33.

Petridou, E., Koussouri, M., Toupadaki, N., Youroukos, N., Papavassiliou, A., Pantelakis, S., Olsen, J., Trichopouls, D. (1998) 'Diet during pregnancy and the risk of cerebral palsy.' *British Journal of Nutrition*, **79**, 407–412.

Petterson, B., Stanley, F., Henderson, D. (1990) 'Cerebral palsy in multiple births in Western Australia: Genetic aspects.' *American Journal of Medical Genetics*, **37**, 346–351.

—— Nelson, K.B., Watson, L., Stanley, F.J. (1993a) 'Twins, triplets, and cerebral palsy at birth in Western Australia in the 1980s.' *British Medical Journal*, **307**, 1239–1243.

—— Stanley, F.J., Garner, B.J. (1993b) 'Spastic quadriplegia in Western Australia. II: Pedigrees and family patterns of birthweight and gestational age.' *Developmental Medicine and Child Neurology*, **35**, 202–215.

—— Blair, E., Watson, L., Stanley, F. (1998) 'Adverse outcome after multiple pregnancy.' *Baillière's Clinical Obstetrics and Gynaecology*, **12**, 1–17.

Pharoah, P.O.D. (1990) 'Incidence and prevalence.' *Archives of Disease in Childhood*, **65**, 471. *(Editorial.)*

—— (1993) 'Incidence and prevalence in cerebral palsy.' *American Journal of Obstetrics and Gynecology*, **169**, 1074. *(Letter.)*

—— (1995) 'Cerebral palsy and perinatal care.' *British Journal of Obstetrics and Gynaecology*, **102**, 356–358.

—— Connolly, K.J. (1987) 'A controlled trial of iodinated oil for the prevention of endemic cretinism: a long-term follow-up.' *International Journal of Epidemiology*, **16**, 68–73.

—— —— (1989) 'Maternal thyroid hormones and fetal brain development.' *In:* DeLong, G.R., Robbins, J., Condliffe, P.G. (Eds.) *Iodine and the Brain*. New York: Plenum Press, pp. 333–354.

—— —— (1995) 'Iodine and brain development.' *Developmental Medicine and Child Neurology*, **37**, 744–748.

—— Cooke, T. (1996) 'Cerebral palsy and multiple births.' *Archives of Disease in Childhood*, **75**, F174–F177.

—— —— (1997) 'A hypothesis for the aetiology of spastic cerebral palsy – the vanishing twin.' *Developmental Medicine and Child Neurology*, **39**, 292–296.

—— Buttfield, I.H., Hetzel, B.S. (1971) 'Neurological damage to the fetus resulting from severe iodine deficiency during pregnancy.' *Lancet*, **1**, 308–310.

—— Connolly, K., Hetzel, B., Ekins, R. (1981) 'Maternal thyroid function and motor competence in the child.' *Developmental Medicine and Child Neurology*, **23**, 76–82.

—— —— Ekins, R.P., Harding, A.G. (1984) 'Maternal thyroid hormone levels in pregnancy and the subsequent cognitive and motor performance of the children.' *Clinical Endocrinology*, **21**, 265–270.

—— Cooke, T., Rosenbloom, I., Cooke, R.W. I. (1987) 'Trends in birth prevalence of cerebral palsy.' *Archives of Disease in Childhood*, **62**, 379–384.

—— —— —— (1989) 'Acquired cerebral palsy.' *Archives of Disease in Childhood*, *64*, 1013–1016.

—— —— Cooke, R.W.I., Rosenbloom, L. (1990) 'Birthweight specific trends in cerebral palsy.' *Archives of Disease in Childhood*, **65**, 602–606.

—— Platt, M.J., Cooke, T. (1996) 'The changing epidemiology of cerebral palsy.' *Archives of Disease in Childhood*, **75**, F169–F173.

—— —— Blair, E., Cooke, T. (1997a) 'Cerebral palsy registers.' *Seminars in Neonatology*, **2**, 203–210.

—— —— Cooke, T. (1997b) 'Increasing prevalence of cerebral palsy amongst low birthweight neonatal survivors 1966–1989.' *Child: Care, Health and Development*, **23**, 201–202.

—— Cooke, T., Johnson, M.A., King, R., Mutch, L. (1998) 'Epidemiology of cerebral palsy in England and Scotland 1984–9.' *Archives of Disease in Childhood*, **79**, F21–F25.

Phelan, J.P., Ahn, M.O., Korst, L.M., Martin, G.I. (1995) 'Nucleated red blood cells: A marker for fetal asphyxia?' *American Journal of Obstetrics and Gynecology*, **173**, 1380–1384.

—— Korst, L.M., Ahn, M.O., Martin, G.I. (1998) 'Neonatal nucleated red blood cell and lymphocyte counts in fetal brain injury.' *Obstetrics and Gynecology*, **91**, 485–489.

Phelps, D.L., Lakato, L., Watts, J.L. (1998) 'D-Penicillamine to prevent retinopathy of prematurity (Cochrane Review).' *In: Cochrane Library. Issue 4*. Oxford: Update Software. (http://www.update-software.com/cochrane.htm)

Pierson, S.H. (1997) 'Outcome measures in spasticity management.' *Muscle and Nerve*, **20**, Suppl. 6, S36–S60.

Pinto-Martin, J.A., Riolo, S., Cnaan, A., Holzman, C., Susser, M.W., Paneth, N. (1995) 'Cranial ultrasound prediction of disabling and nondisabling cerebral palsy at age two in a low birth weight population.' *Pediatrics*, **95**, 249–254.

Piper, M.C., Kunos, V.I., Willis, D.M., Mazer, B.L., Ramsay, M., Silver, K.M. (1986) 'Early physical therapy effects on the high-risk infant: a randomized controlled trial.' *Pediatrics*, **78**, 216–224.

Pollack, R.N., Divon, M.Y. (1992) 'Intrauterine growth retardation: Definition, classification, and etiology.' *Clinical Obstetrics and Gynecology*, **35**, 99–107.

Ponsonby, A-L., Dwyer, T., Kasl, S.V., Cochrane, J.A. (1995) 'The Tasmanian SIDS case–control study: univariable and multivariable risk factor analysis.' *Paediatric and Perinatal Epidemiology*, **9**, 256–272.

Powers, W.F., Kiely, J.L., Fowler, M.G. (1995) 'The role of birth weight, gestational age, race and other infant characteristics in twin intrauterine growth and infant mortality.' *In:* Keith, L.G., Papiernik, E., Keith, D.M., Luke, B. (Eds.) *Multiple Pregnancy: Epidemiology, Gestation and Perinatal Outcome.* New York: Parthenon, pp. 163–174.

Preblud, S.R., Williams, N.M. (1985) 'Fetal risk associated with rubella vaccine: Implications for vaccination of susceptible women.' *Obstetrics and Gynecology*, **66**, 121–123.

Prechtl, H.F.R. (1997) 'State of the art of a new functional assessment of the young nervous system. An early predictor of cerebral palsy.' *Early Human Development*, **50**, 1–11.

Preece, P.M., Tookey, P., Ades, A., Peckham, C.S. (1986) 'Congenital cytomegalovirus infection: predisposing maternal factors.' *Journal of Epidemiology and Community Health*, **40**, 205–209.

Quilligan, E.J., Paul, R.H. (1975) 'Fetal monitoring: is it worth it?' *Obstetrics and Gynecology*, **45**, 96–100.

Quinlivan, J.A., Evans, S.F., Dunlop, S.A., Beazley, L.D., Newnham, J.P. (1998) 'Use of corticosteroids by Australian obstetricians – a survey of clinical practice.' *Australian and New Zealand Journal of Obstetrics and Gynaecology*, **38**, 1–7.

Rantakallio, P. (1985) 'A 14-year follow-up of children with normal and abnormal birth weight for their gestational age.' *Acta Paediatrica Scandinavica*, **74**, 62–69.

—— von Wendt, L., Koivu, M. (1987) 'Prognosis of perinatal brain damage: A prospective study of a one-year birth cohort of 12,000 children.' *Early Human Development*, **15**, 75–84.

—— Oja, H., Koiranen, M. (1991) 'Has the intrauterine weight-gain curve changed in shape?' *Paediatric and Perinatal Epidemiology*, **5**, 201–210.

Razdan, S., Kaul, R.L., Motta, A., Kaul, S., Bhatt, R.K. (1994) 'Prevalence and pattern of major neurological disorders in rural Kashmir (India) in 1986.' *Neuroepidemiology*, **13**, 113–119.

Redline, R.W. (1995) 'Placental pathology: a neglected link between basic disease mechanisms and untoward pregnancy outcome.' *Current Opinion in Obstetrics and Gynecology*, **7**, 10–15.

—— Pappin, A. (1995) 'Fetal thrombolytic vasculopathy: The clinical significance of extensive avascular villi.' *Human Pathology*, **26**, 80–885.

Reed, D.M., Stanley, F.J. (Eds.) (1977) *The Epidemiology of Prematurity.* Baltimore: Urban & Schwarzenberg.

Reilly, S., Poblete, X. (1996) 'Prevalence of feeding problems and oral motor dysfunction in children with cerebral palsy: A community survey.' *Journal of Pediatrics*, **129**, 877–882.

Reisner, D.P., Mahony, B.S., Petty, C.N., Nyberg, D.A., Porter, T.F., Zingheim, R.W., Williams, M.A., Luthy, D.A. (1993) 'Stuck twin syndrome: outcome in thirty-seven consecutive cases.' *American Journal of Obstetrics and Gynecology*, **169**, 991–995.

Reuss, M.L., Paneth, N., Susser, M.W., Southard, C. (1993) 'Hypothyroxinemia of prematurity and risk of cerebral palsy.' *Pediatric Research*, **33**, 82A.

—— —— Pinto-Martin, J.A., Lorenz, J.M., Susser, M. (1996) 'The relation of transient hypothyroxinemia in preterm infants to neurologic development at two years of age.' *New England Journal of Medicine*, **334**, 821–827.

Richmond, S., Niswander, K., Snodgrass, C.A., Wagstaff, I. (1994) 'The obstetric management of fetal distress and its association with cerebral palsy.' *Obstetrics and Gynecology*, **83**, 643–646.

Riikonen, R., Raumavirta, S., Sinivuori, E., Seppala, T. (1989) 'Changing pattern of cerebral palsy in the southwest region of Finland.' *Acta Paediatrica Scandinavica*, **78**, 581–587.

Rizzo, G., Arduini, D., Pennestri, F., Romanini, C., Mancuso, S. (1987) 'Fetal behaviour in growth retardation: its relationship to fetal blood flow.' *Prenatal Diagnosis*, **7**, 229–238.

Robertson, C., Finer, N. (1985) 'Term infants with hypoxic–ischemic encephalopathy: outcome at 3.5 years.' *Developmental Medicine and Child Neurology*, **27**, 473–484.

—— Svenson, L.W., Joffres, M.R. (1998) 'Prevalence of cerebral palsy in Alberta.' *Canadian Journal of Neurological Sciences*, **25**, 117–122.

Robinson, J.S., Hartwich, K.M., Walker, S.K., Erwich, J.J.H.M., Owens, J.A. (1997) 'Early influences on embryonic and placental growth.' *Acta Paediatrica*, Suppl. 423, 159–163.

Roland, E.H., Hill, A. (1997) 'How important is perinatal asphyxia in the causation of brain injury?' *Mental Retardation and Developmental Disabilities Research Reviews*, **3**, 22–27.

Romero, R., Mazor, M., Munoz, H., Gomez, R., Galasso, M., Sherer, D.M. (1994) 'The preterm labor syndrome.' *Annals of the New York Academy of Sciences*, **734**, 414–429.

Rose, J., Medeiros, J.M., Parker, R. (1985) 'Energy cost index as an estimate of energy expenditure of cerebral-palsied children during assisted ambulation.' *Developmental Medicine and Child Neurology*, **27**, 485–490.

Rosenblatt, R.A. (1989) 'The perinatal paradox: doing more and accomplishing less.' *Health Affairs*, **8**, 158–168.

Rosenbloom, L. (1994) 'Dyskinetic cerebral palsy and birth asphyxia.' *Developmental Medicine and Child Neurology*, **36**, 285–289.

Roth, S.C., Edwards, A.D., Cady, E.B., Delpy, D.T., Wyatt, J.S., Azzopardi, D., Townsend, J., Stewart, A.L., Reynolds, E.O.R. (1992) 'Relation between cerebral oxidative metabolism following birth asphyxia, and neurodevelopmental outcome and brain growth at one year.' *Developmental Medicine and Child Neurology*, **34**, 285–295.

Rubin, R., Rosenblatt, C., Balow, B. (1973) 'Psychological and educational sequelae of prematurity.' *Pediatrics*, **52**, 352–363.

Rumeau-Rouquette, C., Du Mazaubrun, C., Verrier, A., Mlika, A. (1994) 'Prévalence des déficiences motrices.' *In: Rumeau-Rouquette, C., Du Mazaubrun, C., Verrier, A., Mlika, A. (Eds.) Prévalence des Handicaps: Évolution dans Trois Générations d'Enfants 1972, 1976, 1981.* Paris: INSERM Unité 149, pp. 40–55.

Russell, D., Rosenbaum, P.L., Cadman, D.T., Gowland, C., Hardy, S., Jarvis, S. (1989) 'The gross motor function measure: a means to evaluate the effects of physical therapy.' *Developmental Medicine and Child Neurology*, **37**, 763–775.

Russell, E.M. (1961) 'Cerebral palsied twins.' *Archives of Disease in Childhood*, **36**, 328–336.

Rutherford, M.A., Pennock, J.M., Cowan, F.M., Dubowitz, L.M.S., Hajnal, J.V., Bydder, G.M. (1997) 'Does the brain regenerate after perinatal infarction?' *European Journal of Paediatric Neurology*, **1**, 13–17.

Saari-Kemppainen, A., Karjalainen, O., Ylostalo, P., Heinonen, O.P. (1990) 'Ultrasound screening and perinatal mortality: controlled trial of systematic one-stage screening in pregnancy.' *Lancet*, **336**, 387–390.

Salisbury, D., Begg, N. (1996) *Immunization Against Infectious Disease.* London: HMSO.

Salokorpi, T., Sajaniemi, N., Hällback, H., Kari, A., Rita, H., von Wendt, L. (1997) 'Randomized study of the effect of antenatal dexamethasone on growth and development of premature children at the corrected age of 2 years.' *Acta Paediatrica*, **86**, 294–298.

Sanderson, D.A., Wilcox, M.A., Johnson, I.R. (1994) 'The individualised birthweight ratio: a new method of identifying intrauterine growth retardation.' *British Journal of Obstetrics and Gynaecology*, **101**, 310–314.

Sathiakumar, N., Yakubu, A.M. (1987) 'Cerebral palsy in Zaria, Northern Nigeria – is it preventable?' *Journal of Tropical Pediatrics*, **33**, 263–265.

Saugstad, O.D. (1998) 'Practical aspects of resuscitating asphyxiated newborn infants.' *European Journal of Pediatrics*, **157**, Suppl. 1, S11–S15.

—— Rootwelt, T., Aalen, O. (1998) 'Resuscitation of asphyxiated newborn infants with room air or oxygen: An international controlled trial: The Resair 2 Study.' *Pediatrics*, **102**, E11–E17.

Savitz, D.A., Blackmore, C.A., Thorp, J.M. (1991) 'Epidemiologic characteristics of preterm delivery: Etiologic heterogeneity.' *American Journal of Obstetrics and Gynecology*, **164**, 467–471.

Scheller, J.M., Nelson, K.B. (1992) 'Twinning and neurologic morbidity.' *American Journal of Diseases of Children*, **146**, 1110–1113.

—— —— (1994) 'Does cesarean delivery prevent cerebral palsy or other neurologic problems of childhood?' *Obstetrics and Gynecology*, **83**, 624–630.

Shy, K.K., Luthy, D.A., Bennett, F.C., Whitfield, M., Larson, E.B., van Belle, G., Hughes, J.P., Wilson, J.A., Stenchever, M.A. (1990) 'Effects of electronic fetal-heart-rate monitoring, as compared with periodic auscultation, on the neurologic development of premature infants.' *New England Journal of Medicine*, **322**, 588–593.

Silverman, W.A. (1980) *Retrolental Fibroplasia: A Modern Parable.* New York: Grune & Stratton.

—— (1998) *Where's the Evidence?* Oxford: Oxford University Press.

Sinclair, J.C. (1992) 'Management of the thermal environment.' *In:* Sinclair, J.C., Bracken, M.B. (Eds.) *Effective Care of the Newborn Infant.* Oxford: Oxford University Press, pp. 40–58.

—— Bracken, M.B. (Eds.) (1992) *Effective Care of the Newborn Infant.* Oxford: Oxford University Press.

Sinha, G., Corry, P., Subesinghe, D., Wild, J., Levene, M.I. (1997) 'Prevalence and type of cerebral palsy in a British ethnic community: the role of consanguinity.' *Developmental Medicine and Child Neurology*, **39**, 259–262.

233

Skari, H., Bjornland, K., Bjornstad-Ostensen, A., Haugen, G., Emblem, R. (1998) 'Consequences of prenatal ultrasound diagnosis: a preliminary report on neonates with congenital malformations.' *Acta Obstetrica et Gynecologica Scandinavica*, **77**, 635–642.

Smaill, F. (1998a) 'Antibiotics vs no treatment for asymptomatic bacteriuria in pregnancy (Cochrane Review).' *In: Cochrane Library. Issue 4.* Oxford: Update Software. (http://www.update-software.com/cochrane.htm)

—— (1998b) 'Intrapartum antibiotics for Group B streptococcal colonisation (Cochrane Review).' *In: Cochrane Library. Issue 4.* Oxford: Update Software. (http://www.update-software.com/cochrane.htm)

Smith, J.M. (Ed.) (1985) *On Being the Right Size and Other Essays. J.B.S. Haldane.* Oxford: Oxford University Press.

Smith, Y. (1985) 'Incidence and outcome: PVL.' *In:* Grant, E.G. (Ed.) *Neurosonography of the Preterm Neonate.* New York: Springer-Verlag, pp. 91–93.

Smithells, R.W. (1970) 'The epidemiology of congenital malformations.' *In:* Apley, J. (Ed.) *Modern Trends in Paediatrics, Vol. 3.* London: Butterworths, pp. 1–22.

Sola, A., Piecuch, R.E. (1994) 'Prevalence of cerebral palsy: estimations, calculations and neonatal care.' *Pediatrics*, **93**, 152–153. *(Letter.)*

Soll, R.F. (1999a) 'Propylactic synthetic surfactant for preventing morbidity and mortality in preterm infants (Cochrane Review).' *In: Cochrane Library. Issue 3.* Oxford: Update Software. (http://www.update-software.com/cochrane.htm)

—— (1999b) 'Synthetic surfactant for respiratory distress syndrome in preterm infants (Cochrane Review).' *In: Cochrane Library. Issue 3.* Oxford: Update Software. (http://www.update-software.com/cochrane.htm)

Sommerfeld, D., Fraser, B.A., Hensinger, R.N., Beresford, L.V. (1981) 'Evaluation of physical therapy sevice for severely mentally impaired students with cerebral palsy.' *Physical Therapy*, **61**, 338–343.

Sonntag, J., Waltz, S., Schollmeyer, T., Schüppler, U., Schröder, H., Weisner, D. (1996) 'Morbidity and mortality of discordant twins up to 34 weeks of gestational age.' *European Journal of Pediatrics*, **155**, 224–229.

Soriani, S., Scarpa, P., Voghenzi, A., De Carlo, L., Cilio, R. (1993) 'Moyamoya disease in childhood: a familial case report.' *Child's Nervous System*, **9**, 215–219.

Souter, D., Harding, J., McCowan, L., O'Donnell, C., McLeay, E., Baxendale, H. (1998) 'Antenatal indomethacin – adverse effects confirmed.' *Australian and New Zealand Journal of Obstetrics and Gynaecology*, **38**, 11–16.

Spencer, J.A.D. (1998) 'Deaths linked to intrapartum asphyxia: largely unexplained but probably preventable.' *British Medical Journal*, **316**, 640.

—— Badawi, N., Burton, P., Keogh, J., Pemberton, P., Stanley, F. (1997) 'The intrapartum CTG prior to neonatal encephalopathy at term: a case–control study.' *British Journal of Obstetrics and Gynaecology*, **104**, 25–28.

Spinillo, A., Stonati, M., Ometto, A., Fazzi, E., Lanzi, G., Guaschino, S. (1993) 'Infant neurodevelopmental outcome in pregnancies complicated by gestational hypertension and intra-uterine growth retardation.' *Journal of Perinatal Medicine*, **35**, 45–54.

—— Capuzzo, E., Stronati, M., Ometto, A., Orcesi, S., Fazzi, E. (1995) 'Effect of preterm premature rupture of membranes on neurodevelopmental outcome: follow up at two years of age.' *British Journal of Obstetrics and Gynecology*, **102**, 882–887.

—— —— Cavallini, A., Stronati, M., De Santolo, A., Fazzi, E. (1998) 'Preeclampsia, preterm delivery and infant cerebral palsy.' *European Journal of Obstetrics, Gynecology, and Reproductive Biology*, **77**, 151–155.

Srivastava, V.K., Laisram, N., Srivastava, R.K. (1992) 'Cerebral palsy.' *Indian Pediatrics*, **20**, 993–996.

Stanley, F.J. (1982) 'Using cerebral palsy in the evaluation of neonatal intensive care: a warning.' *Developmental Medicine and Child Neurology*, **24**, 93–94.

—— (1992) 'Survival and cerebral palsy in low birthweight infants: implications for perinatal care.' *Paediatric and Perinatal Epidemiology*, **6**, 298–310.

—— (1994a) 'Cerebral palsy. The courts catch up with sad realities.' *Medical Journal of Australia*, **161**, 236.

—— (1994b) 'Cerebral palsy trends: implications for perinatal care.' *Acta Obstetrica et Gynecologica Scandinavica*, **73**, 5–9.

—— (1994c) 'The aetiology of cerebral palsy.' *Early Human Development*, **36**, 81–88.

—— (1995) 'Obstetrical responsibility for abnormal fetal outcome.' *In:* Chamberlain, G. (Ed.) *Turnbull's Obstetrics, 2nd Edn.* London: Churchill Livingstone, pp. 833–844.

—— (1997) 'Prenatal determinants of motor disorders.' *Acta Paediatrica*, **86**, Suppl. 422, 92–102.

—— Alberman, E. (Eds.) (1984) *The Epidemiology of the Cerebral Palsies. Clinics in Developmental Medicine No. 87.* London: Spastics International Medical Publications.

—— Blair, E. (1991) 'Why have we failed to reduce the frequency of cerebral palsy?' *Medical Journal of Australia*, **154**, 623–626.

—— —— (1994) 'Cerebral palsy.' *In:* Pless, I.B. (Ed.) *The Epidemiology of Childhood Disorders.* New York: Oxford University Press, pp. 473–498.

—— Chalmers, I. (1989) 'Cerebral palsy, intrapartum care, and a shot in the foot.' *Lancet*, **2**, 1251–1252.

—— English, D.R. (1986) 'Prevalence of and risk factors for cerebral palsy in a total population cohort of low-birthweight (<2000g) infants.' *Developmental Medicine and Child Neurology*, **28**, 559–568.

—— Petterson, B. (1995) 'Cerebral palsy in multiple births: the changing epidemiological patterns.' *In:* Ward, R.H., Whittle, M. (Eds.) *Multiple Pregnancy.* London: RCOG Press, pp. 309–325.

—— Watson, L. (1992) 'Trends in perinatal mortality and cerebral palsy in Western Australia, 1967 to 1985.' *British Medical Journal*, **304**, 1658–1663.

—— Burgar, P.J., Fong, N.W., Milroy, H.M. (1985) 'Congenital rubella syndrome in Western Australia.' *Australian Paediatric Journal*, **21**, 111–114.

—— Blair, E., Hockey, A., Petterson, B., Watson, L. (1993) 'Spastic quadriplegia in Western Australia: a genetic and epidemiological study. I: Case population and perinatal risk factors.' *Developmental Medicine and Child Neurology*, **35**, 191–201.

—— —— Westaway, J. (1994) *Cerebral Palsy: The Role of Obstetric Care in Pregnancy and Delivery.* Perth: Institute for Child Health Research and Confederation of Australian Medical Defence Organisations (CAMDO).

—— Read, A.W., Kurinczuk, J.J., Croft, M.L., Bower, C. (1997) 'A population maternal and child health research database for research and policy evaluation in Western Australia.' *Seminars in Neonatology*, **2**, 195–201.

Steer, P.A., Lucas, A., Sinclair, J.C. (1992) 'Feeding the low birthweight infant.' *In:* Sinclair, J.C., Bracken, M.B. (Eds.) *Effective Care of the Newborn Infant.* Oxford: Oxford University Press, pp. 94–140.

Stephan, M.D., Murray, R.M. (1997) 'Schizophrenia: developmental disturbance of brain and mind?' *Acta Paediatrica*, **86**, Suppl. 422, 112–116.

Stewart, A., Kirkbride, V. (1996) 'Very preterm infants at fourteen years: relationship with neonatal ultrasound brain scans and neurodevelopmental status at one year.' *Acta Paediatrica*, **85**, Suppl. 416, 44–47.

—— Reynolds, E.O., Hope, P.L., Hamilton, P.A., Baudin, Y., Costello, A.M., Bradford, B.C., Wyatt, J.S. (1987) 'Probability of neurodevelopmental disorders estimated from ultrasound appearance of brains of very preterm infants.' *Developmental Medicine and Child Neurology*, **29**, 3–11.

Stine, S.B. (1990) 'Therapy – physical or otherwise – in cerebral palsy.' *American Journal of Diseases of Children*, **144**, 519–520.

Streiner, D.L., Normal, G.R. (1989) *Health Measurement Scales: a Practical Guide to Their Development and Use.* Oxford: Oxford University Press.

Sugimoto, T.,,Woo, M., Nishida, N., Araki, A., Hara, T., Yasuhara, A., Kobayashi, Y., Yamanouchi, Y. (1995) 'When do brain abnormalities in cerebral palsy occur? An MRI study.' *Developmental Medicine and Child Neurology*, **37**, 285–292.

Susser, E., Hoek, H.W., Brown, A. (1998) 'Neurodevelopmental disorders after prenatal famine – The story of the Dutch Famine Study.' *American Journal of Epidemiology*, **147**, 213–216.

Susser, M. (1989) 'The challenge of causality: Human nutrition, brain development and mental performance.' *Bulletin of the New York Academy of Medicine*, **65**, 1032–1049.

—— (1994) 'Timing in prenatal nutrition: a reprise of the Dutch Famine Study.' *Nutrition Reviews*, **52**, 84–94.

—— Susser, E. (1996a) 'Choosing a future for epidemiology: I. Eras and paradigms.' *American Journal of Public Health*, **86**, 668–673.

—— —— (1996b) 'Choosing a future for epidemiology: II. From black box to Chinese boxes and eco-epidemiology.' *American Journal of Public Health*, **86**, 674–677.

Taha, S.A., Mahdi, A.H. (1984) 'Cerebral palsy in Saudi Arabia: a clinical study of 102 cases.' *Annals of Tropical Paediatrics*, **4**, 155–158.

Tardieu, C., Lespargot, A., Tabary, C., Bret, M.D. (1988) 'For how long must the soleus muscle be stretched each day to prevent contracture?' *Developmental Medicine and Child Neurology*, **30**, 3–10.

Tardieu, G., Tardieu, C., Colbeau-Justin, P., Lespargot, A. (1982) 'Muscle hypoextensibility in children with cerebral palsy: II. Therapeutic implications.' *Archives of Physical Medicine and Rehabilitation*, **63**, 103–107.

Tarnow-Mordi, W.O. (1998) 'Room air or oxygen for asphyxiated babies?' *Lancet*, **352**, 341–342.

——— Brocklehurst, P. (1997) 'Randomised controlled trials in perinatal medicine: 1. The need for studies of mortality and major morbidity with adequate power.' *British Journal of Obstetrics and Gynaecology*, **104**, 763–765.

Taudorf, K., Hansen, F.J., Melchior, J.C. (1986) 'Spontaneous remission of cerebral palsy.' *Neuropediatrics*, **17**, 19–22.

Taylor, D.J., Howie, P.W. (1989) 'Fetal growth achievement and neurodevelopmental disability.' *British Journal of Obstetrics and Gynaecology*, **96**, 789–794.

Thacker, S.B., Stroup, D.F. (1998) 'Continuous electronic fetal monitoring during labour (Cochrane Review).' *In: Cochrane Library. Issue 4.* Oxford: Update Software. (http://www.update-software.com/cochrane.htm)

——— ——— Peterson, H. B. (1995) 'Efficacy and safety of intrapartum electronic fetal monitoring: An update.' *Obstetrics and Gynecology*, **86**, 613–620.

Thorarensen, O., Ryan, S., Hunter, J., Younkin, D.P. (1997) 'Factor V Leiden mutation: An unrecognized cause of hemiplegic cerebral palsy, neonatal stroke, and placental thrombosis.' *Annals of Neurology*, **42**, 372–375.

Tirosh, E., Rabino, S. (1989) 'Physiotherapy for children with cerebral palsy: evidence for its efficacy.' *American Journal of Diseases of Children*, **143**, 552–555.

Tito, F. (1996) *Compensation and Professional Indemnity in Health Care: A Final Report.* Canberra: Government Printing Service.

Topp, M., Langhoff-Roos, J., Uldall, P., Kristensen, J. (1996) 'Intrauterine growth and gestational age in preterm infants with cerebral palsy.' *Early Human Development*, **44**, 27–36.

——— ——— ——— (1997a) 'Preterm birth and cerebral palsy – predictive value of pregnancy complications, mode of delivery, and Apgar scores.' *Acta Obstetrica et Gynecologica Scandinavica*, **76**, 843–848.

——— ——— ——— (1997b) 'Validation of a cerebral palsy register.' *Journal of Clinical Epidemiology*, **50**, 1017–1023.

——— Uldall, P., Langhoff-Roos, J. (1997c) 'Trend in cerebral palsy birth prevalence in eastern Denmark: birth-year period 1979–86.' *Paediatric and Perinatal Epidemiology*, **11**, 451–460.

Torfs, C.P., van den Berg, B.J., Oechsli, F.W., Cummins, S. (1990) 'Prenatal and perinatal factors in the etiology of cerebral palsy.' *Journal of Pediatrics*, **116**, 615–619.

Towbin, A. (1986) 'Obstetric malpractice litigation: The pathologist's view.' *American Journal of Obstetrics and Gynecology*, **155**, 927–935.

Trounce, J.Q., Shaw, D.E., Levene, M.I., Rutter, N. (1988) 'Clinical risk factors and periventricular leucomalacia.' *Archives of Disease in Childhood*, **63**, 17–22.

Truffert, P., Goujard, J., Dehan, M., Vodovar, M., Breart, G. (1998) 'Outborn status with a medical neonatal transport service and survival without disability at two years – a population-based cohort survey of newborns of less than 33 weeks of gestation.' *European Journal of Obstetrics, Gynecology, and Reproductive Biology*, **79**, 13–18.

Tyson, J.E. (1992) 'Immediate care of the newborn infant.' *In:* Sinclair, J.C., Bracken, M.B. (Eds.) *Effective Care of the Newborn Infant.* Oxford: Oxford University Press, pp. 21–39.

Uvebrant, P. (1988) 'Hemiplegic cerebral palsy: aetiology and outcome.' *Acta Paediatrica Scandinavica*, Suppl. 345, 1–100.

——— Hagberg, G. (1992) 'Intrauterine growth in children with cerebral palsy.' *Acta Paediatrica*, **81**, 407–412.

van Bogaert, P., Donner, C., David, P., Rodesch, F., Avni, E.F., Szliwowski, H.B. (1996) 'Congenital bilateral perisylvian syndrome in a monozygotic twin with intra-uterine death of a co-twin.' *Developmental Medicine and Child Neurology*, **38**, 166–171.

Vannucci, R.C., Perlman, J.M. (1997) 'Interventions for perinatal hypoxic–ischemic encephalopathy.' *Pediatrics*, **100**, 1004–1014.

Ventriculomegaly Trial Group (1990) 'Randomised trial of early tapping in neonatal posthaemorrhagic ventricular dilatation.' *Archives of Disease in Childhood*, **65**, 3–10.

Villar, J., Carroli, G., Belizan, J.M. (1995) 'Predictive ability of meta-analyses of randomised controlled trials.' *Lancet*, **345**, 772–776.

Ville, Y., Hyett, J., Hecher, K., Nicolaides, K. (1995) 'Preliminary experience with endoscopic laser surgery for severe twin–twin transfusion syndrome.' *New England Journal of Medicine*, **332**, 224–227.

Visser, G., Laurini, R., de Vries, J., Bekedam, D., Prechtl, H. (1986) 'Abnormal motor behaviour in anencephalic fetuses.' *Early Human Development*, **12**, 173–182.

Wald, N., Kennard, A. (1998) 'Routine ultrasound screening for congenital abnormalities.' *Annals of the New York Academy of Sciences*, **847**, 173–180.

Walpole, I., Zubrick, S., Pontre, J. (1990) 'Is there a fetal effect with low to moderate alcohol use before or during pregnancy?' *Journal of Epidemiology and Community Health*, **44**, 297–301.

—— Hodgen, N., Bower, C. (1991a) 'Congenital toxoplasmosis: a large survey in Western Australia.' *Medical Journal of Australia*, **154**, 720–724.

—— Zubrick, S., Pontre, J., Lawrence, C. (1991b) 'Low to moderate maternal alcohol use before and during pregnancy and neurobehavioural outcome in the newborn infant.' *Developmental Medicine and Child Neurology*, **33**, 875–883.

Wang, E., Smaill, F. (1989) 'Infection in pregnancy.' *In:* Chalmers, I., Enkin, M., Keirse, M.J.N.C. (Eds.) *Effective Care in Pregnancy and Childbirth. Vol. I. Pregnancy. Parts I–V.* Oxford: Oxford University Press, pp. 534–564.

Wariyar, U., Richmond, S. (1989) 'Morbidity and preterm delivery: importance of 100% follow-up.' *Lancet*, **1**, 387–388. *(Letter.)*

Watson, L., Stanley, F., Petterson, B. (1996) 'Rates of triplet pregnancies in Western Australia may be beginning to fall.' *British Medical Journal*, **313**, 625–626. *(Letter.)*

Weed, D.L., Hursting, S.D. (1998) 'Biologic plausibility in causal inference: Current method and practice.' *American Journal of Epidemiology*, **147**, 415–425.

Weig, S.G., Marshall, P.C., Abroms, I.F., Gauthier, N.S. (1995) 'Patterns of cerebral injury and clinical presentation in the vascular disruptive syndrome of monozygotic twins.' *Pediatric Neurology*, **13**, 279–285.

Weinberg, C.R. (1993) 'Towards a clearer definition of confounding.' *American Journal of Epidemiology*, **137**, 1–8.

Weindling, A.M., Rochefort, M.J., Calvert, S.A., Fok, T.F., Wilkinson, A. (1985a) 'Development of cerebral palsy after ultrasonographic detection of periventricular cysts in the newborn.' *Developmental Medicine and Child Neurology*, **27**, 800–806.

—— Wilkinson, A.R., Cook, J., Calvert, S.A., Fok, T.F., Rochefort, M.J. (1985b) 'Prenatal events which precede periventricular haemorrhage and leukomalacia in the newborn.' *British Journal of Obstetrics and Gynaecology*, **92**, 1218–1223.

Weindling, M. (1995) 'Periventricular haemorrhage and periventricular leukomalacia.' *British Journal of Obstetrics and Gynaecology*, **102**, 278–281.

Westergaard, T., Wohlfahrt, J., Aaby, P., Melbye, M. (1997) 'Population based study of rates of multiple pregnancies in Denmark, 1980–94.' *British Medical Journal*, **314**, 775–779.

Whitaker, A.H., Feldman, J.F., Van Rossem, R., Schonfeld, I.S., Pinto-Martin, J.A., Torre, C., Blumenthal, S.R., Paneth, N.S. (1996) 'Neonatal cranial ultrasound abnormalities in low birth weight infants: Relation to cognitive outcomes at six years of age.' *Pediatrics*, **98**, 719–729.

WHO (1980) *International Classification of Impairments, Disabilities and Handicaps.* Geneva: World Health Organization.

—— (1999) *ICIDH-2. International Classification of Functioning and Disability. Beta-2 Draft.* Geneva: World Health Organization. (http://www.who.ch/icidh)

Wigfield, R., Gilbert, R., Fleming, P.J. (1994) 'SIDS: Risk reduction measures.' *Early Human Development*, **38**, 161–164.

Wigglesworth, J. (1984) 'Brain development and its modification by adverse influences.' *In:* Stanley, F., Alberman, E. (Eds.) *The Epidemiology of the Cerebral Palsies. Clinics in Developmental Medicine No. 87.* London: Spastics International Medical Publications, pp. 12–26.

—— (1995) 'The placenta in twins.' *In:* Ward, R.H., Whittle, M. (Eds.) *Multiple Pregnancy.* London: RCOG Press, pp. 48–55.

Wild, N.J., Rosenbloom, L. (1986) 'Familial cerebral palsy associated with normal intelligence.' *Postgraduate Medical Journal*, **62**, 827–830.

Williams, B.C. (1994) 'Social approaches to lowering infant mortality: lessons from the European experience.' *Journal of Public Health Policy*, **15**, 18–25.

Williams, C.E., Mallard, C., Tan, W., Gluckman, P.D. (1993) 'Pathophysiology of perinatal asphyxia.' *Clinics in Perinatology*, **20**, 305–325.

Williams, J.C. (Ed.) (1997) *In the Words of Nelson Mandela.* London: Michael Joseph.

Williams, K., Alberman, E. (1998) 'The impact of diagnostic labelling in population-based research into cerebral palsy.' *Developmental Medicine and Child Neurology*, **40**, 182–185.

—— Hennessy, E., Alberman, E. (1996) 'Cerebral palsy: effects of twinning, birthweight, and gestational age.' *Archives of Disease in Childhood*, **75**, F178–F182.

Williams, L.J., Lucci, L.J. (1990) 'Placental examination can help determine cause of brain damage in neonates.' *Texas Medicine*, **86**, 33–38.

Wright, L.L., Papile, L-A. (1997) 'US neonatal databases: methods and uses.' *Seminars in Neonatology*, **2**, 159–169.

Wyatt, J.S., Thoresen, M. (1997) 'Hypothermia treatment and the newborn.' *Pediatrics*, **100**, 1028–1030.

Yokoyama, Y., Shimizu, T., Hayakawa, K. (1995) 'Prevalence of cerebral palsy in twins, triplets and quadruplets.' *International Journal of Epidemiology*, **24**, 943–948.

Yoon, B.H., Jun, J.K., Romero, R., Park, K.H., Gomez, R., Choi, J.H., Kim, I.O. (1997) 'Amniotic fluid inflammatory cytokines (interleukin-6, interleukin-1b, and tumor necrosis factor-a), neonatal brain white matter lesions, and cerebral palsy.' *American Journal of Obstetrics and Gynecology*, **177**, 19–26.

Yow, M.D., Demmler, G.J. (1992) 'Congenital cytomegalovirus disease: 20 years is long enough.' *New England Journal of Medicine*, **326**, 702–703.

Yudkin, P.L., Johnson, A., Clover, L.M., Murphy, K.W. (1994) 'Clustering of perinatal markers of birth asphyxia and outcome at age five years.' *British Journal of Obstetrics and Gynaecology*, **101**, 774–781.

—— —— —— —— (1995) 'Assessing the contribution of birth asphyxia to cerebral palsy in term singletons.' *Paediatric and Perinatal Epidemiology*, **9**, 156–170.

Zupan, V., Gonzalez, P., Lacazw-Masmonteil, T., Boithias, C., d'Allest, A-M., Dehan, M., Gabilan, J-C. (1996) 'Periventricular leukomalacia: risk factors revisited.' *Developmental Medicine and Child Neurology*, **38**, 1061–1067.

INDEX

Delivery
  gestational age, 34–35, 37
  maternal age, 31
  preterm, *33*, 34–35
  timing and intrauterine growth restriction, 164
Delivery mode, 154
  fetal distress, 167–168
Denervation, reversible, 181
Denominators, 25, 26–27
  multiple pregnancy, 110
  postneonatally acquired cerebral palsy, 128
  size, 28
Descriptive studies, 140, *141*
Developed countries
  CNS infection, 131–133
  maternal age, 31
  occurrence, 29–30
  postneonatally acquired cerebral palsy, 128, 131–133
Developing countries
  cerebral infections, 130
  febrile convulsions, 130–131
  occurrence, 30
  postneonatally acquired cerebral palsy, 128, 130–131
Dexamethasone, 152
Diplegia, 15
  chorioamnionitis association, 78
  spastic
    multiple births, 115
    postneonatally acquired cerebral palsy, 134
Disability
  change, 186–187
  severity, *36*, 37–38
Disease recognition, early, 46
Doppler ultrasound, intrauterine growth restriction, 163
Dose dependency, 44
Dyskinesia, 14–15, 21
  postneonatally acquired cerebral palsy, 134

E

Early delivery, iatrogenic, 2
Ecological contexts of causal pathways, 198
Effective Care of the Newborn Infant, 143
Effective Care in Pregnancy and Childbirth, 143
Electrocardiograph, intrapartum fetal, 165
Electromyography (EMG), 176
ELGAN (extremely low gestational age newborn) study, 79
Embryogenesis interruption, 53
Encephalitides, viral, 171
Encephalitis, preterm births, 157–158
Encephalopathy
  hypoxic–ischaemic, 163
  neonatal, 50, 54, 168, 169

birth asphyxia, 100–101, 103, 104
  prenatal clastic, 54
End-points, 71
Enterocolitis, preterm births, 157–158
Epidemiological studies, 140, *141*
  research, 197–200
Epilepsy, 52, 53
Epiphenomenon, 44
  intrauterine growth restriction associated with cerebral palsy, 90–91
  VPTB, 64, 71
Evidence-based practice, 7
Excitatory amino acid transmitter blockade, 169
Exclusions, 11–12
Extracorporeal membrane oxygenation (ECMO), 169
Extremely low birthweight, 33–34
Extremely preterm birth (EPTB), 33–4, *35*, 60

F

Factor V Leiden, 54, 146
Family history, 51–53
Famine, 94
Febrile convulsions, 130–131
Feeding
  difficulties, 23
  very preterm infants, 159
Fetal alcohol syndrome, 59, 94–95
  prevention, 146
Fetal anomalies
  detection, 143
  intrauterine growth restriction, 86
  see also Fetal malformation syndromes; Fetal malformations
Fetal distress, 103
  caesarean section, 167, 168
  delivery mode, 167–168
  ECMO, 169
  forceps delivery, 167–168
  intrapartum, 99, 100, 165
  neonatal encephalopathy, 169
  vacuum extraction, 167–168
Fetal growth
  rate in multiple pregnancies, 117, 119
  slow, 83–84
Fetal heart rate
  birth asphyxia, 101
  electronic monitoring, 107
  see also Heart rate recording
Fetal malformation syndromes, 51, 53–55
Fetal malformations, 51, 104
  see also Fetal anomalies
Fetal monitoring, *see* Fetal heart rate; Heart rate recording
Fetal movement, muscle mass, 96–97
Fetal outcome measures, *see* Outcomes

Fetal size
  multiple births, 87
  see also Birthweight
Fish oil, 163
Folate, dietary, 162
Forceps delivery in fetal distress, 167–168
Frequency
  developed countries, 29–30
  measures, 25–26
Function measures, norm-referenced, 190

G
Gangliosides, 169
Gastrostomy, 23
Gender
  fetal, 87
  multiple pregnancies, 121, 123
  occurrence, 30–31
  postneonatally acquired cerebral palsy, 135–136
Genetic factors, 51–53
Genital tract infection, 73
Germinal matrix haemorrhage, 47, 65, *66*, 67
Gestation duration, risk factor for cerebral palsy, 119
Gestational age
  assessment, 84, 85
  norms for multiple births, 113, 115
  profile, 5
Gestational age at delivery, 34–35, 37, 71, 113
  multiple pregnancies, 119, *120*, 121
  postneonatally acquired cerebral palsy, 136
  pre-eclampsia, 92–93
  subtypes of cerebral palsy, 63–64
Glucocorticoids, 153
Glucose homeostasis, 159
Glutaric aciduria type I, 124
Goals
  end-point, 191
  functional, 186, 190–191
  validity, 191
Goitre, 57
Gonorrhoea, 55
Grey matter
  cerebral, 48
  heterotopia, 50
Gross Motor Function Measure (GMFM), 17, 189, 190
Growth
  norms for multiple births, 113, 115
  preterm twins, 121
  see also Intrauterine growth
Growth hormone, fetal, 162
Growth restriction
  preterm infants, 87
  see also Intrauterine growth restriction
Growth restriction intervention trial (GRIT), 164

H
Haemophilus influenzae meningitis, 133
Haemophilus influenzae type B (Hib) vaccine, 170–171, 197
Haemorrhage
  antepartum, 104–105
  germinal matrix, 47, 65, *66*, 67
  intrapartum, 106
Haemorrhagic disease of the newborn, 173
Handicap, change, 186–187
Head injury
  postneonatally acquired cerebral palsy, 132, 133, 134
  prevention, 172
Heart rate recording
  electronic monitoring, 107
  interpretation, 106
  intrapartum, 165
  see also Fetal heart rate
Height, maternal, 87, 89–90
Hemiplegia, 19
  left, 15
  right, 15
  spastic, 46
    multiple births, 115
    postneonatally acquired cerebral palsy, 134
  see also Quadriplegia
Herpes simplex virus, 55
  neonatal infection, 158
Hib vaccination, 170–171, 197
HIV, 56
Hospital records, 111
Hospitalization with bed rest
  intrauterine growth restriction, 163
  multiple pregnancy, 148–149
Hydranencephaly, 54, 146
Hydrocephalus, 38
Hyperbilirubinaemia, phototherapy, 158
Hypercoagulable state, fetal, 105
Hyperhomocystinaemia mutations, 55
Hypertension, pregnancy-induced, 91–93
  intrauterine growth restriction, 91
  see also Pre-eclampsia
Hypertonicity, reversible denervation, 181
Hypothermia
  apoptosis inhibition, 99
  secondary neuronal damage prevention, 168
Hypotonia, 15
Hypoxia/hypoxic stress
  birth asphyxia, 105
  intrapartum, 99, 100, 108, 163–164
  labour, 96, 108

I
Iatrogenesis, neonatal intensive care, 161–162
Imaging techniques, 3

243

Keywords, 13

L

Labour
  early onset unexplained, 74
  fetal cerebral oxygenation, 100
  hypoxia/hypoxic stress, 96, 108
  preterm and corticosteroids, 150, *151*, 152–153
  tocolysis in second stage, 166
Late interventions, 139
Learning disabilities, 19
Likert scales, 188
Limb-by-limb coding system, 15, 17, *18*, 19
Lissencephaly, 50, 107
Litigation, 5–6
Little Club, 8
Live births, 26, 27
Locking, twins, 117
Long term outcomes, 142
Low birthweight
  meta-analysis, 89–90
  multiple pregnancies, 119

M

Magnesium, dietary, 162
Magnesium sulphate, 149, 150
  antenatal in preterm infants, 153–154
  antenatal prophylaxis of pre-eclampsia, 93
Magnetic resonance imaging (MRI), 3, 51
Malformations
  birth asphyxia, 104
  fetal, 51, 53–55
  see also Fetal anomalies
Malnutrition, 94
Malpresentation, 168
  birth asphyxia, 101, 106
Management, 7.
  neonatal, 37
Management of cerebral palsy, 176
  aims, 185
  carer satisfaction, 187–188
  clinical picture, 181
  communal learning curve, 178–179, 180
  controlled research, 177
  cost effectiveness, 188
  crossover trial design, 193–194
  disability change, 186–187
  evaluation, 176–179
  functional goals, 190–191
  functional outcome, 187, 189
  impairment change, 186–187
  interventions, 182–183
  measurement, 188–189
  N-of-one study, 194
  norm-referenced measures of function, 190
  observers, 192

outcomes, 183–185
  categories, 186–187
  measurement, 189–192
  patient satisfaction, 187–188
  psychological impairment, 181
  quality of life, 185–188
  randomized controlled clinical trials, 193
  research design, 193–194
  subjective factors, 191–192
  subjects, 180–182
    selection for trials, 182
    variability, 181–182
  technical outcome, 187, 189
  therapeutic interventions, 178–179
    components, 179–180
  unquantifiable factors, 191–192
Maternal age
  occurrence, 31
  postneonatally acquired cerebral palsy, 136–137
Maternal causes of intrauterine growth restriction, 89
Maternal characteristics, 1
Maternal health indicators, 139
Maternal nutrition, 89, 90
Maternal shock, birth asphyxia, 106
Measles, vaccination, 171
Measles–mumps–rubella vaccine, 144
Meconium stained liquor, 101
Medical management strategies, 4–5
Medical risk factors, 138–139
Membrane rupture
  aetiology, 80
  premature, 79, *81*
  risk factors, 78, 79–80, *81*
  VPTB, 73, *74*, 79–80, *81*
Meningitis
  postneonatally acquired cerebral palsy, 130, 131, 133
  preterm births, 157–158
Meningococcal disease vaccines, 171
Mental retardation, maternal, 52
Mercury, *see* Methylmercury
Metabolic acidosis, 100
Metabolic errors
  inborn, 89
  inherited defect, 7
  intrauterine growth restriction, 90–91
  postneonatally acquired cerebral palsy, 124
Methylmercury, 58–59
  abnormal motor cortex development, 50
  elimination from food chain, 145
  exposure, 44
  intrauterine growth restriction associated, 90–91
Middle cerebral artery infarcts, *66*, 67
Migration disorders, 54
Molecular epidemiology, 198

247

Prostaglandin inhibitors, 168
Proxy end-points, 71
Psychological impairment, 186
Public health, Cochrane Pregnancy and Childbirth
  Data Base, 141
Pyruvate dehydrogenase deficiency, 124

Q

Quadriplegia, 15
  occurrence, 30
  spastic in postneonatally acquired cerebral palsy,
    134
Quality of life, 185–188
  placebo effect, 186
Quality of upper extremity skills test (QUEST), 190

R

Race, 55
Racially mixed populations, 133–134
Random error, 177–178
Randomized controlled trials, 4, 141, 177, 178,
    202–203
  management, 193
  subjects, 180
Recognition age for cerebral palsy, 5
Recognition of condition, 24, *25*
Recording, data quality, 20
Registers, 8, 195
  age of following, 24
  age limits, 9–10, *210–211*
  collaborative effort, 200–201
  data, 3, 5
  exclusions/inclusions, 11–12
  information range, 201
  international, 204–207
  networks, 200–201
Reproductive disorders, 53
Reproductive tract infections, 55
Rescue, birth asphyxia, 168–169
Research, 197–200
Research, controlled, 177
  blinding, 177
  random error, 177–178
Resolution, 9
Respiratory infections, 23
Resuscitation
  active, 35
  birth asphyxia, 168–169
  requirement, 96
Rhesus factor, 20
Rhesus incompatibility, 41–42, 145–146
Rhesus iso-immunization, 6, 43
Rickets, 138
Risk factors, 20, 197–198
  chorioamnionitis, 77, 78
  medical, 138–139

multiple births, 79
rupture of membranes, 78, 79–80, *81*
SGA babies, 83–84
social, 138–139
VPTB, 73–75, *76*, 77–81
Rubella, 55
  abnormal motor cortex development, 50
  intrauterine growth restriction, 90–91
  maternal vaccination, 55
  vaccination, 144–145
  see also Congenital rubella syndrome

S

Sample size, numerators, 28
Satisfaction expression, 187–188
Schizencephaly, 50
Screening programmes, 144
Seizures, 19, 54
  neonatal, 78
  prevention in pre-eclampsia, 149, 150
Self-esteem, 186
Sensory defects, 19
Septicaemia, preterm births, 157–158
Severity
  codes, 19
  scores, 17
Shoulder dystocia, 106
Single photon emission computed tomography
    (SPECT), 3
Small for gestational age (SGA) babies, 83
  behavioural disturbances, 84
  cognitive defects, 84
  intrauterine growth restriction, 84–86
  measures, 86
  percentiles, 87
  preterm birth, 87
  risk factor, 83–84
Smoking, maternal, 44
  intrauterine growth restriction, 86, 94, 196
Social class, 39
Social conditions, 138–139
  postneonatally acquired cerebral palsy, 133–134
Social contexts of causal pathways, 198
Social factors
  intrauterine growth restriction, 94–95
  VPTB, 74
Social group risk, 55
Social risk factors, 138–139
Social support in pregnancy, 147–148
Spasms, *see* Infantile spasms; Seizures
Spasticity, 14
  distributions, 15, *16*
  numerators, 28
Spinal cord, 49
Statistical analysis, causal pathways, 196
Statistical power, 44, 46

249